Tumors of the Thyroid Gland

Atlas
of
Tumor Pathology

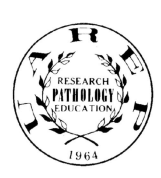

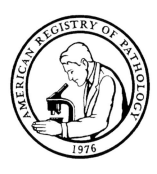

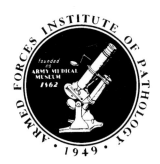

ATLAS OF TUMOR PATHOLOGY

Third Series
Fascicle 5

TUMORS OF THE
THYROID GLAND

by

JUAN ROSAI, M.D.
Department of Pathology
Memorial Sloan-Kettering Cancer Center
New York, New York 10021

MARIA LUISA CARCANGIU, M.D.
Department of Pathology
Yale University School of Medicine
New Haven, Connecticut 06510

and

RONALD A. DELELLIS, M.D.
Department of Pathology
Tufts University School of Medicine
and the New England Medical Center
Boston, Massachusetts 02111

Published by the
ARMED FORCES INSTITUTE OF PATHOLOGY
Washington, D.C.

Under the Auspices of
UNIVERSITIES ASSOCIATED FOR RESEARCH AND EDUCATION IN PATHOLOGY, INC.
Bethesda, Maryland
1992

Accepted for Publication
1990

Available from the American Registry of Pathology
Armed Forces Institute of Pathology
Washington, D.C. 20306-6000
ISSN 0160-6344
ISBN 1-881041-03-4

ATLAS OF TUMOR PATHOLOGY

EDITOR
JUAN ROSAI, M.D.
Department of Pathology
Memorial Sloan-Kettering Cancer Center
New York, New York 10021-6007

ASSOCIATE EDITOR
LESLIE H. SOBIN, M.D.
Armed Forces Institute of Pathology
Washington, D.C. 20306-6000

EDITORIAL ADVISORY BOARD

Jeffrey Cossman, M.D.
Georgetown University School of Medicine
Washington, D.C. 20007

Ronald A. DeLellis, M.D.
Tufts University School of Medicine
Boston, Massachusetts 02111

Glauco Frizzera, M.D.
Armed Forces Institute of Pathology
Washington, D.C. 20306-6000

Leonard B. Kahn, M.D.
Long Island Jewish Hospital
New Hyde Park, New York 11042

Richard L. Kempson, M.D.
Stanford University Medical School
Stanford, California 94305

Paul Peter Rosen, M.D.
Memorial Sloan-Kettering Cancer Center
New York, New York 10021

Robert E. Scully, M.D.
Harvard Medical School and Massachusetts General Hospital
Boston, Massachusetts 02114

Steven G. Silverberg, M.D.
The George Washington University School of Medicine
Washington, D.C. 20037

Sharon Weiss, M.D.
University of Michigan School of Medicine
Ann Arbor, Michigan 48109-0602

EDITORS' NOTE

The Atlas of Tumor Pathology has a long and distinguished history. It was first conceived at a Cancer Research Meeting held in St. Louis in September 1947 as an attempt to standardize the nomenclature of neoplastic diseases. The first series was sponsored by the National Academy of Sciences-National Research Council. The organization of this Sisyphean effort was entrusted to the Subcommittee on Oncology of the Committee on Pathology, and Dr. Arthur Purdy Stout was the first editor-in-chief. Many of the illustrations were provided by the Medical Illustration Service of the Armed Forces Institute of Pathology, the type was set by the Government Printing Office, and the final printing was done at the Armed Forces Institute of Pathology (hence the colloquial appellation "AFIP Fascicles"). The American Registry of Pathology purchased the Fascicles from the Government Printing Office and sold them virtually at cost. Over a period of 20 years, approximately 15,000 copies each of nearly 40 Fascicles were produced. The worldwide impact that these publications have had over the years has largely surpassed the original goal. They quickly became among the most influential publications on tumor pathology ever written, primarily because of their overall high quality but also because their low cost made them easily accessible to pathologists and other students of oncology the world over.

Upon completion of the first series, the National Academy of Sciences-National Research Council handed further pursuit of the project over to the newly created Universities Associated for Research and Education in Pathology (UAREP). A second series was started, generously supported by grants from the AFIP, the National Cancer Institute, and the American Cancer Society. Dr. Harlan I. Firminger became the editor-in-chief and was succeeded by Dr. William H. Hartmann. The second series Fascicles were produced as bound volumes instead of loose leaflets. They featured a more comprehensive coverage of the subjects, to the extent that the Fascicles could no longer be regarded as "atlases" but rather as monographs describing and illustrating in detail the tumors and tumor-like conditions of the various organs and systems.

Once the second series was completed, with a success that matched that of the first, UAREP and AFIP decided to embark on a third series. A new editor-in-chief and an associate editor were selected, and a distinguished editorial board was appointed. The mandate for the third series remains the same as for the previous ones, i.e., to oversee the production of an eminently practical publication with surgical pathologists as its primary audience, but also aimed at other workers in oncology. The main purposes of this series are to promote a consistent, unified, and biologically sound nomenclature; to guide the surgical pathologist in the diagnosis of the various tumors and tumor-like lesions; and to provide relevant histogenetic, pathogenetic, and clinicopathologic information on these entities. Just as the second series included data obtained from ultrastructural (and, in the more recent Fascicles, immunohistochemical) examination, the third series will, in addition, incorporate pertinent information obtained with the newer molecular biology techniques. As in the past, a continuous attempt will be made to correlate, whenever possible, the nomenclature used in the Fascicles with that proposed by the World Health Organization's International Histological Classification of Tumors. The format of the third series has been changed in order to incorporate additional items and to ensure a consistency of style throughout. This includes the dropping of the 's possessive in eponymic terms, in accordance with the WHO and the International Nomenclature of Diseases. Close cooperation between the various authors and their respective liaisons from the editorial board will be emphasized to minimize unnecessary repetition and discrepancies in the text and illustrations.

To its everlasting credit, the participation and commitment of the AFIP to this venture is even more substantial and encompassing than in previous series. It now extends to virtually all scientific, technical, and financial aspects of the production.

The task confronting the organizations and individuals involved in the third series is even more daunting than in the preceding efforts because of the ever-increasing complexity of the matter at hand. It is hoped that this combined effort—of which, needless to say, that represented by the authors is first and foremost—will result in a series worthy of its two illustrious predecessors and will be a suitable introduction to the tumor pathology of the twenty-first century.

Juan Rosai, M.D.
Leslie H. Sobin, M.D.

TUMORS OF THE THYROID GLAND

Contents

Introduction 1

The Normal Thyroid Gland 1
  Embryology 1
  Anatomy 2
  Histology 4
    Architectural Features 4
    The Follicular Cell 6
    The C Cell 7
    Solid Cell Nests 12
  Physiology 12
    Thyroid Hormones 13
    Calcitonin and the Calcitonin Gene–Related Peptide 14

Classification of Thyroid Tumors 19

Follicular Adenoma 21
  Adenoma Variants 31
    Adenoma with Bizarre Nuclei 31
    Hyalinizing Trabecular Adenoma 31
    Adenolipoma and Adenochondroma 38
    Atypical Adenoma 38
    Adenoma with Papillary Hyperplasia 40
    "Toxic" Adenoma 40

Follicular Carcinoma 49
  Minimally Invasive (Encapsulated) Type 50
  Widely Invasive Type 62

Papillary Carcinoma 65
  Papillary Carcinoma Variants 96
    Papillary Microcarcinoma 96
    Encapsulated Variant 100
    Follicular Variant 100
    Encapsulated Follicular Variant and Related Lesions 105
    Solid/Trabecular Variant 109
    Diffuse Sclerosing Variant 109
    Tall and Columnar Cell Variants 114

Poorly Differentiated Carcinoma 123
  Insular Carcinoma 123
  Other Poorly Differentiated Carcinomas 128

Undifferentiated (Anaplastic) Carcinoma 135

Tumors with Oncocytic Features (Hürthle Cell Tumors) 161
  Oncocytic Adenoma (Hürthle Cell Adenoma) 162
  Oncocytic Carcinoma (Hürthle Cell Carcinoma) 173
  Papillary Oncocytic Neoplasms 179

Tumors with Clear Cell Features 183
Tumors with Squamous Features 195
Tumors with Mucinous Features 203
Medullary Carcinoma 207
    Medullary Carcinoma Variants 229
        Tubular (Follicular) Variant 229
        Papillary Variant 230
        Small Cell Variant 231
        Giant Cell Variant 232
        Clear Cell Variant 232
        Melanotic (Pigmented) Variant 233
        Oncocytic (Oxyphilic) Variant 233
        Squamous Variant 233
        Amphicrine (Composite Calcitonin and Mucin-Producing) Variant 237
        Paraganglioma-Like Variant 237
        Encapsulated Medullary Carcinoma 237
    Mixed Medullary-Follicular Carcinoma 238
    Mixed Medullary-Papillary Carcinoma 239
C Cell Hyperplasia 247
Sarcomas 259
    Angiosarcoma 259
Malignant Lymphoma 267
    Other Lymphoid Tumors 275
        Plasmacytoma 275
        Hodgkin Disease 275
Miscellaneous Tumors 279
    Parathyroid Tumors 279
    Paraganglioma 279
    Teratoma 280
    Benign Soft Tissue–Type Tumors 282
    Tumors with Thymic or Related Branchial Pouch Differentiation 282
        Ectopic Cervical Thymoma 282
        Ectopic Hamartomatous Thymoma 282
        Spindle Epithelial Tumor with Thymus-Like Differentiation (SETTLE) 282
        Carcinoma Showing Thymus-Like Differentiation (CASTLE) 284
    Salivary Gland–Type Tumors 285
Secondary Tumors 289
Tumor-Like Conditions 297
    Nodular Hyperplasia 297
    Diffuse Hyperplasia 302
    Dyshormonogenetic Goiter 302
    Hashimoto Thyroiditis 303
    Other Forms of Thyroiditis 305
    Malakoplakia 310
    Radiation Changes 310
    Amyloid Goiter 312
    Histiocytosis X 315

Sinus Histiocytosis with Massive Lymphadenopathy 315
Plasma Cell Granuloma 315
Thyroid Tissue in Abnormal Locations 317
  Ectopia 317
  Mechanical Implantation 320
  Parasitic Nodule 320
  Thyroid Inclusions in Lymph Nodes 323
  Thyroid as a Component of Teratoma 323
Thyroid Tumors–General Considerations 327
  Incidence of Thyroid Carcinoma 327
  Clinical and Laboratory Evaluation of Thyroid Tumors 327
  Thyroid Tumors in Childhood 328
  Thyroid Tumors and Radiation Exposure 329
  Fine-Needle Aspiration Biopsy 329
  Frozen-Section Examination 330
  Procedure for Pathologic Examination 331
  Staging and Grading of Thyroid Carcinoma 332
  Treatment of Thyroid Tumors 334
  Prognosis of Thyroid Tumors 334
  Thyroid Tumors in Animals 335
Index 339

TUMORS OF THE THYROID GLAND

INTRODUCTION

Many changes have occurred in the field of pathology of thyroid tumors since Shields Warren and William A. Meissner wrote the previous two Fascicles on the subject. The morphologic spectrum of papillary carcinoma and medullary carcinoma has expanded considerably, the entity of follicular carcinoma has been redefined according to more restrictive criteria, and several rare types and subtypes of thyroid neoplasms have been described.

As far as format is concerned, we have dealt with the major tumor types composed of follicular cells in separate chapters in the usual fashion, but we have also grouped them according to some particular morphologic feature, such as clear cell or mucinous changes. This has resulted in some duplication, but we think the approach is justified because of the differential diagnostic guidance it has provided. Similar comments apply to the section on General Considerations.

It overlaps considerably with those dealing with specific tumor types, particularly papillary carcinoma, but we think it is worth including for discussion of some clinical and clinicopathologic aspects of thyroid neoplasia in a generic fashion. In most instances, we have followed the terminology proposed in 1988 by the World Health Organization (WHO) Committee on Histologic Typing of Thyroid Tumours. We have departed from it in the few instances in which we thought it justified on the basis of new findings or as the result of our own observations (or possibly biases) and only after stating the reasons for doing so.

The sections on the normal C cell, solid cell nests, calcitonin and the calcitonin gene–related peptide, medullary carcinoma, and C cell hyperplasia were written by Ronald A. DeLellis; all others were written by Juan Rosai and Maria Luisa Carcangiu.

THE NORMAL THYROID GLAND

EMBRYOLOGY

The thyroid *anlage* appears as a bilobate vesicular structure at the foramen cecum of the tongue. It then descends as a component of the thyroglossal duct to reach its definitive position in the neck. After involution of the thyroglossal duct, the thyroid *anlage* begins to expand laterally to form the thyroid lobes (4,9,12).

Microscopically, the initially solid thyroid *anlage* begins to form cords and plates of follicular cells during the ninth week. A small lumen appears within the follicles by the tenth week, with colloid secretion becoming evident by the twelfth week. By the fourteenth week, the gland already consists of well-developed follicles lined by follicular cells and containing thyroglobulin-positive colloid in the lumen (figs. 1, 2).

Labeled amino acid studies have suggested that thyroglobulin synthesis begins at a very early stage, when the thyroid is still a solid mass at the base of the tongue and long before lumen formation

and colloid secretion can be detected (3,11). Both embryologic and histochemical studies have shown that the C cells are probably derived from the neural crest and that these cells ultimately migrate to the ultimobranchial bodies before their incorporation into the thyroid (5–8,10). The ultimobranchial bodies, in turn, derive from branchial pouch complex IV–V (13). In some species, such as birds, the thyroid and ultimobranchial bodies are present as separate structures in the adult, and C cells are confined to the ultimobranchial body.

The development of the ultimobranchial body is divisible into four stages: 1) branchial pouch stage (3–12 mm, 5–7 wks); 2) separation stage (13–17 mm, 7–8 wks); 3) incorporation stage (18–27 mm, 8–9 wks); 4) dissolution stage (28–520 mm, 9 wks to term) (12). In the branchial pouch stage, the ultimobranchial body is a thick-walled stratified epithelial cyst that is in continuity with the primitive pharyngeal cavity. At

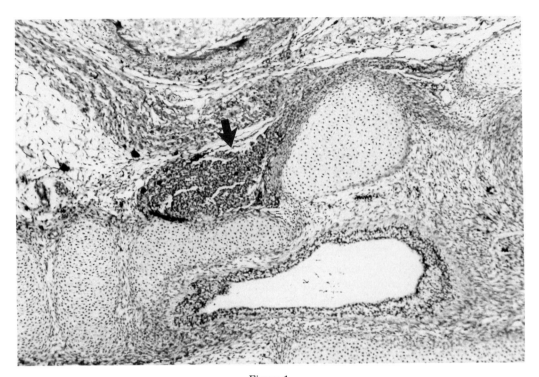

Figure 1
(Figures 1 and 2 are from the same case)
DEVELOPING THYROID GLAND IN A 14-WEEK-OLD FETUS
The thyroid gland (arrow) is located in a groove in front of the laryngotracheal primordium.

the beginning of the separation phase, pouch complex IV–V separates into the parathyroid IV and the ultimobranchial component, which ultimately divides into central and peripheral portions in the dissolution phase. The central portion is represented as a stratified epithelial cyst, whereas the peripheral portion is dispersed into a few cell groups that eventually become cystic.

Additional support for the ultimobranchial origin of the C cells has come from studies of patients with the DiGeorge syndrome (1,2). Affected individuals typically have complete or partial absence of derivatives of pouch complexes III and IV–V. In studies reported by Burke and coworkers (1), only 27 percent of patients with DiGeorge syndrome had C cells within their thyroids. In contrast, the number of bronchopulmonary calcitonin-containing cells was within normal limits. These observations indicate that the bronchopulmonary calcitonin-containing cells develop independently of derivatives of branchial pouches III and IV–V.

ANATOMY

The normal adult thyroid gland is a bilobate structure located in the midportion of the neck, immediately in front of the larynx and trachea. It wraps itself around these two structures and firmly adheres to them. The two lobes extend along either side of the larynx to the midportion of the thyroid cartilage. Their upper and lower extremities are referred to as the *upper* and *lower poles* of the gland, respectively. The two lobes are joined by the isthmus, which lies across the trachea anteriorly, below the level of the cricoid cartilage. Sometimes one lobe (particularly the right) is larger than the other. In some individuals, the isthmus is unusually wide.

The pyramidal lobe is a vestige of the thyroglossal duct; it is found in about 40 percent of normal individuals. It presents as a narrow projection of thyroid tissue extending upward from the isthmus and lying on the surface of the thyroid cartilage. Any diffuse pathologic process

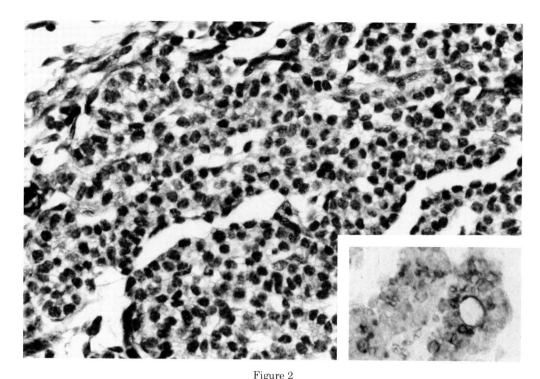

Figure 2
DEVELOPING THYROID GLAND IN A 14-WEEK-OLD FETUS
In this high magnification of the case shown in figure 1, minute follicles are present, some of which have identifiable lumina. The inset shows follicular cells with immunohistochemical positivity for thyroglobulin.

(such as diffuse hyperplasia or Hashimoto thyroiditis) can result in gross enlargement of the pyramidal lobe.

The normal weight of the thyroid in a middle-aged adult is 15 to 25 g in areas without endemic goiter. As an average, each lobe measures 4.0 x 1.5–2.0 x 2.0–4.0 cm, and the isthmus measures 2.0 x 2.0 x 0.2–0.6 cm. However, it should be remembered that there are marked variations related to functional activity, sex, hormonal status, size of the individual, and amount of iodine intake. For instance, the thyroid gland is larger and heavier in women than in men, and it becomes even larger during pregnancy.

The thyroid is completely enveloped by a continuous fibrous capsule, with septa that divide the gland incompletely into lobules. The parathyroid glands are usually located adjacent to the posterior surface of the thyroid lobes. The recurrent laryngeal nerves run in the cleft between the trachea and esophagus just medial to the thyroid lobes.

The thyroid blood supply derives from the right and left superior thyroid arteries (which arise from the external carotid artery) and the right and left inferior thyroid arteries (which arise from the thyrocervical trunk of the subclavian arteries). The thyroid veins drain into the internal jugular, the brachycephalic, and occasionally the anterior jugular veins.

The thyroid gland is endowed with a rich lymphatic network that encircles the follicles and connects both lobes through the isthmus. This network coalesces in the subcapsular region to give rise to collecting trunks that leave the organ in close proximity to the veins (fig. 3). The regional lymph nodes of the thyroid gland are

- the pericapsular nodes (Whole organ sections of the thyroid have shown that the intraglandular lymphatics penetrate the capsule and merge with the pericapsular lymph nodes, which form a plexus around the gland [15].)
- the internal jugular chain nodes
- the pretracheal, paratracheal, and prelaryngeal nodes (The pretracheal node located near the thyroid isthmus is sometimes referred to as the Delphian node.)

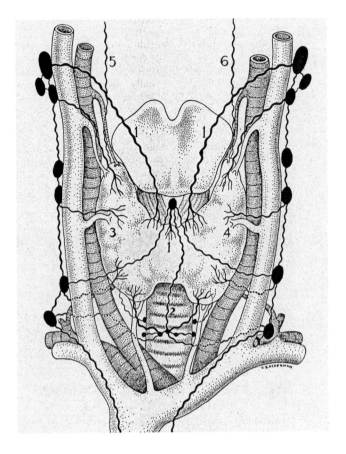

Figure 3
LYMPHATIC DRAINAGE
OF THE THYROID GLAND
This figure illustrates the median superior trunk (1), the median inferior trunk (2), the right and left lateral trunks (3, 4), and the posterosuperior trunks (5, 6). All of these drain to the regional lymph nodes listed in the text. The pericapsular lymph nodes are not illustrated. (Fig. 340 from Del Regato JA, Spjut HJ. Ackerman and Del Regato's Cancer. Diagnosis, treatment, and prognosis. 5th ed. CV Mosby: St. Louis, 1977.)

- the recurrent laryngeal nerve chain nodes
- the retropharyngeal and retroesophageal nodes.

The anterosuperior mediastinal nodes are secondary to the recurrent laryngeal nerve chain and pretracheal groups; however, studies have shown that dye injected into the thyroid isthmus can also drain directly into them (14).

Some correlation exists between the site of a thyroid tumor within a lobe and the location of the initial lymph node metastasis. For instance, involvement of the subdigastric nodes of the internal jugular chain is common with upper pole lesions. However, the degree of anastomosing between these various nodal groups is such that any of them can be found to be the site of disease regardless of the precise location of the primary tumor within the lobe. Even the nodes of the posterior triangle group are affected with some frequency. Conversely, submandibular triangle involvement is rare and usually limited to cases with extensive metastases in other cervical nodal groups. Simi-

larly, involvement of anterosuperior mediastinal nodes is rarely seen in the absence of widespread cervical disease.

HISTOLOGY

Architectural Features

The functional unit of the thyroid gland is the *follicle*, a closed sac lined by a single layer of epithelium. Its average diameter is 200 nm, but there is a considerable size variation, depending on the degree of activity of the gland. The shape of the normal follicle varies from round to oval (fig. 4). Markedly elongated "tubular" and branching follicles are to be regarded as abnormal; they are seen in hyperplastic and neoplastic disorders. A characteristic structure, normally present but accentuated in hyperplastic conditions, is the *Sanderson polster* (see page 301.) The term refers to an architectural arrangement in which collections of small follicles bulge into the lumina of large ones. The lining epithelium

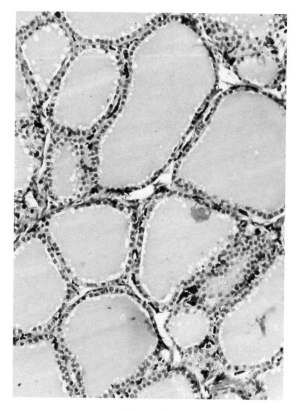

Figure 4
NORMAL ADULT THYROID GLAND
The shape of the follicles in this microscopic field varies
from round to oval.

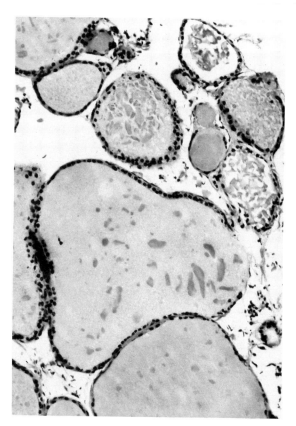

Figure 5
NORMAL THYROID FOLLICLES
Note the flocculent appearance of the colloid in the
lumina of these thyroid follicles. This material was strongly
basophilic on H&E sections. This change is probably of an
artifactual nature and of no pathologic significance.

of the latter is columnar in the area of the bulge but flattened elsewhere.

The lumen of the follicle contains a viscous material known as *colloid*, in which concentrated thyroglobulin is present. This material is eosinophilic, strongly PAS positive, and sometimes focally mucicarminophilic. Its staining quality is somewhat dependent on the degree of activity of the follicles: weakly eosinophilic and flocculent in active follicles and strongly eosinophilic and homogeneous when stored in large inactive follicles (37). Often, darkly staining and elongated clumps appear within it, suggesting an artifactual coagulation-type phenomenon (fig. 5). Anisotropic crystals of calcium oxalate may be present, particularly in older and/or less active glands (pl. I-A) (36).

Each follicle is surrounded by a richly vascularized stroma. A group of 20 to 40 follicles compartmentalized by connective tissue and supplied by a single branch of one of the thyroid

arteries constitutes a *thyroid lobule*, a structure that becomes more apparent in pathologic conditions such as hyperplasia or fibrosis. As already indicated, an intricate lymphatic network between the follicles empties into subcapsular channels, which in turn lead to numerous collecting trunks. Many cross communications exist between the lymph vessels within the thyroid, some of which cross the midline to connect one lobe to the other.

There are a number of variations in the microscopic appearance of the thyroid gland that carry no pathologic significance but that are important to the pathologist because some of them may be confused with lesions of greater significance. They include 1) adipose metaplasia of the interfollicular stroma; 2) intrathyroidal islands of mature cartilage, presumably of branchial pouch derivation (fig. 6) (22); 3) intrathyroidal islands of ectopic thymus; 4) intrathyroidal parathyroid; 5) solid cell nests (see page 12); and 6) intrathyroidal bundles of skeletal muscle (fig. 7). It is also important to realize that microscopically normal thyroid tissue can be found outside the anatomic confines of the gland. In a study of 56 thyroid glands obtained at autopsy from normal individuals between 20 and 40 years old, Hanson and coworkers (26) found thyroid tissue outside the recognizable capsule of the gland in 40 cases and in the skeletal muscles of the neck in 6 cases. This ectopic thyroid tissue can be involved by any of the diseases affecting the main organ, particularly hyperplasia and thyroiditis.

The Follicular Cell

The nucleus of the follicular cell is round to oval. Its chromatin may be finely granular and/or clumped, and there is usually a single nucleolus. In actively secreting cells, the nucleus enlarges and the chromatin undergoes dispersion; this is accompanied by cytoplasmic enlargement, predominantly in the apical half, so that the nucleus acquires a basal position. The cytoplasm may appear pale eosinophilic or amphophilic in H&E preparations. In contrast to parathyroid cells, PAS stain shows little or no glycogen in the cytoplasm of the normal follicular cells; however, this is not necessarily true in neoplastic conditions (see page 31). The amount, shape, and appearance of the follicular cell cytoplasm varies depending on its functional status. Three major types are described, with the understanding that they are part of a continuous morphologic spectrum: flattened (endothelioid), cuboidal, and columnar (cylindrical) (figs. 8, 9). The flattened cells are relatively inactive. Cuboidal cells secrete colloid into the follicular lumen and may contain apical secretory vacuoles. Columnar cells resorb the thyroglobulin-containing colloid, liberate the active hormones, and "excrete" them into blood vessels; they may feature an apical cuticle, apical lipid droplets, and one or more basilar vacuoles (vacuoles of Bensley).

Ultrastructurally, the thyroid follicular cell exhibits numerous microvilli on its luminal surface, particularly during active resorption (29). The cell membranes of adjacent cells interdigitate in a complex fashion and are joined by a junctional

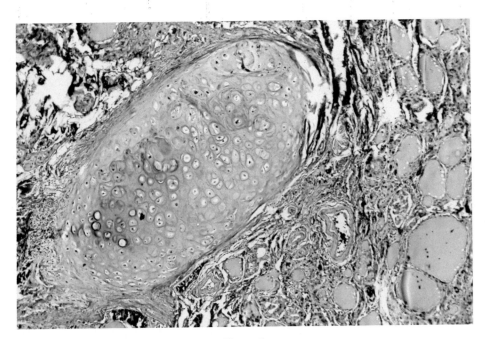

Figure 6
ECTOPIC CARTILAGE IN AN OTHERWISE NORMAL THYROID GLAND
This finding, which is of no clinical significance, probably represents a remnant of the branchial cleft pouch apparatus.

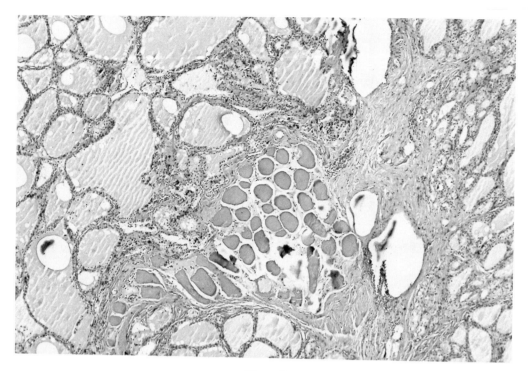

Figure 7
NORMAL SKELETAL MUSCLE WITHIN THE THYROID GLAND
This should not be misinterpreted as invasion of skeletal muscle by a thyroid neoplasm.

complex toward the apex. At the base, a continuous basal lamina separates the follicular cell from the stroma. The cytoplasm contains abundant granular endoplasmic reticulum and a well-developed Golgi apparatus. The latter is located between the nucleus and the luminal surface and becomes prominent in actively secreting cells. Mitochondria are well represented; their length and cytoplasmic location vary according to the functional status of the cell. When mitochondria are unduly numerous, the cell acquires oncocytic features at the light-microscopic level, an abnormality described on page 165. Lysosomes are numerous in actively secreting cells; most are located toward the apical side (fig. 10).

Immunohistochemically, follicular cells are reactive for low–molecular-weight keratins. Some follicular cells also express vimentin, although not as intensely as some tumors derived from them (28). The specific immunohistochemical marker for follicular cells is thyroglobulin, which can be demonstrated by the use of polyclonal or monoclonal antibodies (30,40,41). Thyroglobulin tends to leak out of the cytoplasm of the follicular cells and

to diffuse into the surrounding tissues, where it can then be incorporated into the cytoplasm of other cell types that may be present (e.g., metastatic carcinoma or malignant lymphoma) and cause them to become spuriously positive (38).

The C Cell

C cells are difficult to identify in formalin-fixed, paraffin-embedded sections stained with H&E (17,43). Generally, their nuclei are somewhat larger and paler than those of the follicular cells. Occasionally, C cells may have a clear cytoplasm in formalin-fixed samples, whereas fixation in glutaraldehyde often results in faint cytoplasmic basophilia. In sections stained with argyrophil techniques such as the Grimelius reaction, the cytoplasm of C cells is characterized by the deposition of fine silver granules (21). Lead hematoxylin also stains the cytoplasm of C cells selectively (35). C cells show marked metachromasia with dyes such as toluidine blue and coriophosphine O after acid hydrolysis of tissue sections (35). González-Cámpora and coworkers

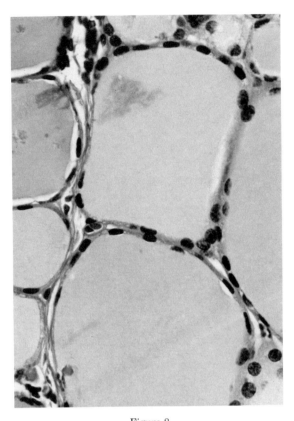

Figure 8
NORMAL THYROID FOLLICLES
These normal thyroid follicles are lined by a flattened (endothelioid) epithelium.

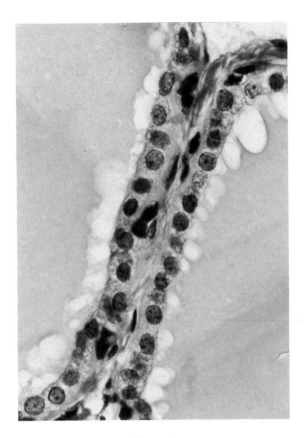

Figure 9
NORMAL THYROID FOLLICLES
These adjacent normal follicles are lined by a cuboidal epithelium having relatively large, vesicular, centrally located nuclei, some of which exhibit a distinct nucleolus. Reabsorption droplets are seen above the apical portion.

(25) have reported that the lectin *Ulex europaeus* agglutinin I reacts selectively with C cells in normal human thyroid glands.

The most reliable procedure for the identification of C cells involves the use of immunofluorescence or immunoperoxidase procedures with polyclonal antisera or monoclonal antibodies to calcitonin (pl. I-B) (18,19,21,31). In addition to calcitonin, C cells also contain katacalcin and the calcitonin gene–related peptide (16). Messenger RNAs (mRNAs) encoding both calcitonin and calcitonin gene–related peptide also have been demonstrated in normal C cells with in situ hybridization techniques (47).

Somatostatin has been identified within C cells of most species (21,39). In the adult rabbit, bat, and guinea pig, most calcitonin-positive cells also contain somatostatin; however, in adult human thyroids, only a small proportion of the calcitonin-positive cells are also somatostatin

positive. Gastrin-releasing peptide and its corresponding mRNA have been identified in most C cells in the human fetus and neonate, whereas studies of adult thyroid have revealed gastrin-releasing peptide in less that 20 percent of C cells (42). Although pro-opiomelanocortin–derived peptides have been found in medullary thyroid carcinomas, their occurrence in normal C cells is still a matter of debate. Similarly, peptides including substance P, vasoactive intestinal peptide, gastrin/cholecystokinin, and neurotensin, which have been demonstrated in some cases of medullary carcinoma, have not been demonstrated in normal C cells. However, helodermin, a peptide that shows considerable homology with vasoactive intestinal peptide, has been demonstrated in normal C cells, where it is colocalized with calcitonin (39).

PLATE I

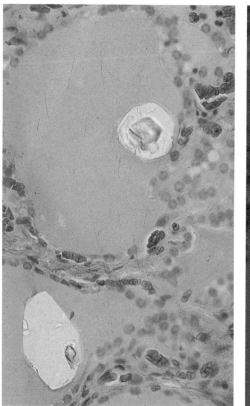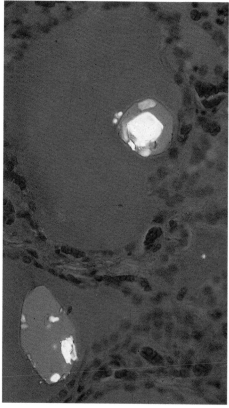

A. CALCIUM OXALATE CRYSTALS IN NORMAL THYROID FOLLICLES

This illustration shows calcium oxalate crystals in the lumina of normal thyroid follicles. The picture on the right was taken with polarizing lenses to show the birefringent quality of the crystals. This finding is said to be associated with decreased function of the gland, such as that induced by suppression.

B. DISTRIBUTION OF C CELLS IN NORMAL ADULT THYROID GLAND

This section was stained for calcitonin with the immunoperoxidase method. C cells are present within follicles. The inset shows individual C cells varying in shape from spindle to polyhedral.

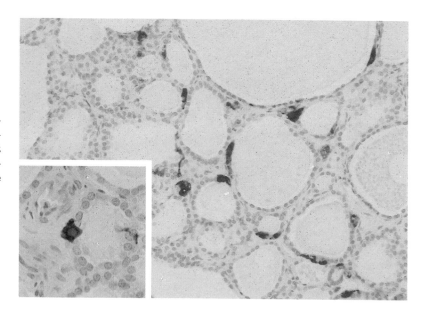

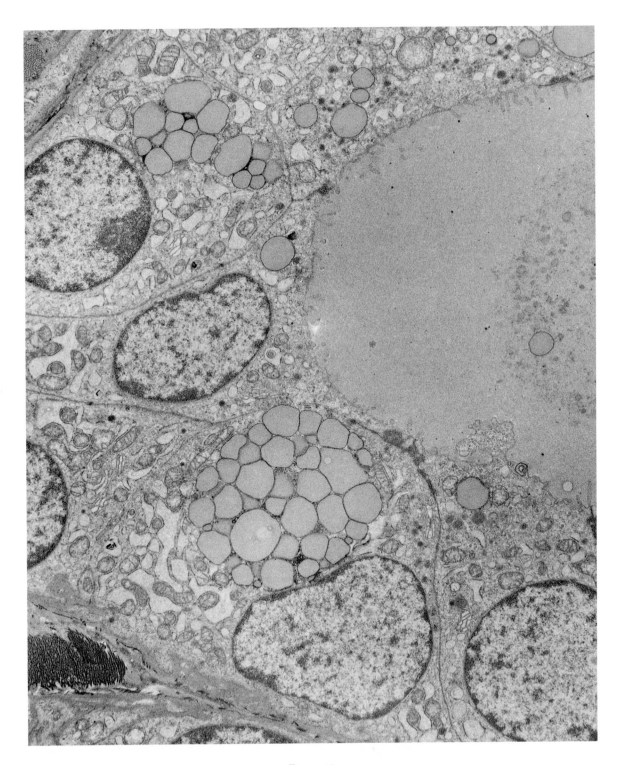

Figure 10
NORMAL THYROID FOLLICLE

The follicular cells in this electron micrograph exhibit microvilli on their luminal surface and are joined by junctional complexes toward the apex. The cytoplasm contains mitochondria, a moderate amount of dilated endoplasmic reticulum, and clusters of large lysosomes. The smaller and darker granules are probably also of lysosomal nature. X6200. (Courtesy of Dr. Robert Erlandson, Memorial Sloan-Kettering Cancer Center, New York, NY.)

In some species, C cells also contain thyrotropin-releasing hormone as determined by immunohistochemical analyses (24). Northern analysis of total thyroid RNA with a pre-prothyrotropin–releasing hormone–specific RNA probe has identified a single hybridizing band that is the same size as thyrotropin-releasing hormone mRNA found in the hypothalamus. These observations support a potential paracrine function for thyrotropin-releasing hormone gene products directly within the thyroid gland (24).

In addition to the regulatory peptide products, C cells also contain a variety of biologically active amines including serotonin (33). Normal C cells express low-molecular-weight cytokeratins but are negative for neurofilament proteins (19, 41). These cells also stain positively for neuron-specific enolase, chromogranin A, and synaptophysin (19,41). Polyclonal antisera to carcinoembryonic antigen (CEA) also react with normal C cells (21).

Detailed immunohistochemical and ultrastructural studies have revealed that C cells occupy an exclusively intrafollicular position and are separated from the thyroid interstitium by the follicular basal lamina (fig. 11) (21,31). C cells are characterized by the presence of variable numbers of secretory granules that range from 60 to 550 nm in diameter (21). Type I granules have an average diameter of 280 nm, with moderately electron-dense, finely granular contents that are closely applied to the limiting membranes of the granules. Type II granules have an average diameter of 130 nm, with more electron-dense contents that are separated from

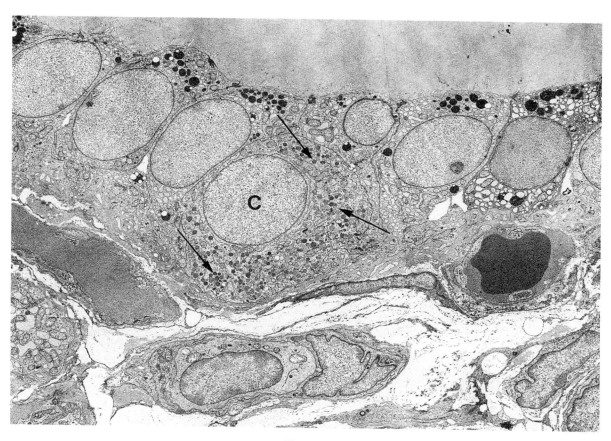

Figure 11
C CELL

The C cell (C) in this electron micrograph is from a patient with mild diffuse C cell hyperplasia. This cell is similar to a normal adult C cell with respect to its intrafollicular location and its content of secretory granules (arrows). The C cell is separated from the luminal colloid by the cytoplasm of adjacent follicular cells and from the interstitium by the follicular basal lamina. X2950.

the limiting membranes by a small but distinct electron-lucent space. In general, normal C cells are filled with type I secretory granules. Immunocytochemical studies performed at the ultrastructural level have revealed that both type I and II secretory granules contain immunoreactive calcitonin (20).

C cells are restricted in their distribution in normal adult and neonatal thyroid glands to a zone in the middle to upper third of the lateral lobes along their central axes. The extreme upper and lower poles and the isthmus are generally devoid of C cells (45,46). In neonates, most C cells are dispersed singly and have a polygonal to spindle shape. Clusters of up to 6 C cells may be present in the neonatal gland, and up to 100 C cells may be seen in a single low-power microscopic field. Prominent populations of C cells may persist until the age of 6 years. C cells are markedly decreased or absent in infants with the DiGeorge syndrome.

C cells in adult thyroid glands are less numerous than they are in neonates. Moreover, adult C cells frequently have a flattened or spindle shape. Early studies of adult thyroids revealed less than 10 C cells per single low-power microscopic field (46). More recent studies, however, have shown that 50 or more C cells per single low-power field may be present in some normal glands (23,34). Gibson and coworkers (23) have demonstrated that occasional normal adult thyroid glands may contain large C cell nodules, particularly after the age of 50 years. These workers have suggested that such C cell nodules may represent age-related hyperplasia or a normal variation in C cell ontogeny. The coexistence of low overall C cell counts and the presence of a large C cell nodule in one of the cases reported by Gibson and coworkers suggest that at least some nodules may result from the partial failure of embryonic C cell migration and dispersion within the gland.

O'Toole and coworkers (34) have examined the influence of age on the distribution of C cells. In their study, thyroid glands from individuals up to age 59 years had relatively constant numbers of C cells with an average of one C cell per millimeter squared. The number of C cells in thyroid glands from individuals older than 60 was extremely variable, with an indication of an age-related increase; however, the number of C cells in these individuals did not differ significantly from that observed in younger individuals.

Solid Cell Nests

Solid cell nests were first recognized as possible remnants of ultimobranchial bodies almost a century ago (27,44). Most solid cell nests measure an average of 0.1 mm in diameter, but occasional nests may measure up to 2 mm. Solid cell nests are composed of cells that are polygonal to oval and contain elongated nuclei with finely granular chromatin (fig. 12). A second cellular component of the solid cell nest has a round nucleus with clear cytoplasm. Ultrastructurally, the cells in these nests have tonofilaments, desmosomes, and intraluminal cytoplasmic projections. Immunohistochemical studies have revealed positive reactions for low–molecular-weight keratins and have established that some of the clear cells contain calcitonin (32). Most solid cell nests are present within the interstitium of the thyroid; however, occasional solid cell nests may be connected to follicular cells forming a so-called "mixed follicle." Occasional cells within such mixed follicles are positive for thyroglobulin. Typically, increased numbers of C cells are evident in the thyroid parenchyma around solid cell nests.

Solid cell nests are found most commonly along the central axis of the middle and upper thirds of the lateral lobes. The probability of finding solid cell nests rises with the numbers of sections studied. They are found in 3 percent of routinely examined thyroids and in 61 percent of glands that have been blocked serially at intervals of 2 to 3 mm (27). Generally, solid cell nests are found in areas of the thyroid that contain the highest concentrations of C cells, as might be expected on the basis of the proposed origin of C cells.

The solid cell nests may contain central lumina lined with Alcian blue and mucicarmine-positive cells with pyknotic nuclei. The cells comprising the solid cell nests are positive for high– and low–molecular-weight keratin proteins. Polyclonal CEA antisera also show a positive reaction.

Solid cell nests must be distinguished from papillary microcarcinomas, micrometastases to the thyroid, and foci of nodular C cell hyperplasia.

PHYSIOLOGY

The function of the thyroid is expressed through the secretion of two separate sets of hormones with completely different functions: (iodinated) thyroid hormones and calcitonin.

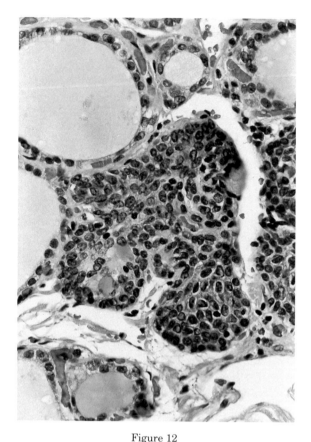

Figure 12
SOLID CELL NEST
Small collections of colloid are present in this otherwise solid nest located between follicles.

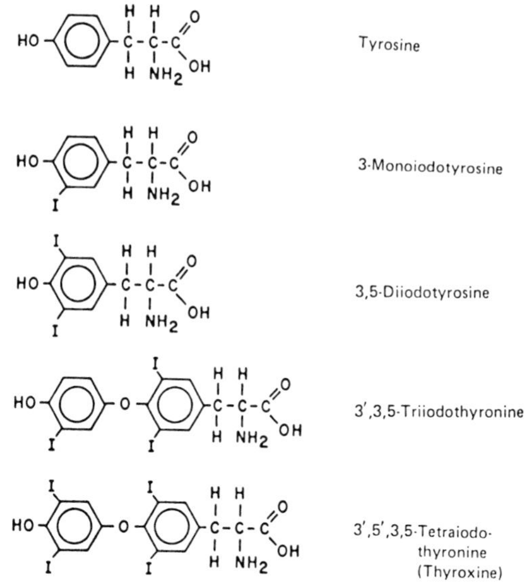

Thyroid Hormones

Biosynthesis of thyroid hormone begins by absorption of ingested iodine into the bloodstream, its transport as iodide into the extracellular fluid compartment, and its energy-dependent concentration in the thyroid. This results in intracellular levels at least 30 times higher than in the peripheral blood. The intrathyroidal iodide is then oxidized to iodine by a peroxidase and bound organically to tyrosine radicals of thyroglobulin to form monoiodotyrosine and diiodotyrosine. Oxidative coupling of diiodotyrosine gives rise to thyroxine (tetraiodothyronine), whereas a similar coupling of monoiodotyrosine and diiodotyrosine gives rise to triiodothyronine (fig. 13). All of these iodothyronines are then incorporated into thyroglobulin. This is a large glycoprotein with a 19S sedimentation coefficient and a molecular weight of 670,000.

Tyrosine

3-Monoiodotyrosine

3,5-Diiodotyrosine

3',3,5-Triiodothyronine

3',5',3,5-Tetraiodothyronine (Thyroxine)

Figure 13
THYROID HORMONES
Molecular structures of major iodoamino acids found in thyroglobulin and their precursers.

It is formed by two identical subunits with a 12S sedimentation coefficient to which many oligosaccharides are linked. Thyroglobulin is encoded by a gene spreading over more than 200 kilobases in the bovine genome (54). The molecular mechanisms involved in the tissue-specific and hormone-dependent expression of the thyroglobulin gene have been studied in follicular cells in primary cultures and cell lines (52,59).

The synthesis of thyroglobulin begins in the endoplasmic reticulum of the follicular cell and continues in the Golgi apparatus, where the end sugars of the carbohydrate site are incorporated. It is then packaged in small apical microvesicles, the contents of which are discharged into the follicular lumen after fusion of the vesicle membranes with the luminal side of the plasma membrane.

Resorption of thyroglobulin takes place through cytoplasmic "streamers," which engulf minute portions of colloid that are then drawn into the cell in the form of membrane-bound colloid droplets. These subsequently fuse with lysosomes, and their content is digested by the lysosomal enzymes. The breakdown products, including thyroxine and triiodothyronine, diffuse through the cell membrane and the basement membrane into the adjacent capillaries, and most of the molecules become bound to a specific carrier protein known as thyroxine-binding globulin (53,57,60).

Thyroid hormone stimulates metabolism, increases oxygen consumption, and causes a rise in heat production, cardiac output, and heart rate. It is essential for normal development, growth, and maturation. The acceleration of growth may result from a direct action on the cells to increase their rate of division, by acting permissively for other hormones or by inducing the synthesis of a variety of growth-promoting hormones (51,57,62–66,69).

Thyroid secretory activity is controlled by the level of thyrotropin (thyroid-stimulating hormone) in the blood. This hormone operates through thyrotropin receptors located on the basolateral surface of the follicular cell membrane and the adenylate cyclase system (50,67). Stimulation of the thyroid gland by thyrotropin increases its secretory activity and vascularity and results in both hypertrophy and hyperplasia of follicular cells, accompanied by reduction of colloid storage. At the functional level, this is reflected by an increase in iodide concentration and organic binding, hormone synthesis, and hormone secretion (60,68,70).

In turn, the release of thyrotropin by the pituitary gland is regulated by thyrotropin-releasing hormone, which is produced by the neurons of the medial-basal hypothalamus and carried into the pituitary gland via the hypophyseal-portal vessels.

Calcitonin and the Calcitonin Gene–Related Peptide

The gene that encodes calcitonin is located on the short arm of chromosome 11 and consists of 6 exons that also encode katacalcin (the C-terminal–flanking peptide of calcitonin) and the calcitonin gene–related peptide (CGRP) (49,61). The primary transcript of the calcitonin gene (calcitonin-CGRP gene) gives rise to two different mRNAs by tissue-specific alternative splicing events that produce calcitonin and CGRP mRNAs (49,61). Detailed molecular studies have revealed a second calcitonin-CGRP gene, which has been designated as the β-gene to distinguish it from the originally described α-calcitonin-CGRP gene (61). The calcitonin-CGRP genes are expressed both in thyroid and nervous tissue, but calcitonin is produced in large quantities only in the thyroid

Both calcitonin and CGRP are synthesized as larger precursors that are cleaved intracellularly to yield the active peptides (58,61). Calcitonin is a 32-amino acid peptide that is released from the thyroid when plasma calcium levels are increased (55). When it is administered to experimental animals with high bone turnover or to patients with Paget disease, calcitonin results in a fall in plasma calcium levels. This effect is mediated by inhibition of osteoclastic activity (61). When calcitonin is administered chronically, as in patients with Paget disease, the number of osteoclasts diminishes progressively. Calcitonin also acts on the kidney to enhance the production of vitamin D_1. The major physiologic role of calcitonin is probably the protection of the skeleton during periods of calcium stress (e.g., growth, pregnancy, lactation) (61). Absence of calcitonin is not associated with hypercalcemia, and a marked excess of the hormone such as that found in patients with medullary thyroid carcinoma does not produce hypocalcemia. Gastrin and cholecystokinin also induce the secretion of calcitonin, as does the chronic administration of estrogenic hormones (61).

In normal adult men, basal calcitonin levels range from 3 to 36 pg/ml (0.9–10.5 pmol/L) (61). Plasma levels in women range from 3 to 17 pg/ml (0.9–5.0 pmol/L). Normal values after pentagastrin stimulation are less than 106 pg/ml (30.9 pmol/L) for men and less than 29 pg/ml (8.5 pmol/L) for women. Katacalcin, the C-terminal–flanking peptide of calcitonin, is a 21–amino acid peptide that is cosecreted with calcitonin in equimolar amounts (48). The function of katacalcin, however, is unknown. CGRP is a 37–amino acid peptide that is an extremely potent vasodilator and also functions as a neuromodulator or neurotransmitter. Circulating CGRP is derived primarily from cardiac and perivascular nerves (56).

REFERENCES

Embryology

1. Burke BA, Johnson D, Gilbert EF, Drut RM, Ludwig J, Wick MR. Thyrocalcitonin-containing cells in the DiGeorge anomaly. Hum Pathol 1987;18:355–60.
2. Conley ME, Beckwith JB, Mancer JF, Tenckoff L. The spectrum of the DiGeorge syndrome. J Pediatr 1979;94:883–90.
3. Gitlin D, Biasucci A. Ontogenesis of immunoreactive thyroglobulin in the human conceptus. J Clin Endocrinol Metab 1969;29:849–53.
4. Hoyes AD, Kershaw DR. Anatomy and development of the thyroid gland. Ear Nose Throat J 1985;64:318–33.
5. Ito M, Kameda Y, Tagawa T. An ultrastructural study of the cysts in chicken ultimobranchial glands, with special reference to C cells. Cell Tissue Res 1986;246:39–44.
6. LeDouarin N, Fontain J, LeLievre C. New studies on the neural crest origin of the avian ultimobranchial glandular cells—interspecific combinations and cytochemical characterization of C cells based on the uptake of biogenic amine precursors. Histochemistry 1974;38:297–305.
7. _____, NM, Teillet MA. The migration of neural crest cells to the wall of the digestive tract in the avian embryo. J Embryol Exp Morphol 1973;30:31–48.
8. Nadig J, Weber E, Hedinger C. C cells in vestiges of the ultimobranchial body in human thyroid glands. Virchows Arch [Cell Pathol] 1978;27:189–91.
9. Norris EH. The early morphogenesis of the human thyroid gland. Am J Anat 1918;24:443–65.
10. Pearse AG, Polak JM. Cytochemical evidence for the neural crest origin of mammalian ultimobranchial C cells. Histochemie 1976;27:96–102.
11. Shepard TH. Onset of function in the human fetal thyroid: biochemical and radioautographic studies from organ culture. J Clin Endocrinol Metab 1967;27:945–58.
12. Sugiyama S. The embryology of the human thyroid gland including ultimobranchial body and others related. Ergeb Anat Entwicklungsgesch 1971;44:6–110.
13. Williams ED, Toyn CE, Harach HR. The ultimobranchial gland and congenital thyroid abnormalities in man. J Pathol 1989;159:135–41.

Anatomy

14. Crile G Jr. The fallacy of the conventional radical neck dissection for papillary carcinoma of the thyroid. Ann Surg 1957;145:317–20.
15. Russell WO, Ibanez ML, Clark RL, White EC. Thyroid carcinoma. Classification, intraglandular dissemination, and clinicopathological study. Cancer 1963;16:1425–60.

Histology

16. Ali-Rachedi A, Varndell IM, Facer P, et al. Immunocytochemical localization of katacalcin, a calcium-lowering hormone cleaved from the human calcitonin precursor. J Clin Endocrinol Metab 1983;57:680–2.
17. Braunstein H, Stephens CL. Parafollicular cells of the human thyroid. Arch Pathol 1968;86:659–66.
18. Bussolati G, Foster GV, Clark MB, Pearse AG. Immunofluorescent localization of calcitonin in medullary (C cell) thyroid carcinoma using antibody to the pure porcine hormone. Virchows Arch [Cell Pathol] 1969;2:234–8.
19. DeLellis RA. Endocrine tumors. In: Colvin RB, Bhan AK, McCluskey RT, eds. Diagnostic immunopathology. New York: Raven Press, 1988:301–38.
20. DeLellis RA, May L, Tashjian AH Jr, Wolfe HJ. C cell granule heterogeneity in man. An ultrastructural immunocytochemical study. Lab Invest 1978;38:263–9.
21. DeLellis RA, Wolfe HJ. The pathobiology of the human calcitonin (C)-cell: a review. Pathol Annu 1981;16(2):25–52.
22. Finkle HI, Goldman RL. Heterotopic cartilage in the thyroid. Arch Pathol 1973;95:48–9.
23. Gibson WC, Peng T-C, Croker BP. C-cell nodules in adult human thyroid. A common autopsy finding. Am J Clin Pathol 1981;75:347–50.
24. Gkonos PJ, Tavianini MA, Liu CC, Roos BA. Thyrotropin-releasing hormone gene expression in normal thyroid parafollicular cells. Mol Endocrinol 1989;3:2101–9.
25. González-Cámpora R, Sanchez Gallego F, Martin Lacave I, Mora Marin J, Montero Linares C, Galera-Davidson H. Lectin histochemistry of the thyroid gland. Cancer 1988;62:2354–62.
26. Hanson GA, Komorowski RA, Cerletty JM, Wilson SD. Thyroid gland morphology in young adults: normal subjects versus those with prior low-dose neck irradiation in childhood. Surgery 1983;94:984–8.
27. Harach HR. Solid cell nests in the thyroid. J Pathol 1988;155:191–200.
28. Henzen-Logmans SC, Mullink H, Ramaekers FC, Tadema T, Meijer CJ. Expression of cytokeratins and vimentin in epithelial cells of normal and pathologic thyroid tissue. Virchows Arch [A] 1987;410:347–54.
29. Klinck GH, Oertel JE, Winship T. Ultrastructure of normal human thyroid. Lab Invest 1970;22:2–22.
30. Kurata A, Ohta K, Mine M, et al. Monoclonal antihuman thyroglobulin antibodies. J Clin Endocrinol Metab 1984;59:573–9.
31. McMillan PJ, Hooker WM, Deftos LJ. Distribution of calcitonin-containing cells in the human thyroid. Am J Anat 1974;140:73–80.

32. Nadig J, Weber E, Hedinger C. C cells in vestiges of the ultimobranchial body in human thyroid glands. Virchows Arch [Cell Pathol] 1978;27:189–91.

33. Nunez EA, Gershon MD. Thyrotropin-induced thyroidal release of 5-hydroxytryptamine and accompanying ultrastructural changes in parafollicular cells. Endocrinology 1983;113:309–17.

34. O'Toole K, Fenoglio-Preiser C, Pushparaj N. Endocrine changes associated with the human aging process: III. Effect of age on the number of calcitonin immunoreactive cells in the thyroid gland. Hum Pathol 1985;16:991–1000.

35. Pearse AG. Common cytochemical and ultrastructural characteristics of cells producing polypeptide hormones (the APUD series) and their relevance to thyroid and ultimobranchial C cells and calcitonin. Proc R Soc Lond B 1968;170:71–80.

36. Reid JD, Choi C-H, Oldroyd NO. Calcium oxalate crystals in the thyroid. Their identification, prevalence, origin, and possible significance. Am J Clin Pathol 1987;87:443–54.

37. Rigaud C, Bogomoletz WV. "Mucin secreting" and "mucinous" primary thyroid carcinomas. Pitfalls in mucin histochemistry applied to thyroid tumours. J Clin Pathol 1987;40:890–5.

38. Rosai J, Carcangiu ML. Pitfalls in the diagnosis of thyroid neoplasms. Pathol Res Pract 1987;182:169–79.

39. Scopsi L, Ferrari C, Pilotti S, et al. Immunocytochemical localization and identification of prosomatostatin gene products in medullary carcinoma of human thyroid gland. Hum Pathol 1990;21:820–30.

40. Stanta G, Carcangiu ML, Rosai J. The biochemical and immunohistochemical profile of thyroid neoplasia. Pathol Annu 1988;23(1):129–57.

41. _____, Carcangiu ML, Rosai J, Marchesi VT. Monoclonal antibodies reveal different thyroglobulin compartmentalization in non-neoplastic thyroid and papillary thyroid carcinoma. (Submitted for publication).

42. Sunday ME, Wolfe HJ, Roos BA, Chin WW, Spindel ER. Gastrin-releasing peptide gene expression in developing, hyperplastic, and neoplastic thyroid C-cells. Endocrinology 1988;122:1551–8.

43. Teitelbaum SL, Moore KE, Shieber W. Parafollicular cells in the normal human thyroid. Nature 1971;230:334–45.

44. Williams ED, Toyn CE, Harach HR. The ultimobranchial gland and congenital thyroid abnormalities in man. J Pathol 1989;159:135–41.

45. Wolfe HJ, DeLellis RA, Voelkel EF, Tashjian AH Jr. Distribution of calcitonin-containing cells in the normal neonatal human thyroid gland: a correlation of morphology with peptide content. J Clin Endocrinol Metab 1975;41:1076–81.

46. _____, Voelkel EF, Tashjian AH Jr. Distribution of calcitonin-containing cells in the normal adult human thyroid gland: a correlation of morphology with peptide content. J Clin Endocrinol Metab 1974;38:688–94.

47. Zajac JD, Penschow J, Mason T, Tregear G, Coghlan J, Martin TJ. Identification of calcitonin and calcitonin gene-related peptide messenger ribonucleic acid in medullary thyroid carcinoma by hybridization histochemistry. J Clin Endocrinol Metab 1986;62:1037–43.

Physiology

48. Ali-Rachedi A, Varndell IM, Facer P, et al. Immunocytochemical localization of katacalcin, a calcium-lowering hormone cleaved from the human calcitonin precursor. J Clin Endocrinol Metab 1983;57:680–2.

49. Amara SG, Jonas V, Rosenfeld MG, Ong SG, Evans RM. Alternative RNA processing in calcitonin gene expression generates mRNAs encoding different polypeptide products. Nature 1982;298:240–4.

50. Atassi MZ, Manshouri T, Sakata S. Localization and synthesis of the hormone-binding regions of the human thyrotropin receptor. Proc Natl Acad Sci USA 1991;88:3613–7.

51. Bernal J, Liewendahl K, Lamberg BA. Thyroid hormone receptors in fetal and hormone resistant tissues. Scand J Clin Lab Invest 1985;45:577–83.

52. Christophe D, Gérard C, Juvenal G, et al. Identification of a cAMP-responsive region in thyroglobulin gene promoter. Mol Cell Endocrinol 1989;64:5–18.

53. Deiss WP, Peake RL. The mechanism of thyroid hormone secretion. Ann Intern Med 1968;69:881–90.

54. De Martynoff G, Pohl V, Mercken L, Van Ommen GJ, Vassart G. Structural organization of the bovine thyroglobulin gene and of its 5'-flanking region. Eur J Biochem 1987;164:591–9.

55. Foster GV. Calcitonin (thyrocalcitonin). N Engl J Med 1968;279:349–60.

56. Girgis SI, MacDonald DW, Stevenson JC, et al. Calcitonin gene related peptide: potent vasodilator and major product of calcitonin gene. Lancet 1985;2:14–6.

57. Green WL. The physiology of the thyroid gland and its hormones. In: Green WL, ed. The thyroid. New York: Elsevier, 1987:1–46.

58. Hurley DL, Katz HH, Tiegs RD, Calvo MS, Barta JR, Heath H III. Cosecretion of calcitonin gene products. J Clin Endocrinol Metab 1988;66:640–4.

59. Lee N-T, Nayfeh SN, Chae C-B. Induction of nuclear protein factors specific for hormone-responsive region during activation of thyroglobulin gene by thyrotropin in rat thyroid FRTL-5 cells. J Biol Chem 1989;264:7523–30.

60. Liddle GW, Liddle RA. Endocrinology. In: Smith LH, Thier SO, eds. Pathophysiology. Philadelphia: WB Saunders, 1981:653–754.

61. MacIntyre I. Calcitonin, physiology, biosynthesis, secretion, metabolism, and mode of action. In: DeGroot LJ, ed. Endocrinology, Vol 2. Philadelphia: WB Saunders, 1989;892–901.

62. Müller MJ, Seitz HJ. Thyroid hormone action on intermediary metabolism. I. Respiration, thermogenesis and carbohydrate metabolism. Klin Wochenschr 1984;62:11–8.

63. _____, Seitz HJ. Thyroid hormone action on intermediary metabolism. II. Lipid metabolism in hyper- and hypothyroidism. Klin Wochenschr 1984;62:49–55.

64. _____, Seitz HJ. Thyroid hormone action on intermediary metabolism. III. Protein metabolism in hyper- and hypothyroidism. Klin Wochenschr 1984;62:97–102.

65. Oppenheimer JH. Thyroid hormone action at the nuclear level. Ann Intern Med 1985;102:374–84.

66. , Samuels HH, Apriletti JW. Molecular basis of thyroid hormone action. New York: Academic Press, 1983.

67. Parmentier M, Libert F, Maenhaut C, et al. Molecular cloning of the thyrotropin receptor. Science 1989;246:1620–2.

68. Pittman JA Jr. Thyrotropin-releasing hormone. Adv Intern Med 1974;19:303–25.

69. Sterling K. Thyroid hormone action at the cell level. N Engl J Med 1979;300:117–23; 173–7.

70. Wilber JF. Thyrotropin releasing hormone: secretion and actions. Annu Rev Med 1973;24:353–64.

❖❖❖

CLASSIFICATION OF THYROID TUMORS

Several classifications of thyroid tumors have been proposed, but none of them is entirely satisfactory. Masson (2) stated in frustration, "No classification is more difficult to establish than that of thyroid epitheliomas. Their pleomorphism is almost the rule; very few are adapted to a precise classification." About the ability to separate benign from malignant tumors, he added, "Of all cancers, thyroid epitheliomas teach, perhaps, the greatest lesson of humility to histopathologists. . . . Many pathologists agree with me in never giving a prognosis on an epithelial thyroid tumor without reservation."

As with many other tumor classifications, those that have been applied to thyroid neoplasms are the result of a haphazard combination of architectural, cytologic, histogenetic, and grading considerations. The most important group, by far, is that of the primary epithelial neoplasms. Because there are only two major types of epithelial cells, the follicular cell and the C cell, we think that the first major division of the corresponding tumors should be into those exhibiting follicular cell differentiation and those featuring C cell differentiation, with a possible third group showing differentiation along both cell lines. This classification scheme, which we have adopted for this Fascicle, differs slightly from that proposed by the WHO (1), in which a behavioral distinction into benign and malignant tumors takes precedence over the above.

There is only one major type of neoplasm exhibiting evidence of C cell differentiation, and this is the malignant tumor that carries the time-honored designation of *medullary carcinoma* (including its variants). For the tumors featuring follicular cell differentiation, the situation is considerably more complex.

Neoplasms of follicular cells are first divided into benign and malignant. The benign tumors are designated as *follicular adenomas*. It follows that their malignant counterparts should be designated as adenocarcinomas. However, this is rarely the case. Instead, the better differentiated members of the group have been traditionally divided into two major categories, *follicular* and *papillary*, on the basis of their architectural features; the lesser differentiated types, whether still recognizable as epithelial or having a sar-coma-like appearance, have been designated as *undifferentiated* or *anaplastic*. The criteria for the recognition of follicular and papillary carcinomas have changed in recent years (papillae are no longer necessary for the diagnosis of papillary carcinoma), but the two names have been retained.

This superficially simple scheme is significantly modified and complicated by two factors. The first is the occurrence in some tumors of follicular cell derivation, whether follicular or papillary, of the following cytoplasmic changes, either singly or in combination: oncocytic, clear, squamous, or mucinous. Some of these changes are inconsequential, but others are associated with definite behavioral connotations and are therefore of consequence.

The other important consideration is that not all follicular or papillary carcinomas are well differentiated tumors. Instead, some exhibit poorly differentiated morphologic features; this is just as important (or perhaps more so) from a prognostic and therapeutic standpoint as whether they belong to one group or another (3). The higher the grade of the tumor, the less significant it becomes to assign it to either a follicular or papillary category: it is important for the better differentiated tumors, less so for the poorly differentiated ones, and unwarranted (and generally not feasible) for the undifferentiated categories. This approach is similar to that which is being adopted in many other sites (e.g., soft tissue tumors), in the sense of considerations based on tumor grading being progressively incorporated into more traditional schemes. Because some of the morphologic features present in these tumors (i.e., clear cell changes) cross classification lines, we thought it useful to list and discuss them separately from the major classification scheme for purposes of differential diagnosis.

As a final comment, it should be pointed out that the terms *goiter* and *struma* simply refer to enlargement of the thyroid gland, whatever the cause. In fact, the terms had been applied in popular language to any type of swelling in the antero-lateral region of the neck, Virchow being the first to suggest that they should be restricted to thyroid swelling. Currently, they are more frequently used for non-neoplastic thyroid conditions (i.e., nodular hyperplasia, Hashimoto thyroiditis). To avoid confusion, these terms should never be used without a qualifier, if at all.

The classification of thyroid neoplasms adopted for this Fascicle follows.

PRIMARY TUMORS

Epithelial Tumors
  Tumors of Follicular Cells
    Benign: follicular adenoma
      conventional
      variants
    Malignant: carcinoma
      differentiated
        follicular carcinoma
        papillary carcinoma
          conventional
          variants
      poorly differentiated
        insular carcinoma
        others
      undifferentiated (anaplastic)
  Tumors of C (and related neuroendocrine) Cells
    medullary carcinoma

others
Tumors of Follicular and C Cells
Sarcomas
Malignant Lymphoma (and related hematopoietic neoplasms)
Miscellaneous Neoplasms

SECONDARY TUMORS

TUMOR-LIKE LESIONS

Cytologic features resulting in special tumor types and subtypes that cross lines in the above classification for the tumors of follicular cells and, to a lesser extent, of C cells include:
  Tumors with oncocytic (Hürthle cell) features
    oncocytic adenoma (Hürthle cell adenoma)
    oncocytic carcinoma (Hürthle cell carcinoma)
    papillary oncocytic (Hürthle cell) tumors
  Tumors with clear cell features
  Tumors with squamous features
  Tumors with mucinous features

REFERENCES

1. Hedinger CE. Histological typing of thyroid tumours. Berlin: Springer-Verlag, 1988. (Hedinger CE, ed. International histological classification of tumours; Vol 11.)
2. Masson P. Human tumors. Histology, diagnosis, and technique. 2nd ed. Detroit: Wayne State Univ, 1970:588–9.
3. Zampi G, Bianchi S, Amorosi A. Attuali criteri classificativi dei tumori della tiroide. Istocitopatologia 1989;110:14–8.

FOLLICULAR ADENOMA

Definition. A benign encapsulated tumor showing evidence of follicular cell differentiation. Sometimes the tumor is simply designated as adenoma without a qualifier, in view of the fact that all of the currently recognized types of thyroid adenoma are of follicular nature. All other adjectives applied to thyroid adenomas refer to subtypes or varieties of follicular adenoma.

General Features. Follicular adenoma is a relatively common neoplasm. The ratio between adenomas and carcinomas, based on surgical specimens, is about 5:1. In a review of 300 consecutive autopsies performed at Yale University on patients aged 20 years or older, 9 adenomas were found, for an incidence of 3 percent (37). In a similar study of 300 cases examined in Sao Paulo, Brazil, the incidence of adenoma was similar: 12 adenomas were found, for an incidence of 4.3 percent (3). There seems to be no relationship between the overall frequency of adenoma and the level of iodine in the diet; however, it has been claimed that solitary autonomously functioning thyroid nodules ("toxic adenomas") are more common in areas of iodine deficiency (2). Thyroid adenomas develop with great frequency in patients with Cowden (multiple hamartoma) syndrome. Thyroid nodular hyperplasia may also occur in this population (5).

Adenomas are nearly always solitary, but instances in which two or more adenomas are seen in the same gland occur, even when strict criteria for their distinction from hyperplastic nodules are applied. Most adenomas occur in otherwise normal glands, but they can also be seen in glands affected by thyroiditis, nodular hyperplasia, or other lesions.

Most adenomas are located in one of the lobes, but a few affect primarily the isthmus. No predilection for one lobe or a portion of a lobe has been noted.

The assumption that follicular adenoma, being a neoplastic process, has a clonal origin has been supported by three studies involving analysis of the X chromosomes: one in mice (39) and two in humans (17,30).

Clinical Features. Most patients with follicular adenomas of the thyroid are middle aged, and women are most often affected. Although indisputable cases of adenomas in children and in the elderly also occur, the chances of an alternative diagnosis, particularly carcinoma, are higher in these two age groups.

Most patients with follicular adenomas are euthyroid and consult because of a painless thyroid lump. Pressure-related symptoms, mainly resulting from tracheal compression, may occur with the larger lesions. Sudden growth, sometimes associated with pain, may be present; this is usually the result of intratumoral hemorrhage. On isotopic scan, the adenoma is usually "cold" (hypofunctional), sometimes "cool" or "warm" (functional), and only exceptionally "hot" (hyperfunctional) (see Clinical and Laboratory Evaluation of Thyroid Tumors). Many patients with follicular adenomas have elevated circulating levels of thyroglobulin (36), but few of the tumors are associated with clinical hyperthyroidism ("toxic" adenomas, see page 40).

Gross Features. Adenomas are usually round or oval. They are characteristically surrounded by a complete fibrous capsule that varies in thickness but is usually thin (pl. II-A and B). The presence of an unduly thick and irregularly shaped capsule should raise the suspicion of follicular carcinoma.

The size of follicular adenomas is highly variable. However, they are rarely described as microscopic findings, perhaps because at this stage their distinction from a hyperplastic nodule is nearly impossible. Most adenomas have a diameter between 1 and 3 cm at the time of excision, but occasional lesions may be considerably larger and weigh several hundred grams. Their consistency is rubbery or firm. In uncomplicated cases, the cut surface is usually homogeneous and without internal lobulation. The color of the adenoma largely depends on the cell composition and amount of colloid present. It is usually grayish white in the trabecular/solid and hyalinizing trabecular varieties and tan in the adenomas showing follicle formation with colloid deposition, the hue being dependent on the relative proportion of cells and colloid and on the degree of vascularity.

Secondary changes that can be seen at the gross level in adenomas, although not as frequently as in hyperplastic nodules, include hemorrhage, fibrosis, calcification, ossification, and cystic degeneration (pl. II-B, C, and D). Fresh tumor necrosis is most unusual as a spontaneous event in adenoma but is now being observed with some frequency as a complication of fine-needle aspiration, especially in the oncocytic type (see page 163).

Microscopic Features. Follicular adenomas exhibit a bewildering variety of architectural patterns, but there is usually a uniform architecture in an individual lesion. Less commonly, an admixture of two or more patterns is seen. Except for the special types listed separately, the variations in architecture mostly depend on the degree of cellularity, presence and size of follicles, and pattern of growth of the nonfollicular portions, if any. Thus, follicular adenomas of conventional types have been traditionally divided among the following categories:

- **Trabecular/solid**
  This tumor subtype is very cellular and grows in either a trabecular or diffuse (solid) fashion, with few or no follicles being formed. It is sometimes also referred to as *embryonal* because of its morphologic resemblance to a developing thyroid in a very early (prefollicular) stage (fig. 14 A,B).
- **Microfollicular**
  In this tumor, neoplastic follicles are formed but are smaller than those of the neighboring gland. The ratio of cells to lumen is greatly altered in the direction of the former, and the amount of colloid present is minimal. This subtype is sometimes designated as *fetal*, following similar embryologic analogies (fig. 14C).
- **Normofollicular (simple)**
  The pattern of growth of this tumor is follicular throughout, and the size of the follicles approaches that of the non-neoplastic gland (fig. 14D).
- **Macrofollicular (colloid)**
  The neoplastic follicles in this tumor are larger and full of colloid, thus resembling those seen in hyperplastic nodules (fig. 14D).

Most follicular adenomas belong to one of the first two categories, either entirely or partially. The larger and more colloid-like the follicles in a benign follicular nodule, the less likely that the lesion is a true neoplasm. Sometimes one or more sharply outlined trabecular/solid nodules are seen in an adenoma with an otherwise normo- or macrofollicular appearance. These have been referred to as *foci of secondary proliferation* (fig. 15).

Although the histologic differences between these subtypes are striking, they are of no clinical importance. Perhaps their only practical value is that the more cellular a follicular nodule is, the more one should search for evidence of malignancy.

The cells of follicular adenoma tend to be polygonal, with normochromatic nuclei that are round to oval. Variations in nuclear size and shape are minimal, except for the special types. Mitoses are usually absent or scanty. Presence of more than an occasional mitosis should raise the index of suspicion. The cytoplasm is acidophilic to amphophilic and moderately abundant. Cell borders are usually well defined.

The lumina of the neoplastic follicles contain variable amounts of colloid that may exhibit an amphophilic or pale eosinophilic staining quality. If the appearance of the colloid is strongly and homogeneously eosinophilic throughout, the alternative possibility that the lesion may be the follicular variant of papillary carcinoma should be considered (see page 100). In rare instances, the lumina of adenomatous follicles are seen to contain calcium oxalate crystals.

The capsule of the adenoma is complete and made of fibrous tissue within which vessels of various sizes are found (fig. 16). It is not uncommon for the capsule to contain almond-shaped or ovoid masses of smooth muscle, probably representing thickened walls of blood vessels (fig. 17) (15). Evans (10) emphasized that the capsule is frequently thin in follicular adenomas, in contrast to that of follicular carcinomas. The interface between the tumor and the inner side of the capsule is usually sharp but can also be irregular due to herniation or entrapment of tumor cells. The adjacent glandular tissues are often compressed and atrophic, particularly with the larger adenomas.

The stromal component is usually more abundant in the central portion of the adenoma, where it tends to exhibit a loose, edematous quality. Degenerative changes such as recent or old hemorrhage, thrombosis, edema, myxoid change, fibrosis and hyalinization, calcification, metaplastic ossification, and cyst formation may occur (figs. 18–20). The fibrosis, if present, tends

PLATE II
FOLLICULAR ADENOMA

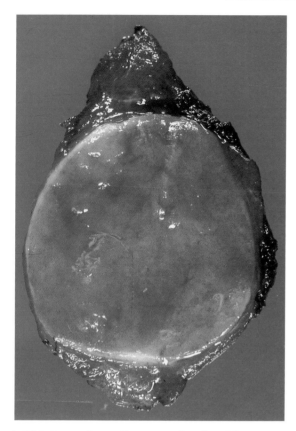

A. This tumor is totally encapsulated and has a relatively homogeneous tan appearance. Compressed residual gland is seen at both poles.

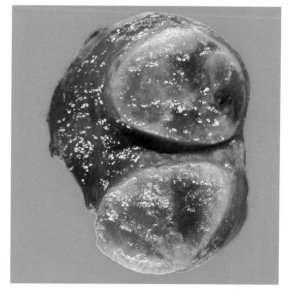

B. The otherwise homogeneous appearance of this bisected adenoma has been altered by the presence of fresh hemorrhage.

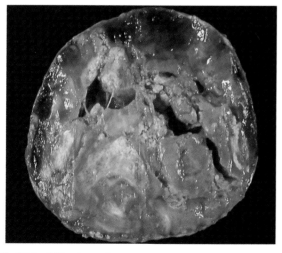

C. This follicular adenoma shows marked necrosis, hemorrhage, and cystic changes.

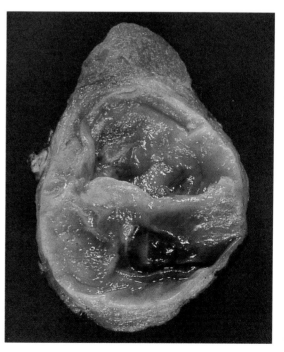

D. Marked cystic degeneration is evident in this tumor. It is likely that most so-called "primary thyroid cysts" represent follicular adenomas exhibiting an extreme form of this phenomenon.

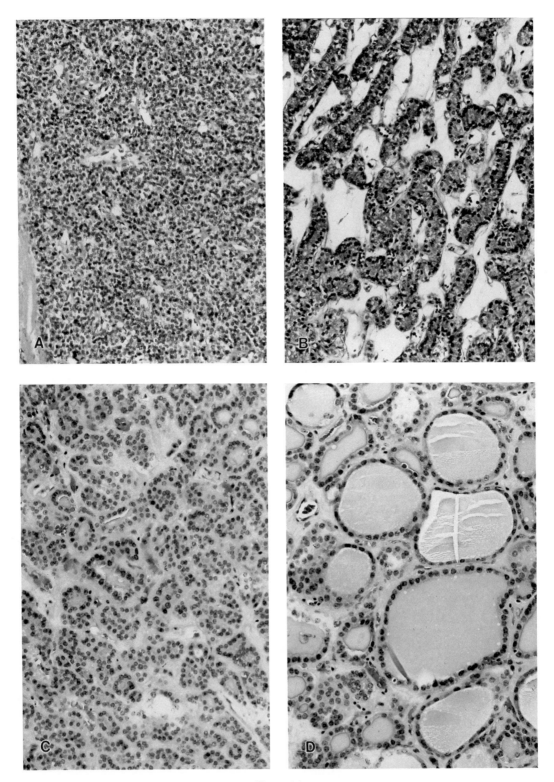

Figure 14
FOLLICULAR ADENOMA
Architecturally, an adenoma may appear solid (A), trabecular (B), microfollicular (C), or normo- or macrofollicular (D). These variations in configuration are of no clinical significance.

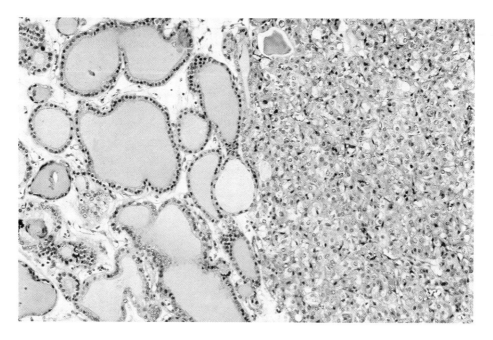

Figure 15
FOLLICULAR ADENOMA
This field shows an admixture of macrofollicular and solid patterns. There is a sharp segregation between the two components.

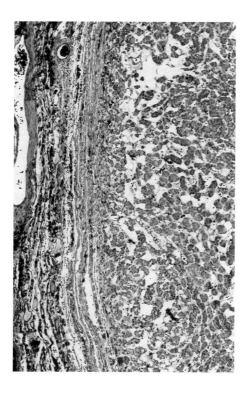
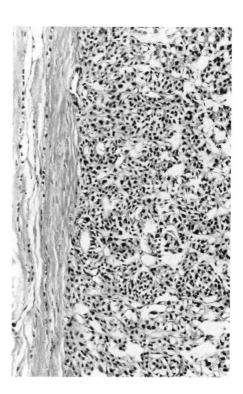

Figure 16
FOLLICULAR ADENOMA
Both of these follicular adenomas show a sharp separation from the surrounding tissue by a relatively thin and uniform fibrous capsule.

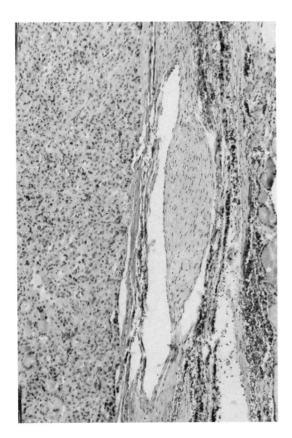

Figure 17
FOLLICULAR ADENOMA
The vessel located in the capsule of this follicular tumor has a cushion of smooth muscle cells along the outer wall. This is a relatively common feature, the significance of which is not clear.

to be centrally located, with a stellate, scar-like configuration.

Squamous metaplasia is exceptionally rare, but it can occur as a focal event, perhaps secondarily to necrosis, whether spontaneous or induced by a fine-needle aspiration (16). Whenever squamous metaplasia is present, the alternative possibility that the tumor is a carcinoma, particularly of papillary type, should be considered.

Similarly, sharply outlined fibrous septa running across the tumor are not a common feature of follicular adenoma. Their presence should raise the possibility of an alternative diagnosis, particularly the follicular variant of papillary carcinoma.

Follicular adenomas are well-vascularized tumors. The intermingling of tumor cells and vessels within the lesion is intimate, and it is not unusual to find isolated follicular cells (or sometimes even small cell clusters) within the vascular lumina. This finding, probably of artifactual nature, is of no diagnostic significance. In some adenomas, the number and prominence of vessels cause them to simulate vascular neoplasms (fig. 21).

Immunohistochemical Features. The immunohistochemical (and enzyme histochemical) profile of follicular adenomas mirrors that of the normal follicle (9). Reactivity for thyroglobulin is the rule. This is more intense in the cytoplasm of the tumor cells but is also evident in the intraluminal colloid, both at a light- and electron-microscopic level (9,24,29). In general, the degree of the thyroglobulin staining in the adenoma is less intense than in the adjacent gland. Positivity is also consistently present for thyroxine and triiodothyronine.

Staining for thyroglobulin is particularly useful diagnostically in the more solid and cellular types of adenomas (as well as in follicular carcinoma). It may show droplet-like foci of positivity in tiny follicles not easily discernible in routinely stained sections.

Keratin reactivity is uniformly present. The keratins expressed in follicular adenomas are the same as those found in the normal follicle. They are of low molecular weight, as befits simple epithelial structures. Thus, Schelfhout and coworkers (34) found consistently high expression of keratins 8 and 18 in both follicular adenomas and normal follicles. The reactivity for keratin 19 in both tissues was only focal and weak. Keratins of high molecular weight are consistently absent. Vimentin is often coexpressed with keratin, the pattern and frequency being similar to those observed in the normal gland and in follicular carcinomas (6,43).

The neoplastic follicles are surrounded by a well-developed basement membrane, which can be demonstrated with the PAS or silver reaction or through immunohistochemical detection of its components, such as laminin and type IV collagen (25,27). This may be useful in delineating small follicles in cellular lesions that appear solid on routinely stained sections.

The enzyme histochemical pattern of follicular adenomas recapitulates that of the normal follicle. There is positivity for 5'-nucleotidase, α-naphthyl acetate esterase, and acid phosphatase and negativity for adenosine triphosphatase and alkaline phosphatase (7).

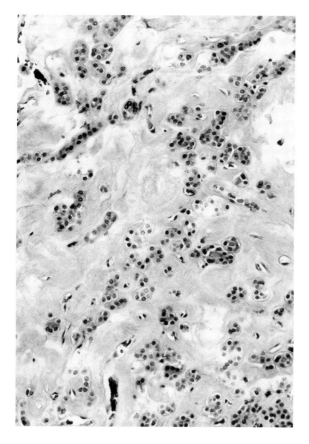

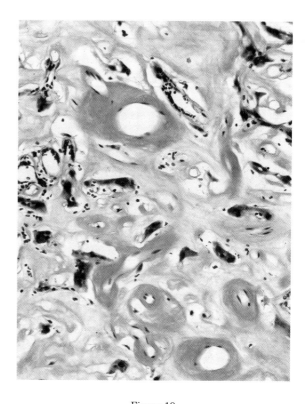

Figure 19
FOLLICULAR ADENOMA
Marked hyaline thickening of the vessel walls associated
with focal calcification. The neoplastic epithelial elements
are not obvious in this photograph.

Figure 18
FOLLICULAR ADENOMA
The follicular adenoma in this illustration shows
marked fibrosis and hyalinization of the stroma.

Figure 20
FOLLICULAR ADENOMA
This tumor shows marked fibrosis,
hyalinization, and calcium deposition.

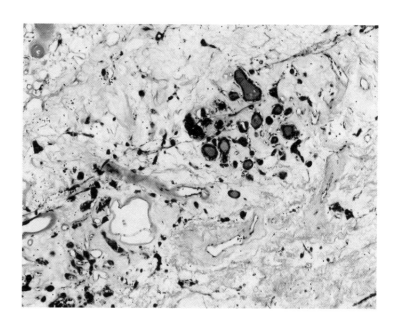

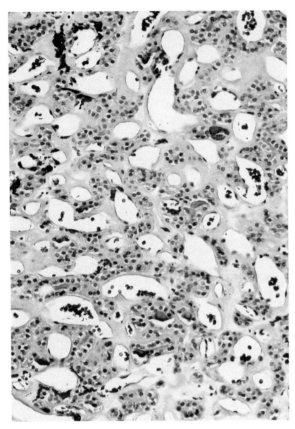

Figure 21
FOLLICULAR ADENOMA
Marked vascularization of this follicular adenoma results in an appearance that can simulate a neoplasm of vascular origin.

The lectin receptors expressed by the cells of follicular adenomas are the same as those of normal follicular cells, but the binding in the neoplastic lesion is said to be significantly stronger (13,33).

Metallothionein, a low–molecular-weight protein thought to be involved in the intracellular storage of essential metals, has been found to be commonly expressed in both benign and malignant tumors of follicular cells but substantially less so by the normal gland (31).

Claims have been made that the following markers are absent or rare in follicular adenoma but consistently expressed by follicular carcinoma: ceruloplasmin, iron-binding proteins (lactoferrin, transferrin, ferritin), tissue polypeptide antigen (1,40,41); tumor associated carbohydrate antigens CA50 and CA19-9 (particularly the former) (44); and Leu-7 antigen

(HNK-1) (10a). Obviously, independent confirmation of these rather surprising results is needed before employing them for differential diagnostic purposes.

Ultrastructural Features. Follicular adenomas have no distinctive features at the ultrastructural level. Their appearance is similar to that of nodular hyperplasia and the normal thyroid gland.

Granular endoplasmic reticulum and Golgi apparatus are well developed, and there are abundant ribosomes and polyribosomes (fig. 22). Accumulations of phagolysosomal bodies are seen in the apical portion of the cytoplasm, and the cell surface is covered with microvilli (fig. 23). Cilia are present in most instances. The follicular cells rest on a continuous basal lamina (38).

Other Special Techniques. Autoradiography has been used to evaluate the functional activity of adenomas and other thyroid lesions. When it is used in whole-organ sections, a correlation with the scintigraphic findings can be made (32).

DNA aneuploidy has been found by flow cytometry in about 25 percent of follicular adenomas of nononcocytic type. This is neither an indicator of clinical malignancy nor of an increased possibility of tumor recurrence (18,20,21). Nevertheless, the fact that it occurs at all raises some disturbing questions, one of them being the possibility that at least some of the lesions currently diagnosed as adenomas are actually noninvasive carcinomas (14). This can neither be proved nor disproved by morphologic studies. If the lesion is shown to be noninvasive after a thorough pathologic evaluation, it will neither recur nor metastasize regardless of its ploidy pattern. Thus, DNA ploidy analysis does not seem to add to the prognostic value of a properly performed microscopic examination (19).

Cytogenetic studies have shown a normal diploid pattern in most adenomas, but complex alterations have been detected in some cases (4,42). This is also the case for follicular carcinomas (20). As in the case of the DNA measurements mentioned above, the significance of these changes is not clear. On the basis of current evidence, they should not be construed as indicators of malignancy.

On flow-cytometric DNA studies, Johannessen and Sobrinho-Simões (22) found that the mean percentage of cells in S phase was higher in

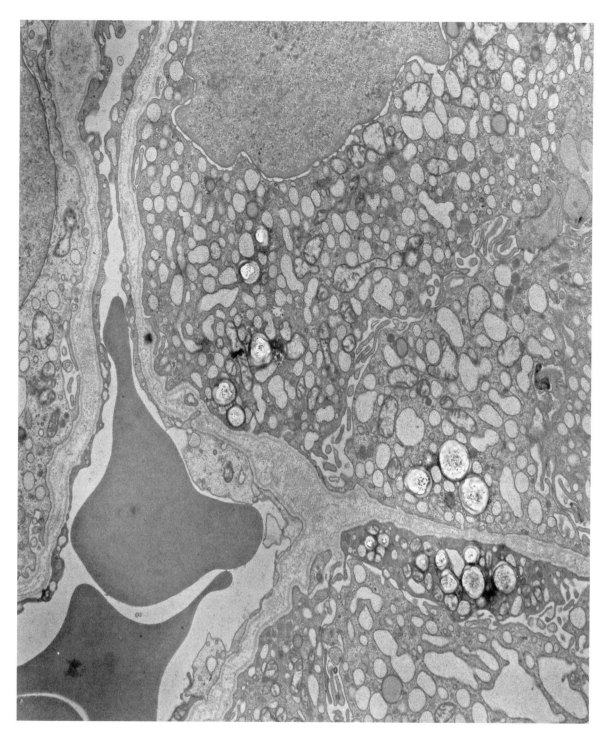

Figure 22
FOLLICULAR ADENOMA

Ultrastructurally, the tumor cells have a small number of mitochondria, abundant and somewhat dilated granular endoplasmic reticulum, scattered lysosomes, and intertwining microvilli. Parallel basal lamina belonging to the follicular epithelial cells and the adjacent endothelial cells from a blood vessel can also be appreciated. X15,925. (Courtesy of Dr. Robert Erlandson, Memorial Sloan-Kettering Cancer Center, New York, NY.)

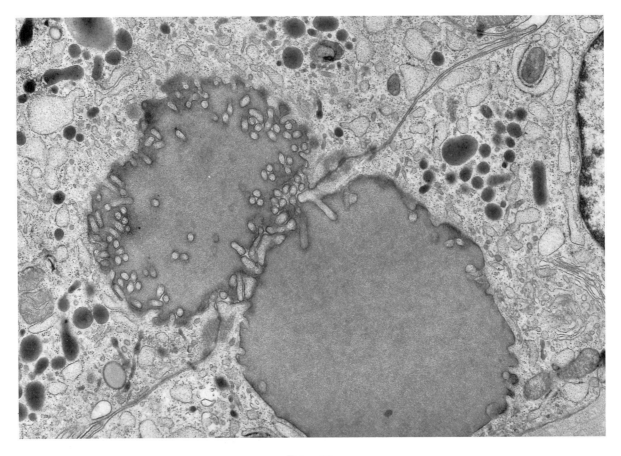

Figure 23
FOLLICULAR ADENOMA
This electron micrograph shows well-developed lumina into which microvilli project. Clusters of lysosomes are visible in the cytoplasm of the tumor cells, together with mitochondria, granular endoplasmic reticulum, and a well-developed Golgi apparatus. X16,625. (Courtesy of Dr. Robert Erlandson, Memorial Sloan-Kettering Cancer Center, New York, NY.)

adenomas than in follicular carcinomas, but that the difference was not significant. Therefore, they concluded that a high percentage of cells in S phase cannot be used as a diagnostic marker for malignancy in thyroid follicular lesions.

The *ras* oncogene p21 antigen has been found to be expressed in follicular adenomas at a level higher than normal thyroid but lower than carcinomas; however, the differences are not diagnostically helpful (23,28).

Differential Diagnosis. The differential diagnosis of follicular adenoma of conventional type includes a dominant hyperplastic nodule, minimally invasive follicular carcinoma (see page 59), and the encapsulated follicular variant of papillary carcinoma (see page 105).

On gross examination, a typical uncomplicated adenoma has a more homogeneous cut surface than nodular hyperplasia and lacks the internal lobulation of the latter. Microscopically, a diagnosis of adenoma should be favored over that of a dominant hyperplastic nodule if the lesion is single, completely encapsulated, leads to compression of the surrounding thyroid, and has a microscopic appearance that is uniform and substantially different from that of the rest of the gland. Statistically, most nodules with a trabecular, solid, or microfollicular pattern of growth are adenomas, whereas most of those with a normo- or macrofollicular pattern of growth are hyperplastic nodules, but exceptions occur in both directions. Features that favor a hyperplastic nodule are presence of inflammation, Sanderson polsters, and papillary projections within dilated follicles Most important, for a nodule to be recognized as hyperplastic, smaller nodules of similar appearance must be detected in the remainder of the gland. However, if the nodule fulfills all the criteria of an adenoma, it should be so designated, even if there is more than one and/or if the rest of the organ shows nodular hyperplastic changes. On some occasions, the distinction between nodular hyperplasia and neoplasia may be impossible, as is also the case in most other endocrine organs.

Cytologic Features. Cytologic specimens from follicular adenomas are cellular and have scanty or no colloid (figs. 24, 25). The cell arrangement is usually microfollicular or trabecular. Some of the aggregates have a syncytium-like configuration. The nuclei are uniformly increased in size, round to oval, with a coarsely granular chromatin that is evenly dispersed and generally uniform and inconspicuous nucleoli. An altered polarity may be noted. The cytoplasm is usually scanty and pale staining (26).

It is generally impossible to distinguish follicular adenomas from well-differentiated follicular carcinomas on the basis of cytologic examination (figs. 26, 27). Whether morphometric analysis will prove helpful in this distinction remains to be determined (8,35). Lesser differentiated follicular carcinomas should be suspected if there is marked nuclear enlargement with crowding and overlapping, a heterogeneous chromatin pattern with very coarse granules, and prominence of nucleoli (fig. 28) (26).

ADENOMA VARIANTS

Several more or less distinct varieties of follicular adenomas have been described, mainly on the basis of microscopic features. Although most of them carry no special clinical significance, their recognition is important to avoid confusion with lesions that have more ominous connotations. Two of these varieties, *oncocytic adenoma* (Hürthle cell adenoma) and *adenoma with clear cell change* (including signet-ring adenoma) are discussed in the chapters on Tumors with Oncocytic Features and Tumors with Clear Cell Features, respectively (see pages 161 and 183).

Adenoma with Bizarre Nuclei

In some adenomas, scattered bizarre nuclei are found that are characterized by huge size (≥10 times that of the adjacent cell), irregular shape, and striking hyperchromasia (figs. 29, 30) (54). These nuclei tend to occur in clusters. They are analogous to nuclei seen in many other endocrine tumors (such as parathyroid adenoma or paraganglioma) and should not be taken by themselves as a sign of malignancy. Actually, they occur more often in follicular adenomas than in carcinomas, as is the case in the parathyroid glands.

Hyalinizing Trabecular Adenoma

Hyalinizing trabecular adenoma is the name recently proposed by Carney and coworkers (48) for a distinctive type of thyroid neoplasm apparently first described by Ward and coworkers (69) as "hyaline cell tumor of the thyroid with massive accumulation of cytoplasmic filaments." Grossly, these tumors are yellow-tan and encapsulated, not significantly different from conventional adenomas. Microscopically, the main distinguishing features are the prominent hyaline appearance (both extracellular due to the perivascular deposition of collagen, and intracellular due to the accumulation of intermediate filaments) and the trabecular arrangement of the tumor cells. The trabecula can be straight or curved in the form of ribbons and festoons (fig. 31). Some of the tumor cells are inserted perpendicularly into the walls of small blood vessels. In other areas, the cells are arranged in compact clusters reminiscent of the "Zellballen" of paraganglioma, hence, the alternative designation of this adenoma variant as *paraganglioma-like* (fig. 32) (46). Follicular formation is minimal or absent; the few follicles present tend to be irregularly shaped and may feature papillary infoldings. The nuclei may be round, oval, or elongated, sometimes markedly. Some of them exhibit grooves, pseudoinclusions, and perinuclear vacuoles (fig. 33) (48). Chan and coworkers (49) have suggested that the latter feature is due to the presence of "nuclear rods," which represent aggregates of intranuclear filaments. Mitoses are usually absent. The cytoplasm can have acidophilic, amphophilic, or clear-staining qualities, and the cell borders are sharply outlined.

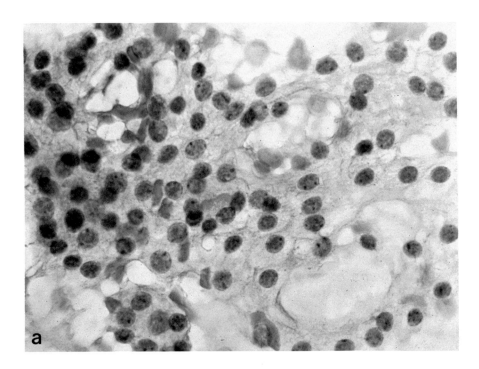

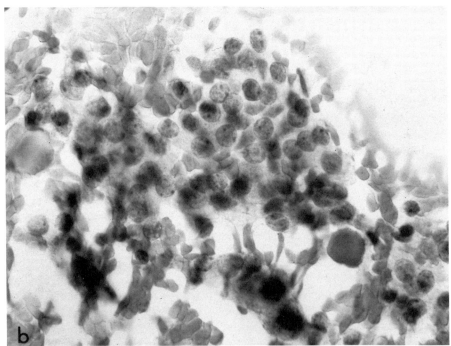

Figure 24
FOLLICULAR ADENOMA WITH MIXED CYTOLOGIC PATTERN
(FINE-NEEDLE ASPIRATION SPECIMEN)

This tumor (A) has regular follicles, solid sheets, and uniform but slightly enlarged nuclei with compact chromatin. Papanicolaou preparation. X497. Another figure from the same case (B) shows a syncytial-type tissue fragment with crowded, overlapped, uniformly enlarged nuclei. Papanicolaou preparation. X497. Whereas the pattern seen in A is also compatible with a nodular hyperplasia, that seen in B is more consistent with a follicular adenoma. (Fig. 6.7a and b from Kini SR. Thyroid. In: Kline TS, ed. Guides to clinical aspiration biopsy; Vol 3. New York: Igaku-Shoin, 1987.)

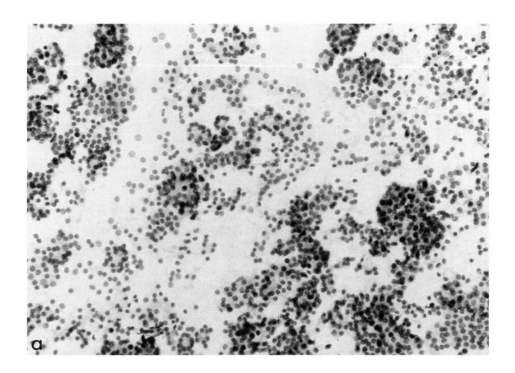

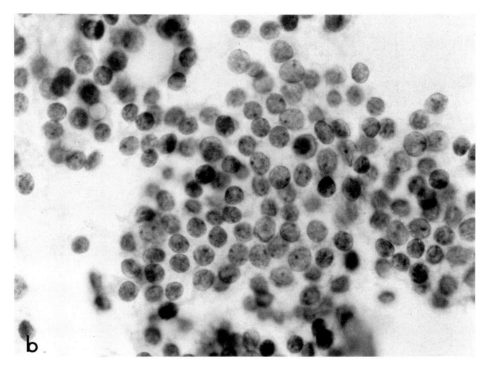

Figure 25
FOLLICULAR ADENOMA (FINE-NEEDLE ASPIRATION SPECIMEN)
Several syncytial-type fragments are seen exhibiting marked crowding and overlapping of uniformly but mildly enlarged nuclei (A). The pattern is microfollicular, and there is no colloid in the background. Papanicolaou preparation. X126. A higher magnification of A shows the follicular pattern of tissue fragments (B). Note the uniformly enlarged nuclei. Papanicolaou preparation. X497. (Fig. 6.9a and b from Kini SR. Thyroid. In: Kline TS, ed. Guides to clinical aspiration biopsy; Vol 3. New York: Igaku-Shoin, 1987.)

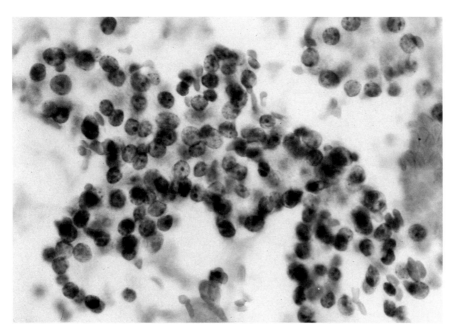

Figure 26
WELL-DIFFERENTIATED FOLLICULAR CARCINOMA
(FINE-NEEDLE ASPIRATION SPECIMEN)
The aspirate is cellular, with syncytial-type tissue fragments that show a microfollicular pattern. The nuclei are crowded and overlapped and have nucleoli. Papanicolaou preparation. X472. (Fig. 6.20 from Kini SR. Thyroid. In: Kline TS, ed. Guides to clinical aspiration biopsy; Vol 3. New York: Igaku-Shoin, 1987.)

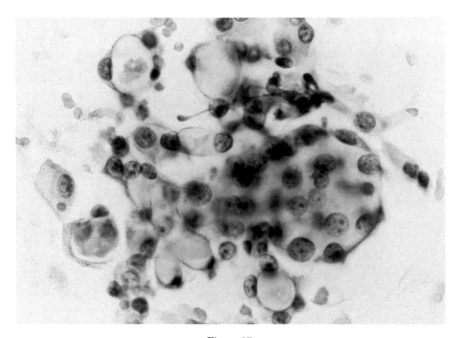

Figure 27
FOLLICULAR CARCINOMA (FINE-NEEDLE ASPIRATION SPECIMEN)
The follicles are markedly irregular. The nuclei are pleomorphic and contain nucleoli. Papanicolaou preparation. X472. (Fig. 6.22 from Kini SR. Thyroid. In: Kline TS, ed. Guides to clinical aspiration biopsy; Vol 3. New York: Igaku-Shoin, 1987.)

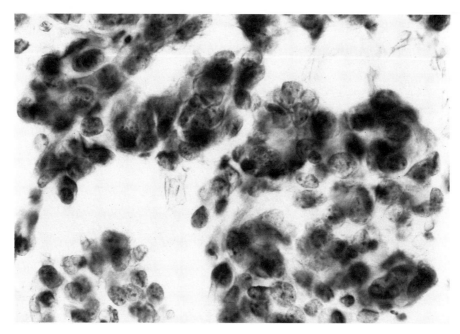

Figure 28
POORLY DIFFERENTIATED FOLLICULAR CARCINOMA
(FINE-NEEDLE ASPIRATION SPECIMEN)

The architectural pattern and nuclear morphology allow an accurate diagnosis of this tumor type. Papanicolaou preparation. X472. (Fig. 6.24 from Kini SR. Thyroid. In: Kline TS, ed. Guides to clinical aspiration biopsy; Vol 3. New York: Igaku-Shoin, 1987.)

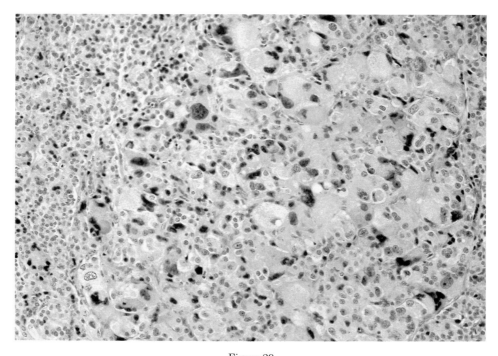

Figure 29
FOLLICULAR ADENOMA WITH BIZARRE NUCLEI

Clusters of cells with bizarre hyperchromatic nuclei are present in a tumor that was otherwise cellular but monomorphic.

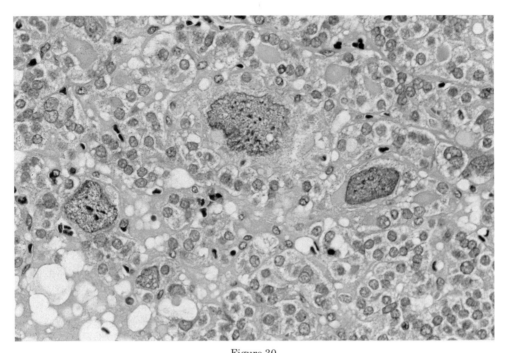

Figure 30
FOLLICULAR ADENOMA WITH BIZARRE NUCLEI
Huge, extremely irregular nuclei with an abnormal chromatin pattern are seen scattered in between smaller nuclei. This feature alone should not be regarded as indicative of malignancy.

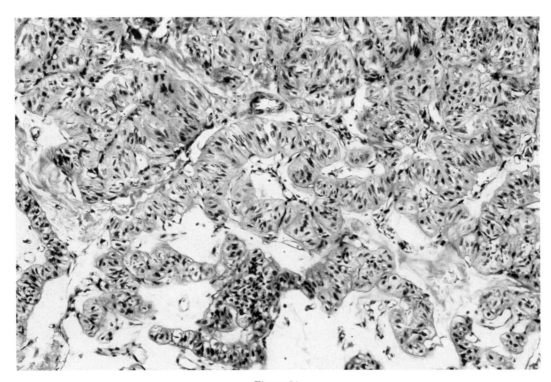

Figure 31
HYALINIZING TRABECULAR ADENOMA
Twisting trabeculae formed by elongated follicular cells are seen in a mildly sclerotic stroma.

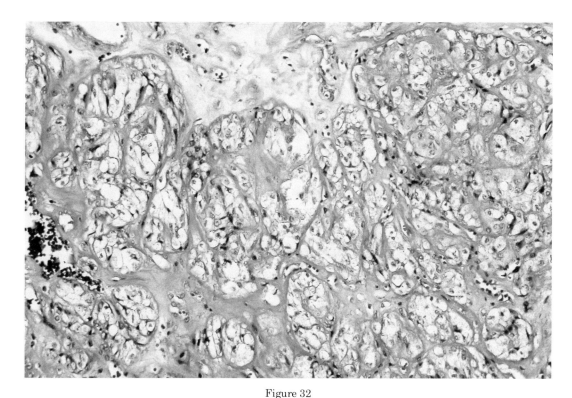

Figure 32
HYALINIZING TRABECULAR ADENOMA
The prominent nesting results in a "Zellballen" appearance that is similar to that seen in paraganglioma.
There is extensive fibrosis and hyalinization, both outside and within the tumor nests.

Hyalinizing trabecular adenoma shares several morphologic features with papillary carcinoma, such as the nuclear features described above and even the occasional occurrence of psammoma body-like formations (fig. 34) (48). We have also seen several examples of papillary carcinoma merging with hyalinizing trabecular adenoma; one of these tumors had metastasized to cervical lymph nodes, and the metastases had focally a hyalinizing trabecular adenoma-like pattern. It is also of interest that several of the reported cases of hyalinizing trabecular adenoma have occurred against a background of Hashimoto thyroiditis or in patients with a history of radiation to the neck, two common antecedents of papillar carcinoma (58). This combination of findings suggests to us that hyalinizing trabecular adenoma and papillary carcinoma are probably related to each other. However, and pending additional studies, it would seem appropriate to regard and treat hyalinizing trabecular adenoma as a benign neoplasm.

Immunohistochemically, the tumor cells are reactive for thyroglobulin and negative for calcitonin, in keeping with their presumed follicular origin (pl. III-A). However, some of these tumors have been found to exhibit argyrophilia and immunohistochemical reactivity for NSE, chromogranin A, neurotensin, and β-endorphin. These findings raise the possibility of a dual follicular and neuroendocrine differentiation (58,62,63). The homogeneous eosinophilic material seen in the stroma in H&E sections reacts immunohistochemically for laminin and type IV collagen, indicating basement membrane accumulation (62). Ultrastructurally, the main features are packing by intermediate filaments of the cytoplasm of the tumor cells and abundance of extracellular basal lamina material (63).

On fine-needle examination, hyalinizing trabecular adenoma resembles papillary carcinoma in many of its cytologic features. The sample is usually hypercellular, with poor cohesion. The cells are oval or spindled and tend to be arranged in parallel arrays with associated hyaline acellular areas (52). All but one of the reported cases of this entity have behaved in a benign fashion, and lobectomy is the preferred therapy (48,62).

Adenolipoma and Adenochondroma

Adenolipoma is the term used for the exceptionally rare type of follicular adenoma in which the neoplastic follicles are separated by islands of mature adipose tissue (fig. 35) (50,56,65). However, the lesion is probably not a mixed tumor with epithelial and mesenchymal components, as the name implies, but rather a follicular adenoma in which the stroma has undergone adipose metaplasia, in a way similar to that seen more frequently in the normal gland, nodular hyperplasia, and papillary carcinoma (51). In one reported case, the adipose tissue within the adenoma had foci of extramedullary hematopoiesis (64).

Adenochondroma has a mixed-tumor appearance analogous to that of adenolipoma, but one in which the stromal component is made up of lobules of mature cartilaginous tissue (pl. III-B; fig. 36) (68,70). The epithelial and cartilaginous components were sharply demarcated in both of the reported cases.

Atypical Adenoma

Hazard and Kenyon (54) proposed the term atypical adenoma for follicular adenomas, having a gross or microscopic appearance which departed from the norm. Specifically, they included in this category (which comprised 2.3 percent of their cases) those adenomas characterized by: 1) closely packed follicles, often lacking lumina; 2) solid columns, often with little intervening stroma; and 3) sheet-like or diffusely cellular masses (fig. 37). In their article, they also illustrated cases in which the tumor cells had spindle-shaped nuclei (figs. 38, 39). Grossly, atypical adenomas are said to be more fleshy and more solid than the usual adenoma. The concept of atypical adenoma thus defined is too broad and imprecise; it merges with the trabecular/solid and microfollicular subtypes of follicular adenoma and perhaps even with the hyalinizing trabecular variety. The WHO Committee describes as atypical those adenomas in which "cellular proliferation is more pronounced and

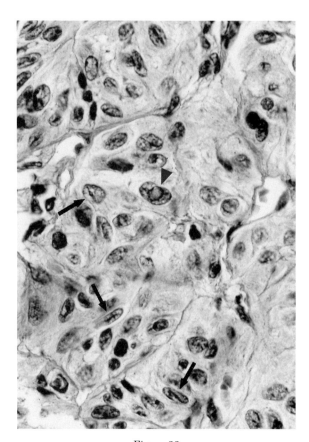

Figure 33
HYALINIZING TRABECULAR ADENOMA
Some of the nuclei in this field contain grooves (arrows) and others feature intranuclear pseudoinclusions (arrowhead).

the architectural and cytological patterns are less regular," thus perpetuating the vague and imprecise connotations of the term (55). As a result, *atypical adenoma* has become for too many pathologists, a wastebasket term in which any adenoma that looks peculiar or worrisome, even for reasons such as spontaneous necrosis or undue mitotic activity, is included. Because hypercellularity seems the most important criterion that authors have used to place a thyroid adenoma into an atypical category (54,59), it would seem better to designate these lesions *hypercellular adenomas* and to delete the term atypical adenoma altogether. In any event, the more "atypical" or cellular an adenoma (regardless of the terminology used), the more important it is to examine it carefully to rule out capsular or vascular invasion.

PLATE III

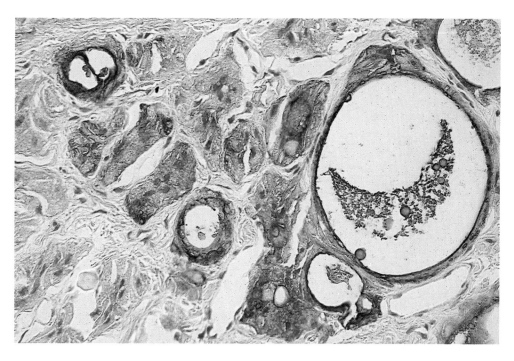

A. HYALINIZING TRABECULAR ADENOMA
Intraluminal and cytoplasmic thyroglobulin positivity is evident.

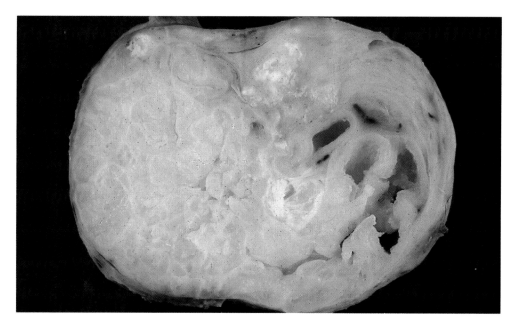

B. FOLLICULAR ADENOMA WITH EXTENSIVE CARTILAGINOUS
METAPLASIA ("ADENOCHONDROMA")
The lobular configuration and shiny white appearance of the cartilaginous element in
this tumor is evident. (Courtesy of Dr. Maurizio Pea, Vicenza, Italy.)

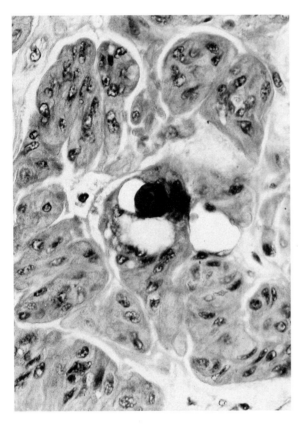

Figure 34
HYALINIZING TRABECULAR ADENOMA
A well-formed psammoma body is seen in the center of the field.

Adenoma with Papillary Hyperplasia

On occasion, otherwise typical follicular adenomas exhibit papillary or pseudopapillary structures that can be confused with those of papillary carcinoma (figs. 35, 40). Most of these adenomas are composed of normal-sized (normofollicular) or large (macrofollicular) follicles. It is characteristic for the papillary formations to be short and blunt and nonbranching and to face the lumina of cystically dilated follicles. A central fibrovascular core is poorly developed or absent. Instead, the stroma is likely to be edematous and to enclose numerous follicles. More important, the follicular cells lining these structures are tall cuboidal or columnar, with basally located nuclei that tend to be perfectly round and normo- or hyperchromatic, i.e., substantially different from those typically seen in papillary carcinoma

(fig. 41) (60). Immunohistochemically, staining for keratin in formalin-fixed, paraffin-embedded material is usually patchy and limited to the low–molecular-weight forms of this marker, in contrast to the diffuse and intense staining usually seen in papillary carcinoma (45).

These papillary structures in adenoma are equivalent in all regards to those seen with higher frequency in hyperplastic nodules and, as in the latter, are probably an expression of localized hyperactivity. Indeed, some of the adenomas featuring these structures are hyperfunctioning ("toxic") (67). The use of the term *papillary adenoma* for these lesions is objectionable on several grounds (67). Many of the formations in question do not qualify morphologically as true papillae. More important, the term papillary adenoma has also been used in the past for an encapsulated papillary lesion with all of the features of papillary carcinoma, including characteristic nuclear changes and psammoma bodies. We regard such lesions as encapsulated papillary carcinomas and therefore exclude them from any category of follicular adenoma (see page 100). It is therefore preferable to designate the type of adenoma described in this section as *adenoma with papillary hyperplasia* (60), as we have done, or as *hyperplastic papillary adenoma* (67).

"Toxic" Adenoma

This lesion, also known as hyperfunctioning adenoma or Plummer adenoma, is a follicular adenoma accompanied by clinical evidence of thyroid hyperfunction, usually of a mild degree. Naturally, such a lesion will appear "hot" on a scintigram. However, the term *toxic* should not be applied to all "hot" adenomas but only to those in which clinical manifestations occur. Thus defined, "toxic" adenoma is a rarity (only ~1 percent of all adenomas) and a clinical rather than pathologic entity. In many clinical papers on "toxic" adenoma, no attempt is made to distinguish the true adenomas from the substantially more frequent hyperplastic nodules on pathologic grounds (57). However, several microscopic correlates of clinically hyperfunctioning thyroid adenomas exist. Such an adenoma is likely to be micro- or normo-follicular and to contain pseudopapillary formations of the type described on page 230 (fig. 42). The lining cells tend to be tall cuboidal

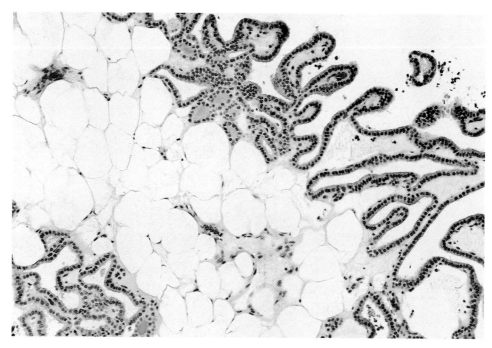

Figure 35
FOLLICULAR ADENOMA WITH PAPILLARY HYPERPLASIA
AND ADIPOSE METAPLASIA OF THE STROMA
Mature adipose tissue is sometimes also found in the stroma of normal glands, follicular adenoma, and papillary carcinoma.

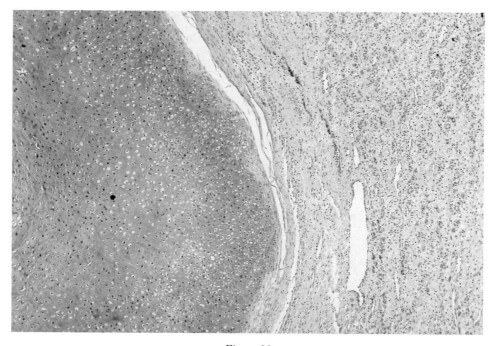

Figure 36
FOLLICULAR ADENOMA WITH CARTILAGINOUS METAPLASIA (ADENOCHONDROMA)
A well-demarcated island of hyaline cartilage is seen adjacent to an epithelial component showing a microfollicular pattern of growth. (Courtesy of Dr. Maurizio Pea, Vicenza, Italy.)

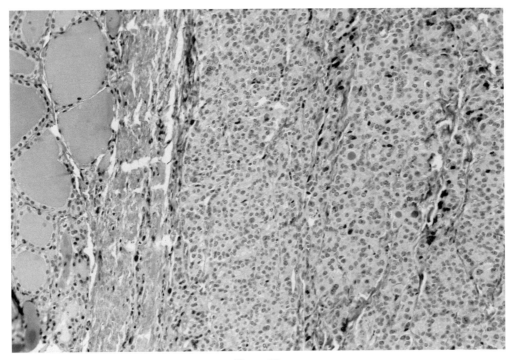

Figure 37
ATYPICAL ADENOMA
This tumor is markedly cellular, the pattern of growth is irregular, and there is mild to moderate pleomorphism. There was no capsular or blood vessel invasion.

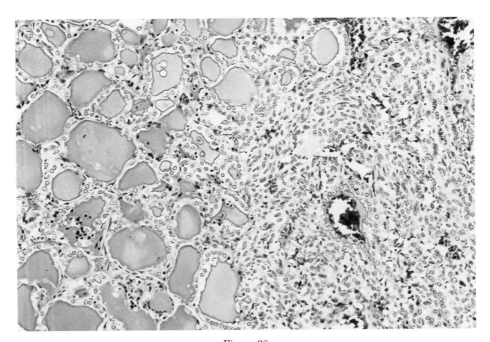

Figure 38
ATYPICAL ADENOMA WITH SPINDLE CELL FEATURES
Well-formed follicles lined by cuboidal cells merge with a solid pattern composed of cells that are oval to spindle shaped with a mesenchymal-like appearance.

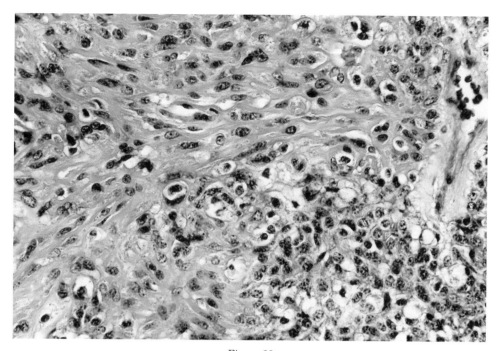

Figure 39
ATYPICAL ADENOMA WITH SPINDLE CELL FEATURES
This high magnification shows an admixture of round cells with clear cytoplasm with others that have a spindled configuration and a mesenchymal-like appearance. There was immunohistochemical positivity for keratin in both cell types.

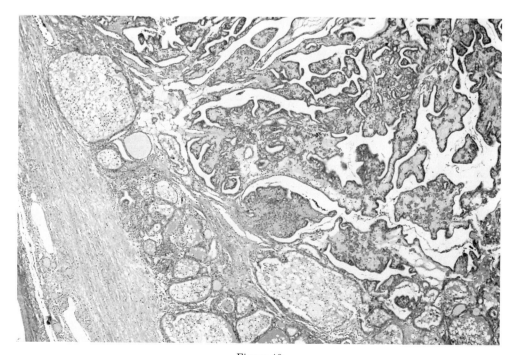

Figure 40
FOLLICULAR ADENOMA WITH PAPILLARY HYPERPLASIA
The papillary formations converge toward the center of the nodule; i.e., they have a centripetal quality.

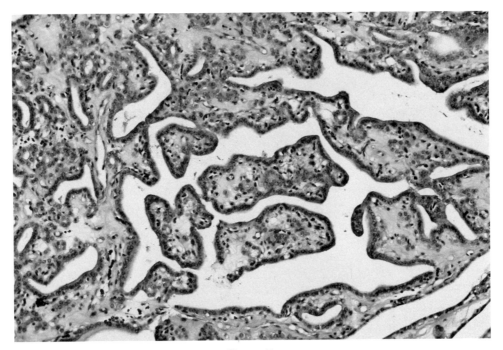

Figure 41
FOLLICULAR ADENOMA WITH PAPILLARY HYPERPLASIA
The lining cells are cuboidal to low columnar, and the nuclei lack the features of those of papillary carcinoma.

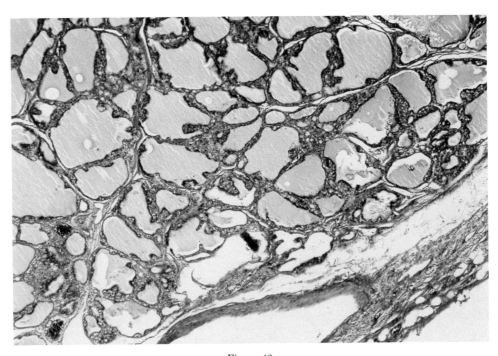

Figure 42
"TOXIC" ADENOMA
This lesion is single and encapsulated. It is formed by irregularly shaped follicles, some of which have small papillary projections within the lumina. The cytoarchitectural features in the individual follicles are indistinguishable from those of a hyperplastic process.

rather than flattened, and the nuclear/cytoplasmic ratio is likely to be decreased due to cytoplasmic prominence (47,53). At the ultrastructural level, the features are those of a very actively secreting follicular cell and comparable to those seen in diffuse hyperplasia (Graves disease) (61). This includes a prominent rough endoplasmic reticulum, well-developed Golgi apparatus, numerous lysosomes, and innumerable slender apical microvilli and pseudopods (66).

Treatment. The standard therapy for follicular adenoma (whether conventional or one of the variants) is surgical removal in the form of lobectomy. Enucleation of the adenoma (nodulectomy) should not be attempted, because if the final diagnosis is that of a minimally invasive follicular or papillary carcinoma, the operation will have been inadequate. The lobectomy is often accompanied by an isthmusectomy for aesthetic reasons, and sometimes a subtotal thyroidectomy is carried out. A total or near-total thyroidectomy is unnecessary for this lesion.

Suppression of the adenoma with L-thyroxine and treatment of the toxic adenoma with ^{131}I have been employed, but in general, the results have been disappointing (11,12).

REFERENCES

Follicular Adenoma

1. Barresi G, Tuccari G. Iron-binding proteins in thyroid tumours. An immunocytochemical study. Pathol Res Pract 1987;182:344–51.
2. Belfiore A, Sava L, Runello F, Tomaselli L, Vigneri R. Solitary autonomously functioning thyroid nodules and iodine deficiency. J Clin Endocrinol Metab 1983;56:283–7.
3. Bisi H, Fernandes VS, Asato de Camargo RY, Koch L, Abdo AH, de Brito T. The prevalence of unsuspected thyroid pathology in 300 sequential autopsies, with special reference to the incidental carcinoma. Cancer 1989;64:1888–93.
4. Bondeson L, Bengtsson A, Bondeson A-G, et al. Chromosome studies in thyroid neoplasia. Cancer 1989;64:680–5.
5. Brownstein MH, Wolf M, Bikowski JB. Cowden's disease: a cutaneous marker of breast cancer. Cancer 1978;41:2393–8.
6. Buley ID, Gatter KC, Heryet A, Mason DY. Expression of intermediate filament proteins in normal and diseased thyroid glands. J Clin Pathol 1987;40:136–42.
7. Cohen MB, Miller TR, Beckstead JH. Enzyme histochemistry and thyroid neoplasia. Am J Clin Pathol 1986;85:668–73.
8. Crissman JD, Kini SR. FNA diagnosis of follicular neoplasms of the thyroid: a morphometric analysis [Abstract]. Lab Invest 1991;64:31A.
9. Davila RM, Bedrossian WM, Silverberg AB. Immunocytochemistry of the thyroid in surgical and cytologic specimens. Arch Pathol Lab Med 1988;112:51–6.
10. Evans HL. Follicular neoplasms of the thyroid. A study of 44 cases followed for a minimum of 10 years, with emphasis on differential diagnosis. Cancer 1984;54:535–40.
10a. Ghali VS, Jimenez EJS, Garcia RL. Distribution of Leu-7 antigen (HNK-1) in thyroid tumors: Its usefulness as a diagnostic marker for follicular and papillary carcinomas. Hum Pathol 1992;23:21-25.
11. Gharib H, James EM, Charboneau JW, Naessens JM, Offord KP, Gorman CA. Suppressive therapy with levothyroxine for solitary thyroid nodules. A double-blind controlled clinical study. N Engl J Med 1987;317:70–5.
12. Goldstein R, Hart IR. Follow-up of solitary autonomous thyroid nodules treated with ^{131}I. N Engl J Med 1983;309:1473–6
13. González-Cámpora R, Sanchez Gallego F, Martin Lacave I, Mora Marin J, Montero Linares C, Galera-Davidson H. Lectin histochemistry of the thyroid gland. Cancer 1988;62:2354–62.
14. Greenebaum E, Koss LG, Elequin F, Silver CE. The diagnostic value of flow cytometric DNA measurements in follicular tumors of the thyroid gland. Cancer 1985;56:2011–8.
15. Hazard JB. Nomenclature of thyroid tumors. In: Inman DR, Young S, eds. Thyroid neoplasia; proceedings of the 2nd Imperial Cancer Research Fund symposium held in London in April, 1967. London: Academic Press, 1968.
16. _____, Kenyon R. Atypical adenoma of the thyroid. Arch Pathol 1954;58:554–63.
17. Hicks DG, LiVolsi VA, Neidich JA, Puck JM, Kant JA. Clonal analysis of solitary follicular nodules in the thyroid. Am J Pathol 1990;137:553–62.
18. Hostetter AL, Hrafnkelsson J, Wingren SO, Enestrom S, Nordenskjöld B. A comparative study of DNA cytometry methods for benign and malignant thyroid tissue. Am J Clin Pathol 1988;89:760–3.
19. Hruban RH, Huvos AG, Traganos F, Reuter V, Leiberman PH, Melamed MR. Follicular neoplasms of the thyroid in men older than 50 years of age. A DNA flow cytometric study. Am J Clin Pathol 1990;94:527–32.
20. Jenkins RB, Hay ID, Herath JF, et al. Frequent occurrence of cytogenetic abnormalities in sporadic nonmedullary thyroid carcinoma. Cancer 1990;66:1213–20.

21. Joensuu H, Klemi P, Eerola E. DNA aneuploidy in follicular adenomas of the thyroid gland. Am J Pathol 1986;124:373–6.

22. Johannessen JV, Sobrinho-Simões M. Well differentiated thyroid tumors. Problems in diagnosis and understanding. Pathol Annu 1983;18(Pt. 1):255–85.

23. Johnson TL, Lloyd RV, Thor A. Expression of *ras* oncogene p21 antigen in normal and proliferative thyroid tissues. Am J Pathol 1987;127:60–5.

24. Kawaoi A, Okano T, Nemoto N, Shikata T. Production of thyroxine (T_4) and triiodothyronine (T_3) in nontoxic thyroid tumors. An immunohistochemical study. Virchows Arch [A] 1981;390:249–57.

25. Kendall CH, Sanderson PR, Cope J, Talbot IC. Follicular thyroid tumours: a study of laminin and type IV collagen in basement membrane and endothelium. J Clin Pathol 1985;38:1100–5.

26. Kini SR. Thyroid. In: Kline TS, ed. Guides to clinical aspiration biopsy; Vol 3. New York: Igaku-Shoin, 1987: 57–95.

27. Miettinen M, Virtanen I. Expression of laminin in thyroid gland and thyroid tumors: an immunohistologic study. Int J Cancer 1984;34:27–30.

28. Mizukami Y, Nonomura A, Hashimoto T, et al. Immunohistochemical demonstration of *ras* p21 oncogene product in normal, benign, and malignant human thyroid tissues. Cancer 1988;61:873–80.

29. Nakayama I, Noguchi S, Yamashita H, et al. Immunoelectron microscopic localization of thyroglobulin in human follicular adenoma. Acta Pathol Jpn 1983;33:1139–50.

30. Namba H, Matsuo K, Fagin JA. Clonal composition of benign and malignant human thyroid tumors. J Clin Invest 1990;86:120–5.

31. Nartey N, Cherian MG, Banerjee D. Immunohistochemical localization of metallothionein in human thyroid tumors. Am J Pathol 1987;129:177–82.

32. Risberg B, Eneström S, Lennquist S, Bergman C. Evaluation of thyroid scintigraphic lesions by whole-organ sections and autoradiography. Acta Pathol Microbiol Immunol Scand [A] 1982;90:19–26.

33. Sasano H, Rojas M, Silverberg SG. Analysis of lectin binding in benign and malignant thyroid nodules. Arch Pathol Lab Med 1989;113:186–9.

34. Schelfhout LJ, Van Muijen GN, Fleuren GJ. Expression of keratin 19 distinguishes papillary thyroid carcinoma from follicular carcinomas and follicular thyroid adenoma. Am J Clin Pathol 1989;92:654–8.

35. Schürman G, Mattfeldt T, Feichter G, Koretz K, Möller P, Buhr H. Stereology, flow cytometry, and immunohistochemistry of follicular neoplasms of the thyroid gland. Hum Pathol 1991;22;179–84.

36. Shlossberg AH, Jacobson JC, Ibbertson HK. Serum thyroglobulin in the diagnosis and management of thyroid carcinoma. Clin Endocrinol (Oxf) 1979;10:17–27.

37. Silverberg SG, Vidone RA. Adenoma and carcinoma of the thyroid. Cancer 1966;19:1053–62.

38. Sobrinho-Simões M, Nesland JM, Johannessen JV. Ultrastructural features of neoplastic lesions of the thyroid gland. In: Russo J, Sommers SC, eds. Tumor diagnosis by electron microscopy. New York: Field, Rich, and Associates, 1989:53–92.

39. Thomas GA, Williams D, Williams ED. The clonal origin of thyroid nodules and adenomas. Am J Pathol 1989;134:141–7.

40. Tuccari G, Barresi G. Immunohistochemical demonstration of ceruloplasmin in follicular adenomas and thyroid carcinomas. Histopathology 1987;11:723–31.

41. _____, Barresi G. Tissue polypeptide antigen in thyroid tumours of follicular cell origin: an immunohistochemical re-evaluation for diagnostic purposes. Histopathology 1990;16:377–81.

42. van den Berg E, Oosterhuis JW, de Jong B, et al. Cytogenetics of thyroid follicular adenomas. Cancer Genet Cytogenet 1990;44:217–22.

43. Viale G, Dell'Orto P, Coggi G, Gambacorta M. Coexpression of cytokeratins and vimentin in normal and diseased thyroid glands. Lack of diagnostic utility of vimentin immunostaining. Am J Surg Pathol 1989;13: 1034–40.

44. Vierbuchen M, Schröder S, Uhlenbruck G, Ortmann M, Fischer R. CA 50 and CA 19-9 antigen expression in normal, hyperplastic, and neoplastic thyroid tissue. Lab Invest 1989;60:726–32.

Adenoma Variants

45. Bennett WP, Bhan AK, Vickery AL Jr. Keratin expression as a diagnostic adjunct in thyroid tumors with papillary architecture [Abstract]. Lab Invest 1988;58:9A.

46. Bronner MP, LiVolsi VA, Jennings TA. Plat: paraganglioma-like adenomas of the thyroid. Surg Pathol 1988;1:383–9.

47. Campbell WL, Santiago HE, Perzin KH, Johnson PM. The autonomous thyroid nodule: correlation of scan appearance and histopathology. Radiology 1973;107:133–8.

48. Carney JA, Ryan J, Goellner JR. Hyalinizing trabecular adenoma of the thyroid gland. Am J Surg Pathol 1987;11:583–91.

49. Chan JK, Tse CC, Chiu HS. Hyalinizing trabecular adenoma-like lesion in multinodular goitre. Histopathology 1990;16:611–14.

50. DeRienzo D, Truong L. Thyroid neoplasms containing mature fat: a report of two cases and review of the literature. Mod Pathol 1989;2:506–10.

51. Gnepp DR, Ogorzalek JM, Heffess CS. Fat-containing lesions of the thyroid gland. Am J Surg Pathol 1989;13:605–12.

52. Goellner JR, Carney JA. Cytologic features of fine-needle aspirates of hyalinizing trabecular adenoma of the thyroid. Am J Clin Pathol 1989;91:115–9.

53. Hamburger JI. Solitary autonomously functioning thyroid lesions. Diagnosis, clinical features and pathogenetic considerations. Am J Med 1975;58:740–8.

54. Hazard JB, Kenyon R. Atypical adenoma of the thyroid. Arch Pathol 1954;58:554–63.

55. Hedinger CE, Williams ED, Sobin LH. Histological typing of thyroid tumours. In: Hediger CE, ed. International histological classification of tumours, Vol 11. 2nd ed. Berlin: Springer-Verlag, 1988.

56. Hjorth L, Thomsen LB, Nielsen VT. Adenolipoma of the thyroid gland. Histopathology 1986;10:91–6.

57. Horst W, Rösler H, Schneider C, Labhart A. 306 cases of toxic adenoma: clinical aspects, findings in radioiodine diagnostics, radiochromatography and histology; results of 131I and surgical treatment. J Nucl Med 1967;8:515–28.

58. Katoh R, Jasani B, Williams ED. Hyalinizing trabecular adenoma of the thyroid. A report of three cases with immunohistochemical and ultrastructural studies. Histopathology 1989;15:211–24.

59. Lang W, Georgii A, Stauch G, Kienzle E. The differentiation of atypical adenomas and encapsulated follicular carcinomas in the thyroid gland. Virchows Arch [A] 1980;385:125–41.

60. LiVolsi VA. Surgical pathology of the thyroid. In: Bennington JL ed. Major problems in pathology; Vol 22. Philadelphia: WB Saunders, 1990.

61. Panke TW, Croxson MS, Parker JW, Carriere DP, Rosoff L Sr, Warner NE. Triiodothyronine-secreting (toxic) adenoma of the thyroid gland: light and electron microscopic characteristics. Cancer 1978;41:528–37.

62. Sambade C, Franssila K, Cameselle-Teijeiro J, Nesland J, Sobrinho-Simões M. Hyalinizing trabecular adenoma: a misnomer for a peculiar tumor of the thyroid gland. Endocr Pathol 1991;2:83–91.

63. _____, Sarabando F, Nesland JM, Sobrinho-Simões M. Hyalinizing trabecular adenoma of the thyroid (case of the Ullensvag course). Hyalinizing spindle cell tumor of the thyroid with dual differentiation (variant of the so-called hyalinizing trabecular adenoma). Ultrastruct Pathol 1989;13:275–80.

64. Schmid C, Beham A, Seewann HL. Extramedullary haematopoiesis in the thyroid gland. Histopathology 1989;15:423–5.

65. Schröder S, Böcker W, Hüsselmann H, Dralle H. Adenolipoma (thyrolipoma) of the thyroid gland. Virchows Arch [A] 1984;404:99–103.

66. Sobrinho-Simões M, Nesland JM, Johannessen JV. Ultrastructural features of neoplastic lesions of the thyroid gland. In: Russo J, Sommers SC, eds. Tumor diagnosis by electron microscopy. New York: Field, Rich, and Associates, 1989:53-92.

67. Vickery AL Jr. Thyroid papillary carcinoma. Pathological and philosophical controversies. Am J Surg Pathol 1983;7:797–807.

68. Visoña A, Pea M, Bozzola L, Stracca-Pansa V, Meli S. Follicular adenoma of the thyroid gland with extensive chondroid metaplasia. Histopathology 1991;18:278–9.

69. Ward JV, Murray D, Horvath E, Kovacs K, Baumal R. Hyaline cell tumor of the thyroid with massive accumulation of cytoplasmic microfilaments [Abstract]. Lab Invest 1982;46:88A.

70. Wolvos TA, Chong FK, Razvi SA, Tully GL III. An unusual thyroid tumor: a comparison to a literature review of thyroid teratomas. Surgery 1985;97:613–7.

❖❖❖

FOLLICULAR CARCINOMA

Definition. A malignant epithelial tumor showing evidence of follicular cell differentiation and not belonging to any of the other distinctive types of thyroid malignancy.

General Considerations. Generically, any malignant thyroid tumor with features of follicular cell differentiation (and, specifically, making follicles) could be regarded as follicular carcinoma. The difficulty with this approach is that it results in lumping into one category tumor types that vary considerably in their morphologic appearance and, more important, natural history. It would thus obscure the important differences that exist among them and could result in inappropriate therapeutic and prognostic determinations. Tumors that have enough distinctive features to be excluded from the category of follicular carcinoma "not otherwise specified" and that are therefore discussed in other sections of this Fascicle include the following entities:

- *Follicular variant of papillary carcinoma.* This tumor belongs to the papillary family of neoplasms despite its predominantly or exclusively follicular configuration (see page 100).
- *Follicular carcinoma, oncocytic type.* Most oncocytic thyroid tumors have follicular features, although they are often admixed with trabecular and/or solid areas. We believe that these lesions differ enough from other follicular tumors to justify considering them separately (see page 173).
- *Poorly differentiated "insular" carcinoma.* Most of these tumors probably represent poorly differentiated types of follicular carcinoma; however, others with a similar appearance have been found to have a close link with papillary carcinoma. Because of these histogenetic considerations and the unfavorable prognostic connotations associated with this pattern, we prefer to place it in a category of its own (see page 123).

General Features. In series originating from non–iodine-deficient areas, the frequency of follicular carcinoma among thyroid malignancies has ranged from 5 to 15 percent (3,9,10). Unfortunately, not much weight can be given to these figures considering the lack of consistency with which the term follicular carcinoma is used. In any event, it seems established that, in iodine-deficient areas, the relative incidence of this tumor type is increased, reaching up to 30 to 40 percent of all thyroid cancers (3,9,10). Interestingly, iodide addition to the diet results in a relative increase in papillary carcinoma and a corresponding decrease in follicular carcinoma (4,5,9).

Whether thyroid nodular hyperplasia not related to iodine deficiency is associated with a higher incidence of follicular carcinoma remains a controversial issue. If there is indeed an increased incidence, it seems to be of such a minimal nature that it becomes insignificant from a therapeutic standpoint.

Even more controversial is the alleged relationship between follicular carcinoma and dyshormonogenetic goiter. Here the difficulty is compounded by the fact that, in this group of diseases, the gland may acquire multinodular, hypercellular, atypical, and pseudoinvasive features (see page 302) (8). Therefore, some writers would not accept a diagnosis of follicular carcinoma arising in a dyshormonogenetic gland unless the tumor had metastasized. We think that this is an unreasonably restrictive approach. We believe that the criteria for malignancy should be the same regardless of whether the gland is the site of this genetically determined abnormality or not. In any event, enough metastasizing thyroid carcinomas arising under these circumstances are now on record to indicate that their frequency may indeed be increased (2,8).

Clinical Features. Follicular carcinoma is more prevalent in women; the average age of occurrence is 10 years older than for papillary carcinoma (6). It typically presents as a solitary thyroid nodule that is nearly always "cold" on scintigraphic examination and unaccompanied by cervical adenopathy. It is exceptionally rare for follicular carcinoma to result in clinically evident signs of hyperthyroidism, but several well-documented cases are on record (7). Occasionally, distant metastases (particularly to the bone) are the first manifestations of the disease. In contrast to papillary carcinoma, it is unusual for follicular carcinoma to be clinically occult (1).

Classification. Once the special types of carcinoma listed on page 49 have been eliminated, there remains a relatively homogeneous form of thyroid malignancy to which the term *follicular carcinoma* is well suited. Still, from a morphologic and prognostic standpoint, this tumor can be divided into two major categories on the basis of the degree of invasiveness: 1) minimally invasive or encapsulated and 2) widely invasive. Oddly, there is little overlap between these two widely disparate types, of which the former is by far the most common.

MINIMALLY INVASIVE (ENCAPSULATED) TYPE

Gross Features. The gross appearance of this tumor does not differ appreciably from that of a follicular adenoma. It is generally round and of variable size (although almost always >1 cm in diameter) and is light-tan to brown with a solid, bulging cut surface (pl. IV-A). Secondary hemorrhagic, cystic, and fibrotic changes occur as frequently as in adenomas (pl. IV-B). The capsule that surrounds the tumor tends to be thicker and more irregular than in adenomas (pl. IV-C) (16). It is unusual for capsular or blood vessel invasion to be identifiable on gross examination.

Microscopic Features. The cytoarchitectural features of minimally invasive follicular carcinoma resemble those of its benign counterpart. However, the carcinomas have a greater representation of hypercellular forms (corresponding to the embryonal, fetal, and atypical form of the adenoma), and few exhibit a normofollicular or macrofollicular (colloid) appearance. Therefore, the index of suspicion should be raised whenever encountering a follicular neoplasm with a solid, trabecular, microfollicular, or atypical pattern of growth (figs. 43, 44) (17,21,27). This is also the case when mitotic figures are easily encountered and/or the nuclei are large and have conspicuous nucleoli (fig. 45) (29). The fact still remains that, in this tumor type, the diagnosis of malignancy depends primarily on the demonstration of unequivocal capsular and/or vascular invasion. Because of the crucial significance of these two features, a detailed description is in order.

Capsular invasion. A tumor must penetrate the entire thickness of the capsule to be regarded as having unequivocal capsular invasion (figs. 46, 47). Irregularities of contour along the inner border or clusters of follicular cells embedded within the capsule are not sufficient (fig. 48). A more serious interpretive problem is created by the presence of a small nodule of tumor cells lying immediately outside an intact capsule. Two possible explanations for this phenomenon are invasion of the capsule not apparent at that particular level (which would imply the diagnosis of carcinoma) and occurrence of an independent follicular nodule adjacent to the larger one (which would not). Irregular outlines and similarity of cytoarchitectural features favor the former interpretation, which could be explained as a narrow focus of capsular invasion with a more expansile (mushroom-like) extracapsular component. The opposite features, together with the presence of additional similar nodules in the remaining thyroid, would be more in keeping with the latter interpretation. In any event, demonstration of a capsular break through serial sectioning or submission of additional material is necessary before labeling the tumor as malignant. It should be kept in mind that when a follicular carcinoma invades into and through the capsule, it usually does not permeate the surrounding parenchyma; instead, a new fibrous capsule is formed at the leading edge (figs. 46, 50). When the expansile extracapsular component becomes very large but is covered by this newly formed capsule, the tumor may resemble a dumbbell or may appear as an irregular nodule partially divided in two by an apparent septum.

As already mentioned in the section on Gross Features, the fibrous capsule tends to be thicker and more irregular in carcinomas than in adenomas (figs. 49, 50) (16,40). This seemingly paradoxical finding could perhaps be explained by viewing the capsule of an adenoma as the result of the condensation of preexistent stromal fibers by the expanding mass and the carcinoma having, in addition, a component of newly laid down collagen fibers as an expression of host response to the malignancy.

Vascular invasion. As the WHO Committee stated (23), vascular invasion is a much more reliable sign of malignancy than capsular invasion. The criteria for its recognition, therefore, need to

PLATE IV

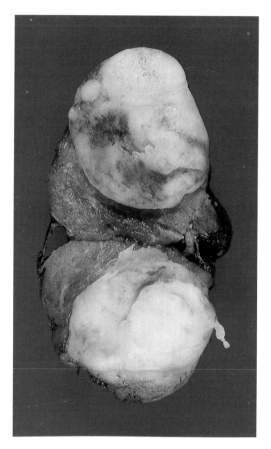

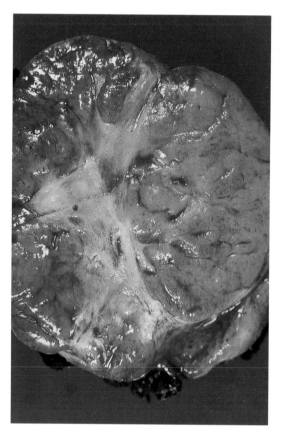

A. FOLLICULAR CARCINOMA

The tumor is encapsulated, has a relatively homogeneous light-tan appearance, and contains small foci of hemorrhage. The features are indistinguishable from those of a cellular follicular adenoma.

B. MINIMALLY INVASIVE FOLLICULAR CARCINOMA

The tumor has a fleshy appearance and an irregularly shaped central scar.

C. MINIMALLY INVASIVE FOLLICULAR CARCINOMA

It is common for this type of tumor to have a capsule that is thicker and more irregular than that of adenomas, as shown in this case. This particular tumor metastasized to the iliac bone.

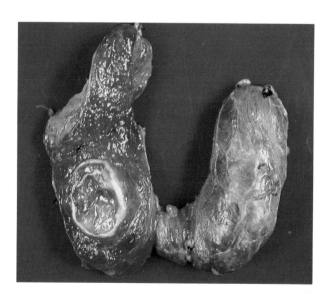

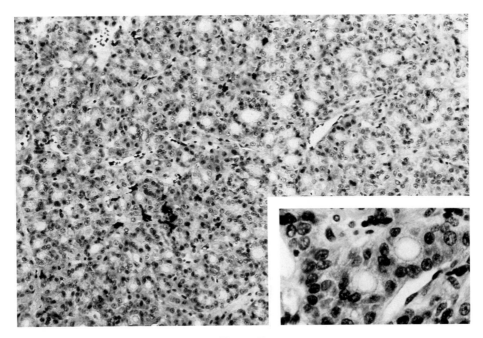

Figure 43
FOLLICULAR CARCINOMA
The tumor is composed of small, closely packed follicles. The inset highlights the hyperchromatic nuclear features and nucleolar prominence of the tumor cells. This tumor exhibited both capsular and blood vessel invasion.

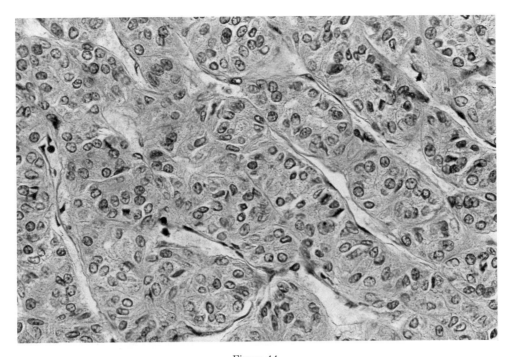

Figure 44
FOLLICULAR CARCINOMA WITH TRABECULAR PATTERN OF GROWTH
It has been claimed that follicular carcinomas with this pattern tend to run a more aggressive clinical course. In this case the cells have a granular cytoplasm resembling that of oncocytes.

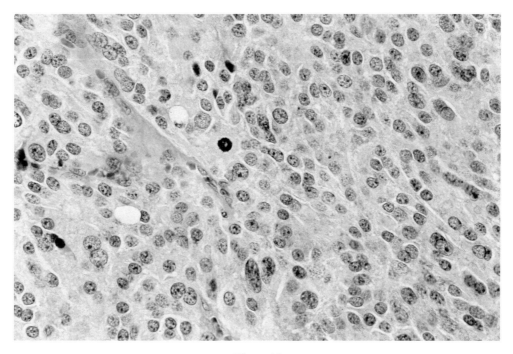

Figure 45
FOLLICULAR CARCINOMA
This tumor is solid and exhibits a moderate to marked degree of pleomorphism, with an abnormal chromatin pattern and occasional mitotic activity. This combination of cytologic features should alert the pathologist to the possibility of malignancy and lead to a careful search for capsular and/or blood vessel invasion.

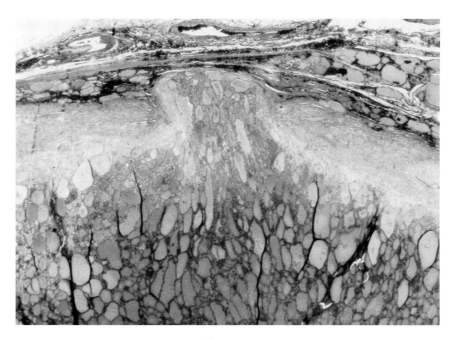

Figure 46
MINIMAL CAPSULAR INVASION IN FOLLICULAR CARCINOMA
There is penetration of the thick fibrous capsule by neoplastic follicles.

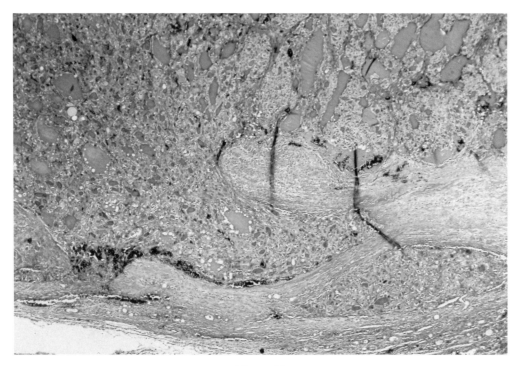

Figure 47
MARKED CAPSULAR INVASION IN FOLLICULAR CARCINOMA
The cluster of tumor cells in the lower right corner of this field probably represents vascular invasion.

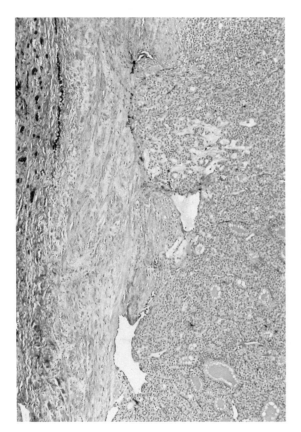

Figure 48
FOLLICULAR CARCINOMA
This follicular neoplasm is surrounded by a thick, fibrous capsule. The interface between the tumor and the inner side of the capsule is irregular, and there is protrusion of tumor cells within subcapsular vessels. Although these features are suggestive of minimally invasive follicular carcinoma, they are not diagnostic by themselves. Obvious capsular invasion was present elsewhere in this tumor.

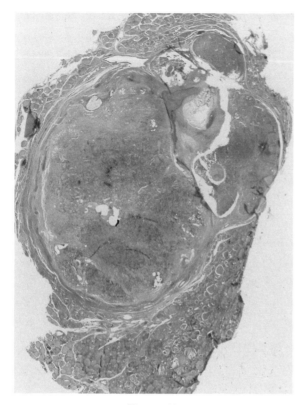

Figure 49
(Figures 49 and 50 are from the same patient)
MINIMALLY INVASIVE FOLLICULAR CARCINOMA
This tumor is surrounded by a thick and irregular fibrous capsule with focal osseous metaplasia. It invaded into the capsule and metastasized to the skeletal system.

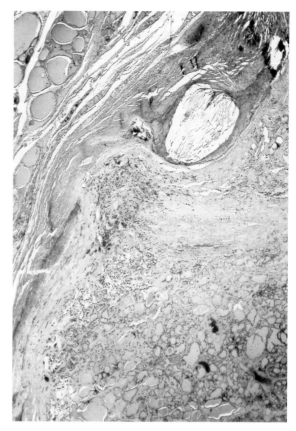

Figure 50
MINIMALLY INVASIVE FOLLICULAR CARCINOMA
This is a closer view of an area of capsular invasion by the same tumor shown in figure 49. Regressive changes are prominent, indicating the long-standing nature of this process.

be just as stringent or more so (17,21,22, 26,38,39). The vessel should be located within the capsule or immediately outside it (rather than within the tumor itself). It should be of large (i.e., venous rather than capillary) caliber and should have an identifiable wall and endothelial lining. The intravascular cells should have a clear-cut epithelial appearance (sometimes simulated by plump endothelial cells in areas of organizing thrombosis) (figs. 51–54). They should project into the vessel lumen in a thrombus-like fashion, in such a way that they partly or completely obliterate it. Most important, they should be attached at some point to the vessel wall. A cluster of follicular cells found floating in the vascular lumen may be the result of artifactual detachment at surgery or gross examination and should therefore be discounted. Another feature to be regarded as insufficient

evidence of vascular invasion is the close intermingling of follicular cells and vessels within the capsule. This may be the result of the labyrinthine configuration of those vessels coupled with the sometimes marked irregularity of the interface between tumor cells and capsule.

There is some controversy regarding the significance of the endothelial layer sometimes seen over the protruding tumor nests. Some observers consider this evidence that vascular invasion has not yet occurred, arguing that one component of the vessel wall is still present between the tumor cells and the vascular lumen. Others, ourselves included, not only regard its presence as compatible with a diagnosis of vascular invasion but view it as corroborating evidence for this occurrence (17). It has been suggested that the reason for its presence is analogous to that operating in

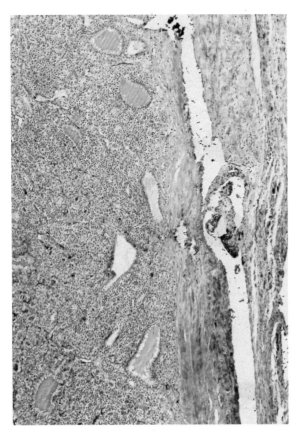

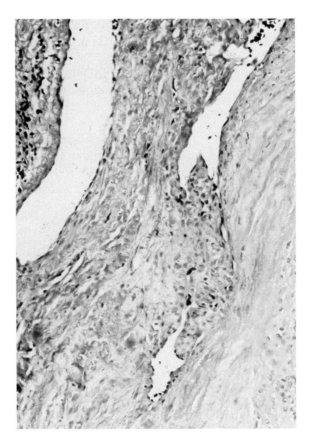

Figure 51
VASCULAR INVASION IN
FOLLICULAR CARCINOMA
The involved vessel is typical of this situation, in that it is located in the capsule and endowed with a wide lumen and thin wall. The tumor thrombus is focally attached to the wall, an important requirement for its identification as such.

Figure 52
MINIMAL VASCULAR INVASION IN
FOLLICULAR CARCINOMA
A capsular vessel shows growth of neoplastic follicular cells in the wall, some of them resulting in a polypoid projection within the lumen, which is covered by endothelial cells. The adjacent blood vessel is normal.

ordinary thrombi, i.e., an attempt at organization and recanalization.

Because it is sometimes difficult to decide whether an intracapsular nest of tumor cells is located within a vessel or not, attempts have been made to facilitate this determination with the use of special stains. In general, the results have been disappointing, mostly because of the peculiar nature of the capsular vessels. Despite their large caliber, the walls are partially or sometimes completely devoid of a continuous smooth muscle layer or an elastic lamina (pl. V-A) (17). As a result, elastic tissue stains, trichrome stains, or immunocytochemical reactions for actin are often of no avail. Immunostains for endothelial cells, such as factor VIII–related antigen and *Ulex*

europaeus agglutinin I have proved more useful (pl. V-B; fig. 55), but their utility is limited because the results are sometimes completely negative in structures indubitably representing vessels, whether for technical reasons, delayed fixation, or true lack of expression (18,19,34).

Immunohistochemical and Ultrastructural Features. In general, the immunohistochemical and ultrastructural features of follicular carcinoma do not differ from those of follicular adenoma (fig. 56) (see pages 26–28). Some intriguing immunohistochemical differences between the two have been described by some groups, but independent confirmation of these claims is needed (11,35–37).

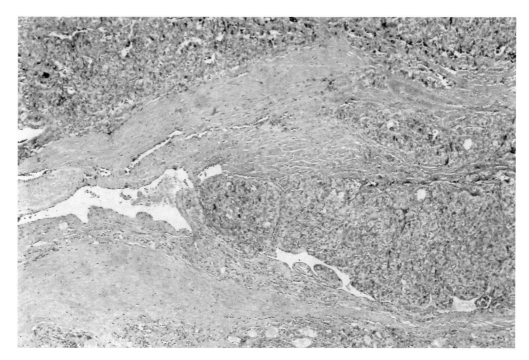

Figure 53
MASSIVE VASCULAR INVASION IN FOLLICULAR CARCINOMA
The lumen is almost totally obliterated by a solid tumor growth of follicular cells.

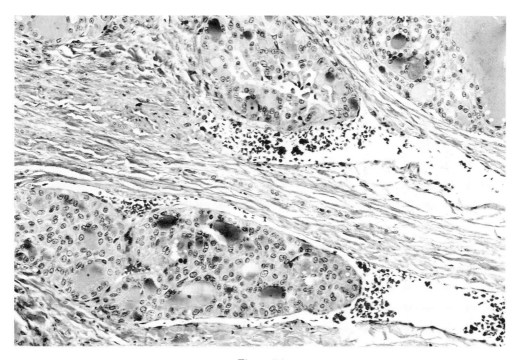

Figure 54
MASSIVE VASCULAR INVASION IN FOLLICULAR CARCINOMA
The tumor thrombi, which are composed of relatively well-differentiated cells and form small follicles, are covered by flattened endothelial cells.

PLATE V

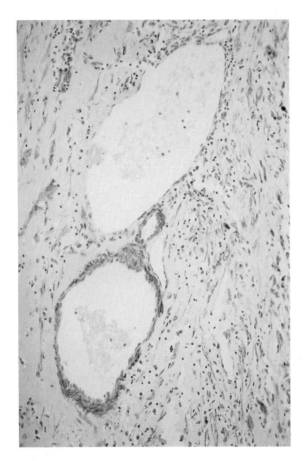

A. ENCAPSULATED FOLLICULAR NEOPLASM

This illustration shows actin staining of vessels located in the capsule of an encapsulated follicular neoplasm. Whereas some of the vessels have a continuous and well-developed smooth muscle coat, others (e.g., the one at the top) lack it completely, thus minimizing the utility of actin stain for the detection of vascular invasion.

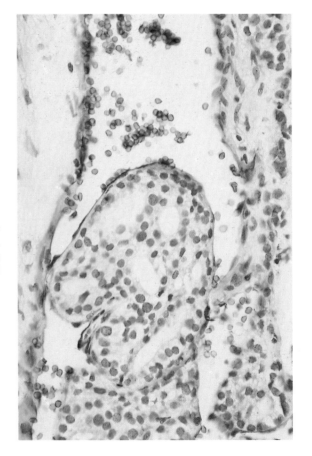

B. INVASIVE FOLLICULAR CARCINOMA

Blood vessel invasion in follicular carcinoma is confirmed with staining for *Ulex europaeus* agglutinin I. There is positivity in the endothelial cells, including those covering the tumor thrombus. The intravascular red blood cells are also reactive.

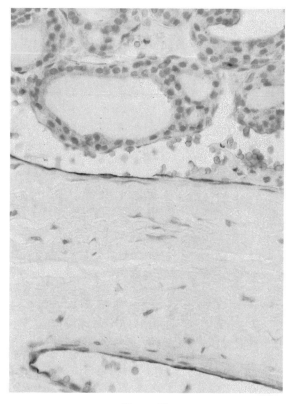

Figure 55
VASCULAR INVASION IN
FOLLICULAR CARCINOMA
The vascular invasion is documented by strong immunoreactivity for factor VIII-related antigen in the endothelial
cells of the invaded vessel. A normal vessel located at the
bottom of the photograph serves as a built-in control.

Other Special Techniques. Most of the
other special techniques related to follicular neoplasms are discussed in the chapter on Follicular
Adenoma (see page 28). Suffice to say that all of
the DNA ploidy studies carried out so far indicate
that the diagnostic utility of this technique is
limited. Specifically, it cannot be used to separate
follicular adenomas from well-differentiated follicular carcinomas, inasmuch as some of the former are aneuploid and many of the latter are
diploid. After studying 44 follicular thyroid neoplasms by DNA flow cytometry, Hruban and coworkers (24) concluded that, "although ploidy
does correlate with outcome, it does not significantly add to the information provided by the
histologic assessment of capsular and vascular
invasion" and added that "histologic findings
were in fact a better predictor of which neoplasm
would metastasize."

Differential Diagnosis. The differential diagnosis of minimally invasive follicular carcinoma includes follicular adenoma, a dominant
nodule of nodular hyperplasia, the follicular variant of papillary carcinoma, and the tubular (follicular) variant of medullary carcinoma. Of these,
the most common and most difficult is the distinction with follicular adenoma. This is not too surprising because many features are shared by the
two neoplasms. As already mentioned, the distinction is based almost exclusively on the detection of capsular and/or blood vessel invasion in
the carcinoma. Thus, there are two issues of
practical importance that need to be addressed.

The first issue is whether it is possible to make
the diagnosis of carcinoma in an encapsulated
follicular neoplasm lacking evidence of capsular
and/or blood vessel invasion and/or distant metastases. Generally, the answer is no. Only when
a noninvasive encapsulated follicular tumor
shows clear-cut signs of malignancy in the form
of high mitotic activity (including atypical
forms), widespread nuclear atypia with undue
nucleolar prominence (rather than the occasional bizarre hyperchromatic nucleus), and necrosis should this diagnosis be considered (figs. 43,
45). When thus defined, the occurrence is exceptional indeed. The few cases we have seen have
approached the nuclear/cytoplasmic features of
poorly differentiated (insular) carcinoma, and we
suspect that a more thorough sampling would
have revealed the presence of invasion.

The second issue concerns what to do with cases
in which an exhaustive search for evidence of
capsular and/or vascular invasion provides only
suspicious or doubtful rather than definite evidence. We recommend (particularly when only
questionable *capsular* invasion is featured) a conservative approach, in terms of both nomenclature
and therapy. Specifically, we propose to designate
them *follicular neoplasms of undeterminate malignant behavior* and treat them similarly to adenomas. Others use the term *atypical adenoma* in a
similar context.

Cytologic Features. These are discussed
under Follicular Adenoma (page 31).

Spread and Metastasis. Because a minimal
degree of invasiveness is a sine qua non for the
diagnosis of this tumor, it follows that direct
extension into the surrounding gland or perithyroid tissue is never a feature at the time of

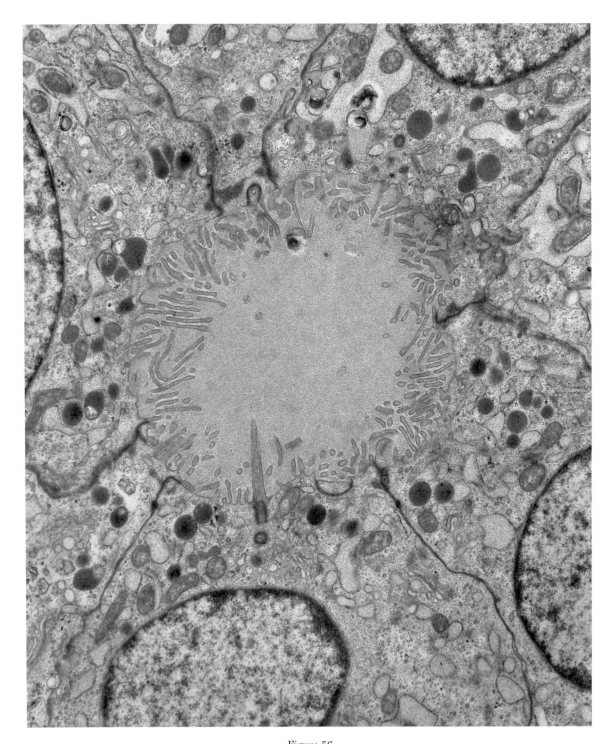

Figure 56
WELL-DIFFERENTIATED FOLLICULAR CARCINOMA
The follicular tumor cells shown in this electron micrograph converge toward a central lumen that contains a moderately electron-dense granular material consistent with colloid. Numerous long microvilli are seen on the luminal side of the tumor cells, as well as single cilia. Other features include junctional complexes, lysosomes, and a moderately well developed endoplasmic reticulum. The appearance is indistinguishable from that of a follicular adenoma. X15,037. (Courtesy of Dr. Robert Erlandson, Memorial Sloan-Kettering Cancer Center, New York, NY.)

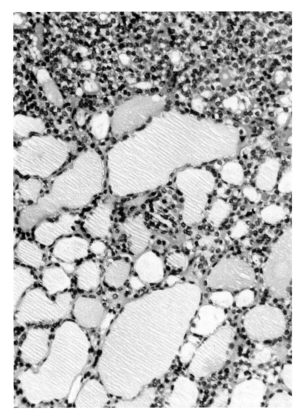

Figure 57
FOLLICULAR CARCINOMA METASTATIC
TO THE ILIAC BONE
Some areas are solid or microfollicular, but in others, the degree of differentiation results in a normo- and/or macrofollicular appearance indistinguishable from that of an adenoma or a non-neoplastic condition.

These bone metastases can feature follicular structures so well differentiated as to closely simulate those of non-neoplastic thyroid. This is the source for the picturesque but incorrect and deservedly obsolete expression *benign metastasizing goiter* (fig. 57). The high degree of differentiation is also demonstrated by the ability of the follicular structures to incorporate radioactive iodine, a feature that is exploited for diagnostic and therapeutic purposes.

Treatment. The optimal therapy for minimally invasive follicular carcinoma remains just as controversial as that for papillary carcinoma. Some authors advocate the performance of total thyroidectomy followed by the administration of radioactive iodine (14,20). Others, ourselves included, have the impression that a more conservative approach, i.e., a lobectomy or subtotal thyroidectomy without radioactive iodine administration, will result in similar if not identical survival curves (32,33). In the absence of prospective randomized studies, the issue remains open.

Metastatic disease is generally treated with radioactive iodine. Excision or external radiation therapy can also be used, depending on the site and number of metastases. Bone metastases are rarely cured, but excellent long-term palliation can be achieved (20).

Prognosis. The overall prognosis of minimally invasive follicular carcinoma is excellent, perhaps as good as that of papillary carcinoma. This is not immediately apparent when evaluating the extant literature on the subject. The main problem is that, in most of these papers (particularly those published in surgical journals), the term follicular carcinoma is used in a generic sense, thereby including neoplasms with a distinctly less favorable outcome, such as oncocytic, widely invasive, and poorly differentiated (insular) carcinoma (12). An additional source of difficulty is that, in some series, no distinction is made among the patients who developed metastases after thyroidectomy and those who already had them at the time of the initial diagnosis, i.e., those who presented with stage III disease (16).

The few studies that have dealt exclusively with the minimally invasive type of follicular carcinoma that was limited to the thyroid at the time of surgery have shown a cure rate of over 95 percent (15,27). This figure has reached 100

presentation. Recurrence in the residual gland after lobectomy is also distinctly rare. Lymph node metastases to the neck are the exception. Whenever they are observed in a tumor presumed to be follicular carcinoma, the alternative possibilities of follicular variant of papillary carcinoma, oncocytic carcinoma, and poorly differentiated (insular) carcinoma should be considered.

The most common sites for metastases in follicular carcinoma are lung and bone, particularly the latter (28). Sometimes these bone metastases (which are usually osteolytic) are the first manifestation of the disease. A pathologic fracture of a long bone due to a metastasis of a heretofore silent follicular thyroid carcinoma is a well-known form of presentation. Bones most often involved are long bones (such as femur) and flat bones (particularly pelvis and sternum but also skull) (30).

percent in some series in which capsular invasion was the sole criterion for malignancy, leading some authors to question the diagnostic significance of the latter finding (13,25). It is because of these figures, which have been mirrored by our own experience, that we have taken an increasingly conservative approach to this tumor type, and avoided using the word carcinoma for those neoplasms in which the evidence of capsular or blood vessel invasion is questionable.

In cases of metastatic disease to lung and/or bone, adverse prognostic factors are said to include multiplicity of sites, older patient age at the time of discovery of the metastases, and absence of radioactive iodine uptake by the metastases. In one series (which also included some "moderately differentiated" types and probably some widely invasive tumors), the overall survival rates were 53 percent at 5 years, 38 percent at 10 years, and 30 percent at 15 years (31).

WIDELY INVASIVE TYPE

As the name indicates, this tumor shows extensive areas of invasion at the gross and microscopic level, and therefore, the differential diagnosis with adenoma is nonexistent. Often, the mass lacks evidence of preexisting encapsulation altogether. Lang and coworkers (42) have suggested including in this category those encapsulated follicular neoplasms in which four or more capsular vessels are invaded, a criterion that we find rather arbitrary.

Microscopically, some of these tumors look similar to their minimally invasive counterpart. However, most exhibit features suggestive of malignancy at the cytoarchitectural level, such as a solid, nesting, or trabecular pattern of growth; high mitotic activity; marked nuclear hyperchromasia; and necrosis. These features overlap considerably with those of poorly differentiated (insular) carcinoma (see page 123). This similarity is also maintained at the behavioral level, in the sense that widely invasive follicular carcinoma is associated with a distant metastatic rate (mainly to lung and bone but also brain and liver) and a mortality rate roughly comparable to those for poorly differentiated (insular) carcinoma (41). Thus, Lang and coworkers (42) found that 80 percent of their patients with widely invasive carcinomas developed metastases and that about 20 percent died of tumor. Woolner and coworkers found a 50 percent death rate for widely invasive tumors, as opposed to only 3 percent for those with minimal invasion (43,44).

The incidence of widely invasive follicular carcinoma relative to that of the minimally invasive type greatly depends on the liberality of the pathologist in making the former diagnosis. In our experience, widely invasive follicular carcinoma is an uncommon neoplasm.

REFERENCES

Follicular Carcinoma

1. Boehm T, Rothouse L, Wartofsky L. Metastatic occult follicular thyroid carcinoma. JAMA 1976;235:2420–1.
2. Cooper DS, Axelrod L, DeGroot LJ, Vickery AL Jr, Maloof F. Congenital goiter and the development of metastatic follicular carcinoma with evidence for a leak of nonhormonal iodide: clinical, pathological, kinetic, and biochemical studies and a review of the literature. J Clin Endocrinol Metab 1981;52:294–306.
3. Cuello C, Correa P, Eisenberg H. Geographic pathology of thyroid carcinoma. Cancer 1969;23:230–9.
4. Harach HR, Escalante DA, Oñativia A, Lederer Outes J, Saravia Day E, Williams ED. Thyroid carcinoma and thyroiditis in an endemic goitre region before and after iodine prophylaxis. Acta Endocrinol (Copenh) 1985;108:55–60.
5. Hofstadter F. Frequency and morphology of malignant tumours of the thyroid before and after the introduction of iodine prophylaxis. Virchows Arch [A] 1980;385:263–70.
6. Lang W, Choritz H, Hundeshagen H. Risk factors in follicular thyroid carcinomas. A retrospective follow-up study covering a 14-year period with emphasis on morphological findings. Am J Surg Pathol 1986;10:246–55.
7. Paul SJ, Sisson JC. Thyrotoxicosis caused by thyroid cancer. Endocrinol Metab Clin North Am 1990;19:593–612.
8. Vickery AL Jr. The diagnosis of malignancy in dyshormonogenetic goitre. Clin Endocrinol Metab 1981;10:317–35.
9. Williams ED. Pathology and natural history. In: Duncan W, ed. Thyroid cancer. Berlin: Springer-Verlag, 1980:47–55. (Duncan W, ed. Recent results in cancer research; Vol 73.)
10. _____, Doniach I, Bjarnason O, Michie W. Thyroid cancer in an iodide rich area: histopathologic study. Cancer 1977;39:215–22.

Minimally Invasive (Encapsulated) Type

11. Barresi G, Tuccari G. Iron-binding proteins in thyroid tumours. An immunocytochemical study. Pathol Res Pract 1987;182:344–51.
12. Brennan MD, Bergstralh EJ, van Heerden JA, McConahey WM. Follicular thyroid cancer treated at the Mayo Clinic, 1946 through 1970: initial manifestations, pathologic findings, therapy, and outcome. Mayo Clin Proc 1991;66:11–22.
13. Cady B, Rossi R, Silverman M, Wool M. Further evidence of the validity of risk group definition in differentiated thyroid carcinoma. Surgery 1985;98:1171–8.
14. Clark OH. Total thyroidectomy: the treatment of choice for patients with differentiated thyroid cancer. Ann Surg 1982;196:361–70.
15. Elsner B, Curutchet HP, Bellotti MS, Degrossi OJ, Kerman A. Carcinoma folicular de la glándula tiroides. Estudio clinicopatológico. Medicina [Buenos Aires] 1980;40:501–10.
16. Evans HL. Follicular neoplasms of the thyroid. A study of 44 cases followed for a minimum of 10 years, with emphasis on differential diagnosis. Cancer 1984;54:535–40.
17. Franssila KO, Ackerman LV, Brown CL, Hedinger CE. Follicular carcinoma. Semin Diagn Pathol 1985;2:101–22.
18. González-Cámpora R, Montero C, Martin-Lacave I, Galera-Davidson H. Demonstration of vascular endothelium in thyroid carcinomas using *Ulex europaeus* I agglutinin. Histopathology 1986;10:261–6.
19. Harach HR, Jasani B, Williams ED. Factor VIII as a marker of endothelial cells in follicular carcinoma of the thyroid. J Clin Pathol 1983;36:1050–4.
20. Harness JK, Thompson NW, McLeod MK, Eckhauser FE, Lloyd RV. Follicular carcinoma of the thyroid gland: trends and treatment. Surgery 1984;96:972–80.
21 Hazard JB, Kenyon R. Atypical adenoma of the thyroid. Arch Pathol 1954;58:554–63.
22. _____, Kenyon R. Encapsulated angioinvasive carcinoma (angioinvasive adenoma) of the thyroid gland. Am J Clin Pathol 1954;24:755–66.
23. Hedinger CE, Williams ED, Sobin LH. Histological typing of thyroid tumors. In: Hedinger CE, ed. International histological classification of tumours; Vol 11. Berlin: Springer-Verlag, 1988.
24. Hruban RH, Huvos AG, Traganos F, et al. Follicular neoplasms of the thyroid in men older than 50 years of age. A DNA flow cytometric study. Am J Clin Pathol 1990;94:527–32.
25. Iida F. Surgical significance of capsule invasion of adenoma of the thyroid. Surg Gynecol Obstet 1977;144:710–2.
26. Kahn NF, Perzin KH. Follicular carcinoma of the thyroid: an evaluation of the histology criteria used for diagnosis. Pathol Annu 1983;18:221–53.
27. Lang W, Choritz H, Hundeshagen H. Risk factors in follicular thyroid carcinomas. A retrospective follow-up study covering a 14-year period with emphasis on morphological findings. Am J Surg Pathol 1986;10:246–55.
28. Massin J-P, Savoie J-C, Garnier H, Guiraudon G, Leger FA, Bacourt F. Pulmonary metastases in differentiated thyroid carcinoma. Study of 58 cases with applications for the primary tumor treatment. Cancer 1984;53:982–92.
29. Mazzaferri EL, Oertel JE. The pathology and prognosis of thyroid cancer. In: Kaplan EL, ed. Surgery of the thyroid and parathyroid glands. Clinical Surgery International, Vol 6. Edinburgh: Churchill Livingstone, 1983:23–5.
30. Nagamine Y, Suzuki J, Katakura R, Yoshimoto T, Matoba N, Takaya K. Skull metastasis of thyroid carcinoma. Study of 12 cases. J Neurosurg 1985;63:526–31.
31. Schlumberger M, Tubiana M, De Vathaire F, et al. Long-term results of treatment of 283 patients with lung and bone metastases from differentiated thyroid carcinoma. J Clin Endocrinol Metab 1986;63:960–7.
32. Schroder DM, Chambors A, France CJ. Operative strategy for thyroid cancer. Is total thyroidectomy worth the price? Cancer 1986;58:2320–8.
33. Starnes HF, Brooks DC, Pinkus GS, Brooks JR. Surgery for thyroid cancer. Cancer 1985;55:1376–81.
34. Stephenson TJ, Griffiths DW, Mills PM. Comparison of *Ulex europaeus* I lectin binding and factor VIII-related antigen as markers of vascular endothelium in follicular carcinoma of the thyroid. Histopathology 1986;10:251–60.
35. Tuccari G, Barresi G. Immunohistochemical demonstration of ceruloplasmin in follicular adenomas and thyroid carcinomas. Histopathology 1987;11:723–31.
36. _____, Barresi G. Tissue polypeptide antigen in thyroid tumours of follicular cell origin: an immunohistochemical re-evaluation for diagnostic purposes. Histopathology 1990;16:377–81.
37. Vierbuchen M, Schröder S, Uhlenbruck G, Ortmann M, Fischer R. CA 50 and CA 19-9 antigen expression in normal, hyperplastic, and neoplastic thyroid tissue. Lab Invest 1989;60:726–32.
38. Warren S. Invasion of blood vessels in thyroid cancer. Am J Clin Pathol 1956;26:64–5.
39. _____, Significance of invasion of blood vessels of the thyroid gland. Arch Pathol 1931;11:255–7.
40. Yamashina M. Follicular neoplasms of the thyroid. Total circumferential evaluation of the fibrous capsule. Am J Surg Pathol 1992;16(4):392–400.

Widely Invasive Type

41. Carcangiu ML, Zampi G, Rosai J. Poorly differentiated (insular) thyroid carcinoma. A reinterpretation of Langhans' "wuchernde Struma." Am J Surg Pathol 1984;8:655–68.
42. Lang W, Choritz H, Hundeshagen H. Risk factors in follicular thyroid carcinomas. A retrospective follow-up study covering a 14-year period with emphasis on morphological findings. Am J Surg Pathol 1986;10:246–55.
43. Woolner LB. Thyroid carcinoma: pathologic classification with data on prognosis. Semin Nucl Med 1971;1:481–502.
44. _____, Beahrs OH, Black BM, McConahey WM, Keating FR Jr. Classification and prognosis of thyroid carcinoma. Am J Surg 1961;102:354–87.

PAPILLARY CARCINOMA

Definition. A malignant epithelial tumor showing evidence of follicular cell differentiation and characterized by the formation of papillae and/or a set of distinctive nuclear features.

General Features. Papillary carcinoma is the most common type of thyroid cancer (~65 to 80 percent in the United States) (72). It has been claimed that its relative incidence compared with that of follicular carcinoma is even greater in areas of high iodine intake (56,124).

There is a well-documented association between radiation exposure to the neck and subsequent development of papillary thyroid carcinoma (13,53,103,126). In most of the cases, the radiation was given during childhood, and the average interval until the development of malignancy has been about 20 years (14). Cases have also been reported of papillary thyroid carcinoma that developed shortly after the administration of high-dose radiation to the neck for malignant disease (see page 329) (5,7, 49,81,115,118). In two large series, the number of patients with thyroid papillary carcinoma who gave a history of previous irradiation to the area were 6.0 and 6.6 percent, respectively (14,78).

It has been suggested that there might be an increased incidence of papillary carcinoma in Graves disease, but this has not been conclusively proven (33,34,82,83,95,108). The incidence of Graves disease in patients with papillary carcinoma is 4 percent. It has been hypothesized that, in those patients with Graves disease who develop thyroid carcinoma, the thyroid-stimulating antibodies that are responsible for the disease may play a role in the genesis of the tumor (35).

Papillary carcinoma is also said to be more common in glands affected by lymphocytic/Hashimoto thyroiditis (fig. 58) (22,91,106). We find the reported evidence for this claim to be more convincing than that for Graves disease but feel that a definite statistical relationship remains to be proven. Hyperplastic nodules or adenomas are present in about 40 percent of the glands harboring papillary carcinomas, but the two events are probably unrelated (14).

Cases of papillary carcinoma have been reported in a familial setting (74), in patients with ataxia-telangiectasia (87), as part of a type of multiple endocrine neoplasia (MEN) syndrome (55), and in association with parathyroid tumors (52), carotid body tumors (2), and a variety of colorectal abnormalities. The latter include sporadic adenocarcinoma, polyposis coli, Gardner syndrome, and Cowden syndrome (94). Whether the coexistence of these neoplasms is significant or coincidental is not clear (70). Some of the cases of synchronous papillary carcinoma and parathyroid adenoma have occurred in patients with a history of previous irradiation to the neck (52).

Clinical Features. Papillary carcinoma is more common in women. The ratio of women to men in most series ranges between 2:1 and 3:1 (14,36,48,77,109,127) but is substantially higher in Japan (9:1 to 13:1). The mean age at the time of diagnosis ranges from 31 to 49 years in the various series. Several authors noted a shift to a younger range in recent years, perhaps due to earlier diagnosis (11,28). Papillary carcinoma constitutes 90 percent or more of all cases of thyroid carcinoma in childhood (109). A possible congenital case has been described (84).

Nearly all patients present with clinically evident disease in the neck (50,76,77). In one series, this was located in the thyroid gland alone in 67 percent, in the thyroid gland plus cervical nodes in 13 percent, and in cervical nodes alone in 20 percent of the cases (14).

Gross Features. Grossly, the typical papillary carcinoma presents as an invasive neoplasm of ill-defined margins, firm consistency, and a granular cut surface (pl. VI; fig. 59). The color is usually whitish, and calcifications may be present. The size is extremely variable, with the mean diameter between 2 and 3 cm (51). The percentage of tumors measuring 1.5 cm or less in diameter ranges in the various series from 13.7 percent (116) to 64 percent (37). This wide variation probably reflects either the type of material examined or the tendency of some patient populations to consult late in the course of the disease. Most of the variations in the gross appearance of the tumor are related to its variants and are discussed with them. This applies to the well-circumscribed and fleshy appearance resembling adenoma that can be exhibited by the

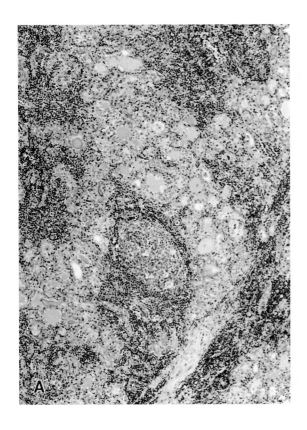

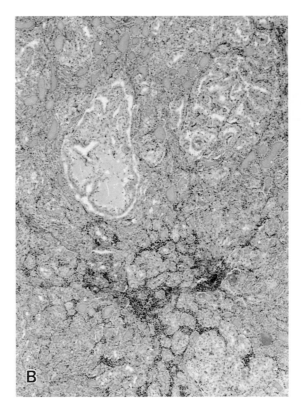

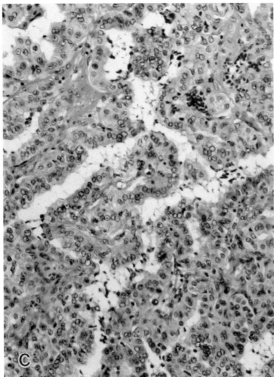

Figure 58
PAPILLARY CARCINOMA IN
HASHIMOTO THYROIDITIS
This composite figure taken from the same case illustrates the typical appearance of Hashimoto thyroiditis (A), the low-power appearance of papillary carcinoma (B), and the high-power appearance of the same tumor (C). The branching papillary formations and ground-glass nuclei of this tumor can be readily seen.

PLATE VI

PAPILLARY CARCINOMA

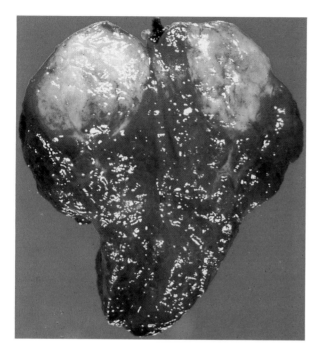

A. This bisected thyroid lobe shows papillary carcinoma at one pole. The tumor is relatively well circumscribed but not encapsulated, bulges on the surface, and has a granular solid appearance.

B. This large papillary carcinoma shows invasive features and a predominantly solid appearance, with marked granularity suggestive of papillary formations. The uninvolved thyroid gland is seen in the upper left corner.

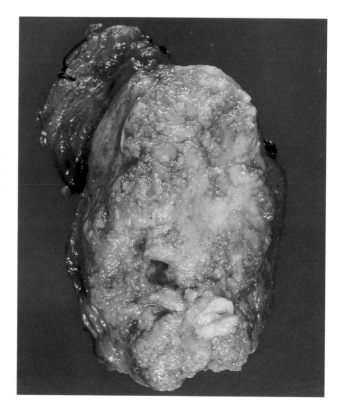

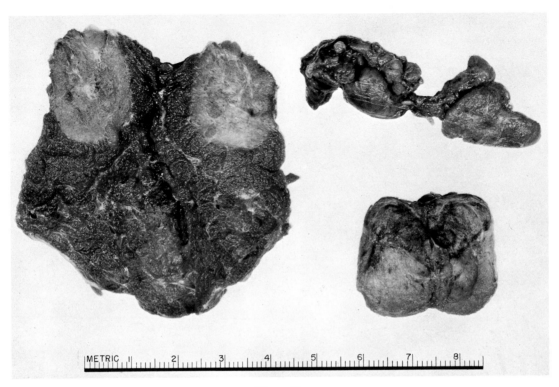

Figure 59
PAPILLARY CARCINOMA

This papillary carcinoma, located in the upper portion of a thyroid lobe, has metastasized to the cervical lymph nodes, as seen on the right side of the photograph. Some of the lymph nodes were larger than the primary tumor. (Fig. 68 from Fascicle 4, Second Series.)

follicular variant and the partial or complete cystic change that can be seen in some of the encapsulated types (formerly designated papillary cystadenocarcinomas).

Fresh tumor necrosis is exceptional in papillary carcinoma. Its presence should suggest an alternative diagnosis or the emergence of a more aggressive (i.e., poorly differentiated or undifferentiated) component within.

Microscopic Features. The two morphologic features that best characterize typical papillary carcinoma are the papillae and the nuclear changes.

Papillae. As in papillary tumors in other locations, the papillae of papillary thyroid carcinoma are formed by a central fibrovascular stalk covered by a neoplastic epithelial lining (figs. 60–62). The better developed papillae are long, with a complex arborizing pattern. Some of these papillae are straight and slender, arranged in a parallel, regimented fashion; others are short and stubby, standing in a "picket-fence" configuration from a

straight base. In some instances, the papillae are tightly packed, resulting in glomeruloid and pseudosolid configurations (fig. 63). When the latter areas are cut perpendicular to the long axis of the papillae, the resulting images resemble rosettes. A most unusual configuration, perhaps secondary to fusion of individual papillae, is a cribriform pattern resembling that seen in intraductal carcinoma of the breast (16,18).

The thickness and composition of the papillary stalk is variable. In most instances, it is made up of loose connective tissue and variously sized thin-walled vessels. In some cases, it is swollen by edema fluid or occupied by an abundant acellular hyaline material (fig. 64). Sometimes it is infiltrated by lymphocytes or clusters of macrophages, some of which may be foamy or hemosiderin laden (fig. 65). Psammoma bodies (to be discussed below) and other calcific concretions may be present. In exceptionally rare instances, it may contain mature adipose tissue (119). Finally, it is not unusual

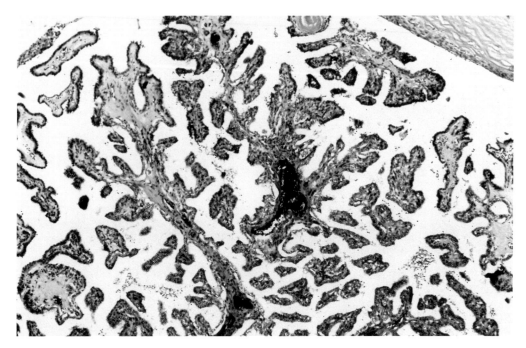

Figure 60
PAPILLARY CARCINOMA
This figure illustrates the typical low-power appearance of papillary carcinoma. The papillae are complex and branching and contain a central fibrovascular core.

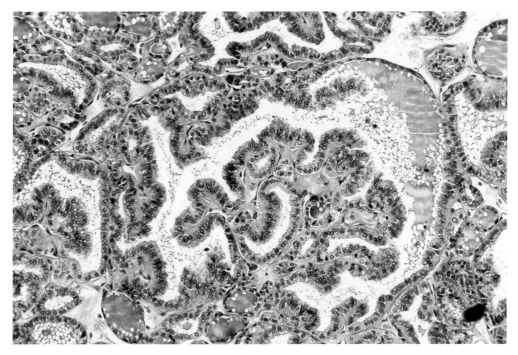

Figure 61
PAPILLARY CARCINOMA
This figure illustrates the typical growth pattern of papillary carcinoma. The complex branching configuration of the papillae is evident, particularly at the center. A few neoplastic follicles are seen within the papillary cores.

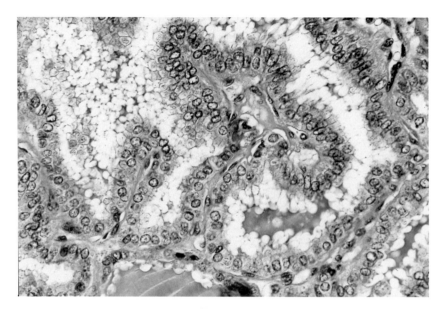

Figure 62
PAPILLARY CARCINOMA
The papillae are lined by a layer of cuboidal to low columnar cells, with irregularly distributed vesicular nuclei. The colloid shows prominently scalloped edges.

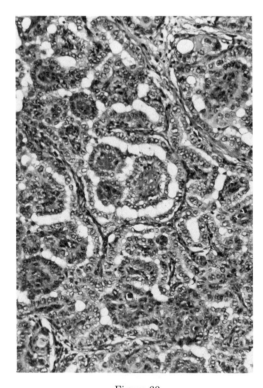

Figure 63
PAPILLARY CARCINOMA
The complex arrangement and tight packing of the papillae in this papillary carcinoma result in glomeruloid formations.

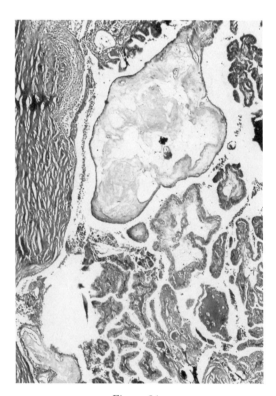

Figure 64
PAPILLARY CARCINOMA
Some of the papillae of this tumor show striking hyalinization of the stroma.

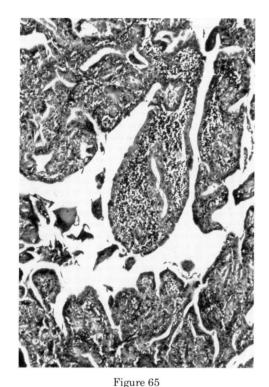

Figure 65
PAPILLARY CARCINOMA
Heavy lymphocytic infiltration of the stroma is evident in this tumor.

to find round structures with the appearance of follicles, containing colloid in their lumina, within these stalks (fig. 61).

It has often been stressed that, for papillae to qualify as such they need to contain a central fibrovascular stalk, in contrast to the infolding epithelium of benign lesions. This requirement is sound, but exceptions exist on both sides. The "abortive" papillae of some variants of papillary carcinoma are devoid of a stalk, but they may represent the first clue to the diagnosis. Conversely, in some benign conditions such as diffuse hyperplasia, nodular hyperplasia, or adenoma with papillary hyperplasia, the papillary structures within them may contain fibrovascular stalks.

In its most characteristic form, papillary carcinoma shows a great predominance of papillary structures throughout the tumor. However, it is rare for it to be composed exclusively of papillae (73a). In most cases, the papillae are interspersed with neoplastic follicles that have similar nuclear features (fig. 66). The proportion of papillae to follicles varies greatly from case to case. This distinction

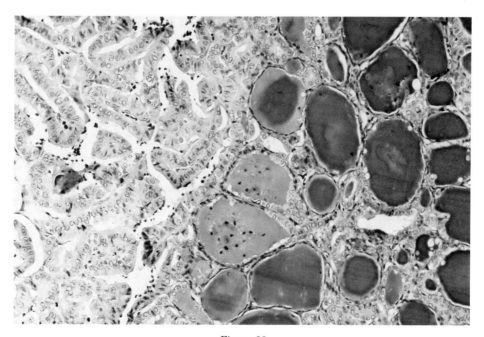

Figure 66
PAPILLARY CARCINOMA
The left half of this photograph shows a typical papillary configuration, whereas the right half shows a follicular pattern of growth. The cellular features are similar on both sides. These tumors should be designated as papillary carcinomas rather than mixed (papillary-follicular) carcinomas.

can be indicated by the expressions *with papillary predominance* or *with follicular predominance,* depending on the case, although this is probably unnecessary. The term *mixed carcinoma* should not be used for these tumors. As long as the cells in the follicles partake of the nuclear features seen in the papillae, the natural history of the tumor will be that of a papillary carcinoma. When the follicular predominance over the papillae is complete, the tumor should be placed into the follicular variant but still regarded as a papillary neoplasm (see page 100).

Nuclear features. The nuclei of the papillary carcinoma cells usually have a distinctive appearance, which in recent years has acquired a diagnostic significance at least comparable to that of the papillae. The shape of the nuclei is round or slightly oval. The contours may appear smooth on superficial examination of a thick section; however, close inspection of thinner preparations reveals subtle irregularities in the form of indentations, crenellations, and folds (fig. 67A). These nuclear irregularities may manifest in the form of pseudoinclusions or grooves. The former arise from deep cytoplasmic invaginations and result in nuclear acidophilic, inclusion-like round structures, sharply outlined and slightly eccentric, with a crescent-shaped rim of compressed chromatin on one side (fig. 67B) (1,62). They are similar in appearance (and probably in their mechanism of formation) to those seen in other neoplasms, such as glioblastoma multiforme and malignant melanoma. The nuclear grooves are more common in the oval nuclei and are usually parallel to the long axis of the nuclei. Sometimes two or more grooves are seen in the same nucleus, running side by side; they are similar to those seen in granulosa cell tumors of the ovary and in the cells of histiocytosis X, among others (fig. 67C) (19).

Another peculiar and constant feature of the nucleus of papillary carcinoma cells is represented by an empty appearance of the nucleoplasm, which seems almost totally devoid of chromatin strands (fig. 67D,E). The inner aspect of the nuclear membrane is irregularly thickened by the apposition of chromatin material. The nucleolus, which may be prominent, has often been pushed aside against the nuclear membrane. These nuclei have been variously described as pale, clear, optically clear, watery, empty, ground glass, and "Orphan Annie's eyes." Nuclei with these alterations are enlarged

and often have an overlapping quality, even in thin sections. Their appearance has been likened to that of tiles on a roof or an egg-basket (fig. 67E) (42). The ground-glass appearance is well shown in fixed, paraffin-embedded material (regardless of the fixative used) but is inconspicuous or absent in frozen sections or smears from the same cases (pl. VII) (15,21). This led to the conclusion that it represents an artifact of fixation and/or embedding. Even if this were the case, we strongly suspect that it reflects some intrinsic physicochemical alteration of the chromatin structure or associated nuclear proteins.

Mitotic figures are exceptional or absent in papillary carcinoma, a feature that correlates with their low proliferative activity as measured by bromodeoxyuridine labeling (129a). Their presence in more than an occasional number should suggest the emergence of a poorly differentiated neoplasm (see page 123) (69).

In contrast to the highly distinctive nuclear qualities, the cytoplasm of papillary carcinoma cells is nondescript. In most instances, it is modest in amount, slightly to moderately eosinophilic to amphophilic, and cuboidal. Variations include pale cells, cells with a finely granular cytoplasm (due to richness of mitochondria), and cells with a diffusely acidophilic cytoplasm (due to cytoplasmic filaments). The latter may result in a squamoid appearance.

Other morphologic features. In addition to the papillary and follicular patterns, papillary carcinoma can grow in solid or trabecular formations. Solid areas are detected in about 25 percent of the cases (36). Usually this is a focal change, but it may involve most or all of the neoplasm (fig. 68). This should not be taken as evidence that the tumor has become undifferentiated or even poorly differentiated, as long as the typical nuclear features of papillary carcinoma persist in it. Squamous metaplasia is also common in this tumor, having been recorded in 20 to 40 percent of the cases (14,36). It can be focal or extensive. In its most characteristic form, squamous metaplasia presents as concentric whorls of keratinized cells surrounded by papillary foci. Squamous metaplasia is most common in tumor foci surrounded by abundant stromal tissue.

Another structure classically associated with papillary carcinoma is the *psammoma body,* which refers to round calcific concretions that

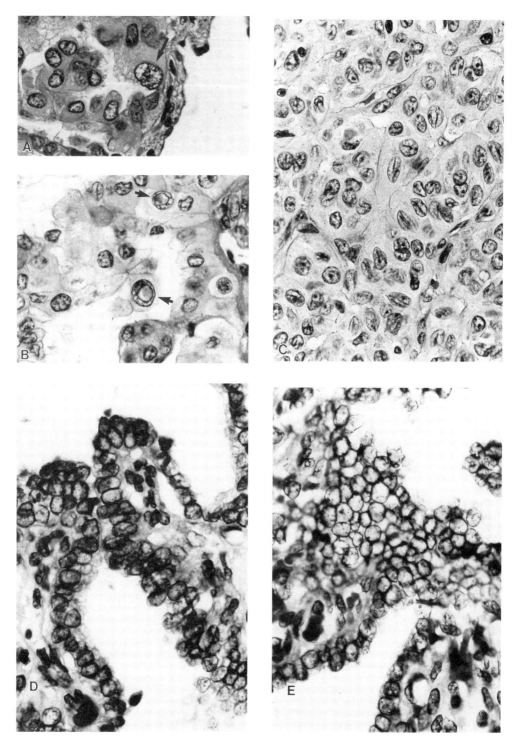

Figure 67
PAPILLARY CARCINOMA

This series of illustrations shows the typical nuclear features of papillary carcinoma cells. The large nucleus located in the center of the photograph has a finely irregular (serrated) appearance (arrow) (A). Two large nuclear pseudoinclusions are evident (arrows) (B). Many of the nuclei show prominent longitudinal grooves (C). Typical ground-glass nuclei show marked overlapping (D). The "egg-basket" appearance results from tangential sectioning of ground-glass nuclei (E).

PLATE VII

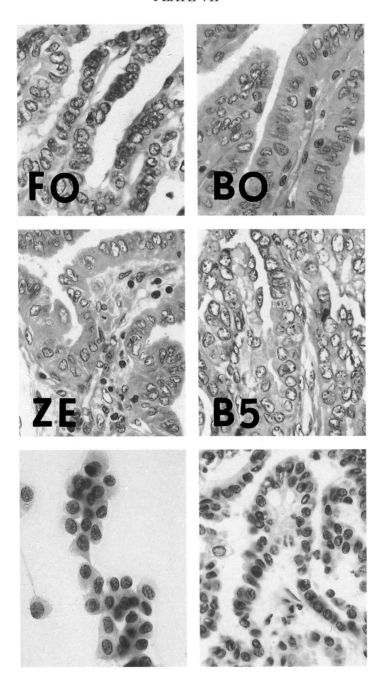

PAPILLARY CARCINOMA

This photograph illustrates the nuclear features of tumor cells from the same case of papillary carcinoma, as seen after various procedures. The ground-glass appearance of the nuclei is evident in the paraffin-embedded material, regardless of whether the fixation was carried out in buffered formalin (FO), Bouin's fluid (BO), Zenker's fluid (ZE), or B-5; however, it is not appreciable in a touch preparation (bottom left) or frozen section (bottom right).

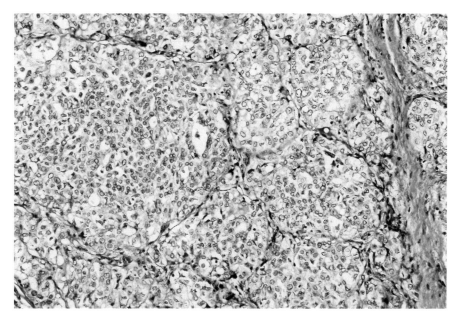

Figure 68
PAPILLARY CARCINOMA WITH A PREDOMINANTLY SOLID GROWTH PATTERN
A well-defined fibrous band is seen on the right side. Most of the nuclei have a ground-glass appearance.

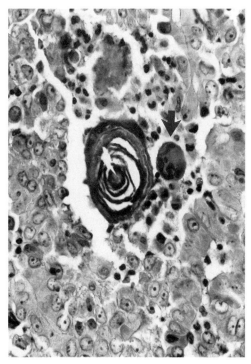

Figure 69
PSAMMOMA BODY IN PAPILLARY CARCINOMA
A typical psammoma body within papillary carcinoma is illustrated. The structure is heavily calcified and shows well-defined concentric laminations. A foreign-body–type giant cell is seen adjacent to it (arrow).

exhibit concentric lamination (figs. 69, 70). Psammoma bodies are found in about 50 percent of the cases and are particularly common in tumors that feature a predominantly papillary growth pattern. Their mechanism of formation is controversial, but we find appealing the hypothesis that the nidus for their genesis is a single necrotic tumor cell, upon which successive layers of calcium salt have deposited (pl. VIII; fig. 71) (63). Psammoma bodies are not entirely specific for papillary carcinoma; however, they are so exceptionally rare in benign thyroid diseases that their detection should immediately suggest the presence of such a neoplasm lurking in the background (68,92). If found in an area of inflammation and dense fibrosis, they probably represent the residua ("fossils" or "tombstones") of a papillary cancer that has regressed at that site (fig. 72). If found in an otherwise normal thyroid, chances are high that a papillary carcinoma is present a few microns away (fig. 73). If present in an otherwise normal cervical lymph node, there is a high probability that the node is involved by a metastatic papillary carcinoma that is not apparent in that particular level.

Although the most characteristic location of psammoma bodies is near the tip of the papillary

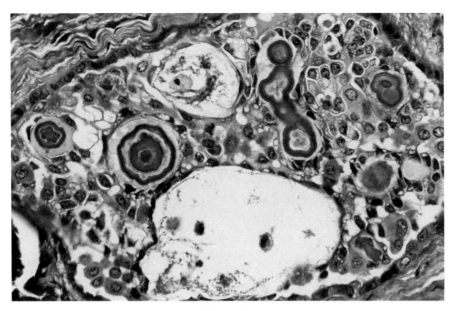

Figure 70
PSAMMOMA BODIES
This illustration shows numerous psammoma bodies in various stages of formation within a papillary carcinoma. In some of them, a necrotic tumor cell is evident at the center.

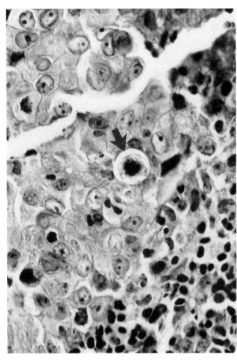

Figure 71
PAPILLARY CARCINOMA
This field contains a single necrotic cell in papillary carcinoma with beginning calcification, which probably represents the nidus for early psammoma body formation (arrow).

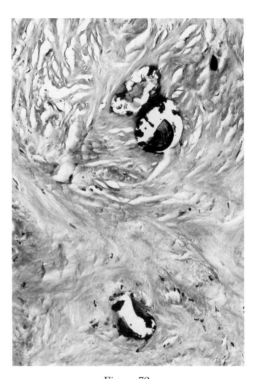

Figure 72
PSAMMOMA BODIES
These psammoma bodies embedded in dense, fibrous tissue show a characteristic cracking artifact. This represents an area of papillary carcinoma that has undergone total regression, leaving the psammoma bodies as the tumor's "fingerprints."

PLATE VIII

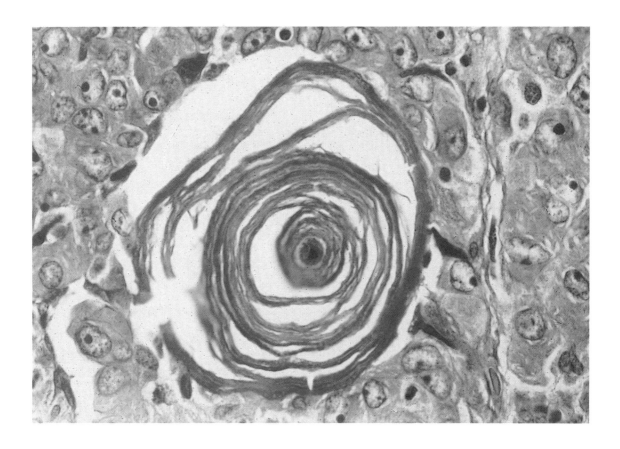

PSAMMOMA BODY IN PAPILLARY CARCINOMA
There is a single necrotic tumor cell in the center of this structure that probably acts as the nidus for its formation.

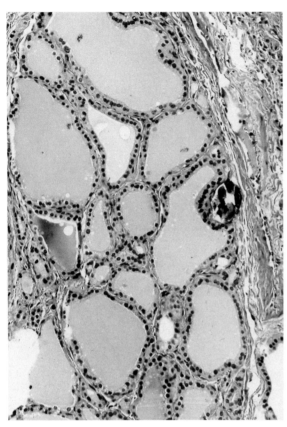

Figure 73
PSAMMOMA BODY IN
OTHERWISE NORMAL THYROID
A papillary carcinoma was present nearby.

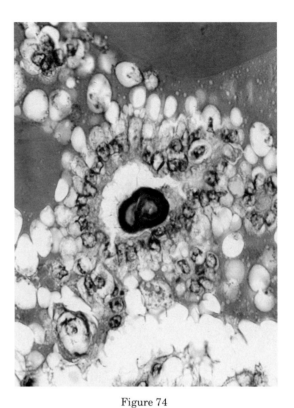

Figure 74
PSAMMOMA BODY
This psammoma body is located in the center of a papilla
of papillary carcinoma shown in cross section.

Figure 75
PSAMMOMA BODY
This psammoma body appears in a papillary carcinoma with a
predominantly solid pattern of growth. The clue to the real nature of
this tumor is provided not only by the psammoma body but also by
the ground-glass nuclear features, and the sharply outlined fibrous
bands which divide the tumor incompletely into lobules.

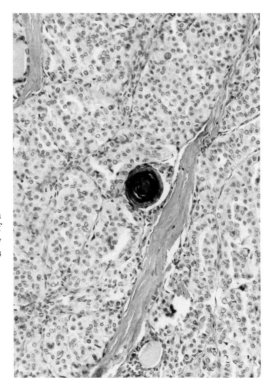

stalk (fig. 74), they are also numerous in intrathyroid tumor emboli within lymph vessels. They can also be found in the stroma between neoplastic follicles or in the midst of a solid epithelial component (fig. 75). Psammoma body-like formations located in the lumina of follicles should be disregarded. In most instances, they are the result of inspissated secretion and are more commonly seen in connection with oncocytic neoplasms (see page 162).

Psammoma bodies have also been described in cases of follicular carcinoma, but we suspect that most of these cases would be classified as the follicular variant of papillary carcinoma, according to current criteria. They can also occur in medullary carcinoma (see page 226) and have even been described in carcinoma metastatic to the thyroid (99). Other types of calcification can be seen in association with papillary carcinoma, sometimes accompanied by metaplastic ossification, but these phenomena do not carry a diagnostic significance similar to that of the psammoma body.

The presence of an abundant fibrous stroma is a common feature of papillary carcinoma (fig. 76) (73a). In most instances, it presents in the form of wide hyaline bands that traverse the tumor and divide it incompletely into irregularly shaped and often angulated lobules. The fibrosing tendencies of this tumor are particularly evident at the advancing edge. Some of this stromal reaction has a very cellular ("desmoplastic") appearance. In a few cases, it acquires a nodular fasciitis-like or fibromatosis-like quality and is so abundant that it obscures the neoplastic component (pl. IX; fig. 77) (17,86a). In other cases, a prominent myxoid change may be encountered (90).

Approximately one third of papillary carcinomas show a lymphocytic infiltration that is moderate to marked. This change tends to be more pronounced at the tumor periphery and within the fibrovascular papillary stalks. In most instances, it probably represents a host reaction to the tumor; in others, it may be the expression of a preexisting autoimmune thyroiditis (66,107).

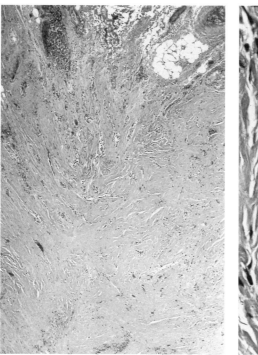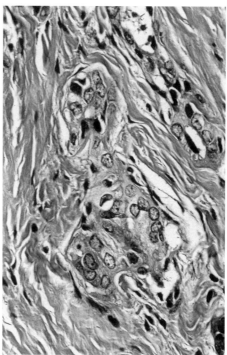

Figure 76
MARKED FIBROSCLEROTIC CHANGES IN PAPILLARY CARCINOMA
The high magnification in the right photograph shows a cluster of tumor cells embedded in the fibrous stroma.

PLATE IX

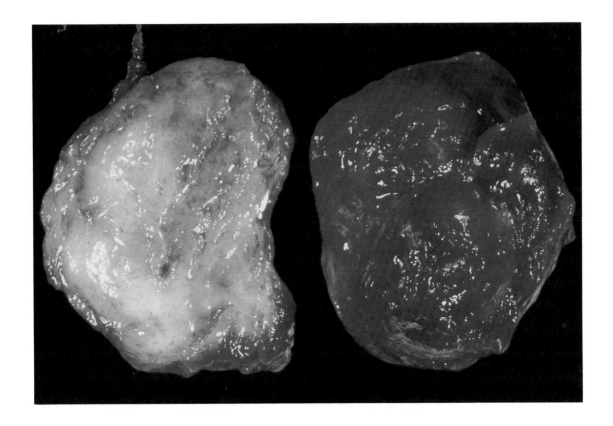

PAPILLARY CARCINOMA

Outer aspect and cut surface of this papillary carcinoma accompanied by abundant nodular fasciitis-like stroma. The bulk of the mass was formed by this exuberant myofibroblastic proliferation.

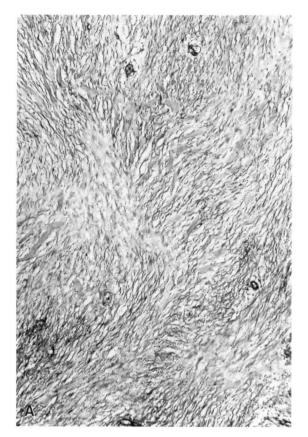

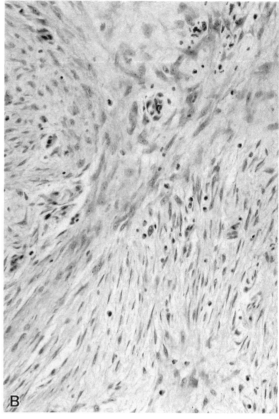

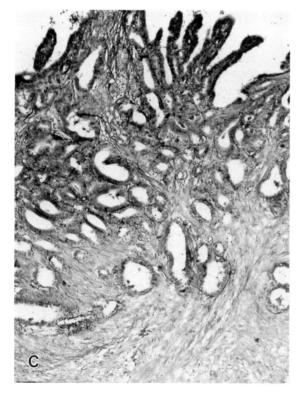

Figure 77
PAPILLARY CARCINOMA WITH
NODULAR FASCIITIS-LIKE STROMA
This tumor shows an exuberant myofibroblastic prolif-
eration associated with deposition of dense bands of colla-
gen, which obscures the neoplastic nature of the process
(A and B). An area of papillary carcinoma merging with
the desmoplastic stroma is shown in C.

The stroma of papillary carcinoma may also contain aggregates of cells immunoreactive for S-100 protein, which have been interpreted as Langerhans and/or reticulum cell type (see also the section on Prognosis, page 95) (105).

Secondary cystic changes are common. The more papillary the tumor, the more likely that the changes will be present. Most of these cysts are lined by papillary formations diagnostic of the entity, but others are covered by a very attenuated, single-layered, flat epithelium with a deceptively benign appearance.

Blood vessel invasion is not as common or as diagnostically important as in the follicular carcinoma, but it certainly does occur; it is found in about 7 percent of the cases (fig. 78) (14). Invasion of lymph vessels is a much more common phenomenon, but it is not always easy to detect. When lymphatic invasion is extensive, the possibility of the tumor belonging to the diffuse sclerosing variant should be considered. The issue of multicentricity is discussed in the section on Spread and Metastases (see page 90).

Microscopic Grading. The overwhelming majority of papillary carcinomas have the nuclear and architectural features already described. A few

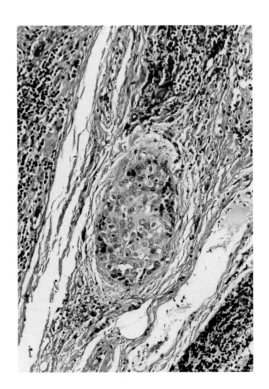

Figure 78
BLOOD VESSEL INVASION
IN PAPILLARY CARCINOMA
This is an unusual finding in this tumor type.

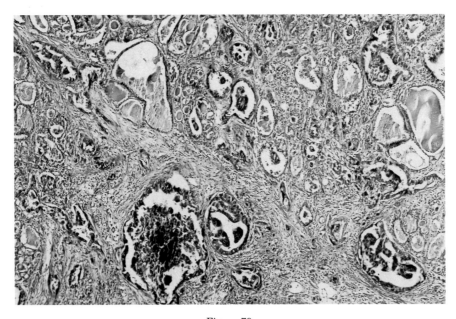

Figure 79
HIGH-GRADE PAPILLARY CARCINOMA
There is necrosis, and the tumor cells feature hyperchromatic nuclei. Mitotic figures were also present.

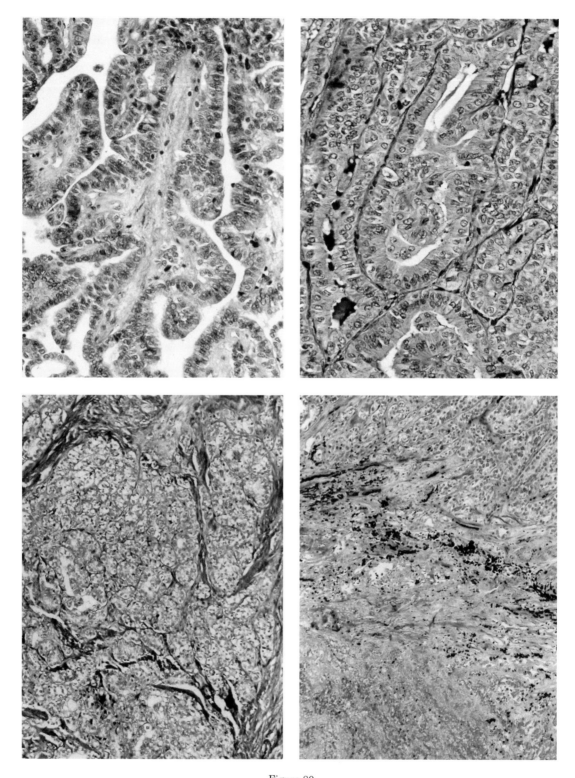

Figure 80
HIGH-GRADE (POORLY DIFFERENTIATED) PAPILLARY CARCINOMA
The clinically aggressive behavior that this tumor is likely to manifest can be predicted by the tall appearance
of the epithelium (top), nesting (insular) pattern of growth (bottom left), and presence of necrosis (bottom right).

will exhibit nuclear pleomorphism, hyperchromasia, mitotic activity, foci of necrosis, and other features (figs. 79, 80). Such tumors have been designated *high-grade* or *poorly differentiated papillary carcinomas* and are described further in the next chapter. In the Mayo Clinic experience, papillary carcinoma thought to have a microscopic grade higher than I comprised 6.2 percent of the cases (79).

Ultrastructural Features. The characteristic nuclei of papillary carcinoma cells exhibit a finely dispersed chromatin, highly folded nuclear membrane, and an apparent paucity of nuclear pores (fig. 81) (6,62,64). The nuclear folds may result in large invaginations within the nucleus that correspond to the inclusion-like formations seen with the light microscope, both in histologic and cytologic preparations. The cytoplasm is rich in mitochondria, lysosomes, and filaments. The latter are particularly numerous in foci of squamous metaplasia, in which they may be accompanied by keratohyalin granules. The apical surface exhibits microvillous differentiation (fig. 82).

Immunohistochemical Features. Papillary carcinoma cells are consistently positive for thyroglobulin, although, as a rule, the intensity of the reaction is less pronounced than in follicular neoplasms (pl. X-A) (93,112). The tumor cells are also immunoreactive for keratin and vimentin (10,54, 125). There is often a coexpression of these two markers in the same cell (120). The keratins expressed are not only of the low–molecular-weight type present in the normal thyroid but also those

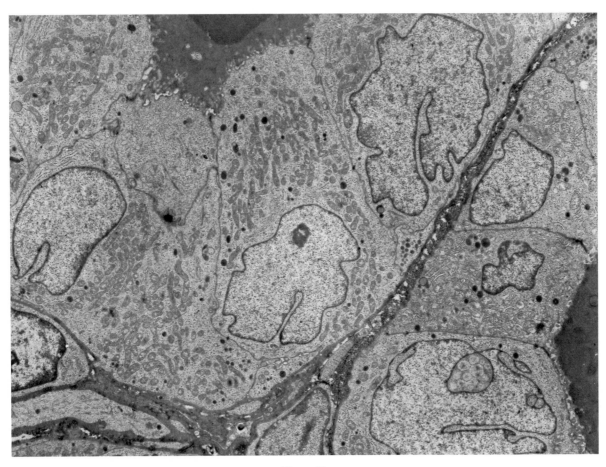

Figure 81
PAPILLARY CARCINOMA
The cells lining the papillae in this electron micrograph are tall cuboidal. The cytoplasm contains a relatively large number of mitochondria and scattered lysosomes. The nucleus is characteristically indented. This corresponds to the grooves seen in light-microscopic preparations. X7812. (Courtesy of Dr. Robert Erlandson, Memorial Sloan-Kettering Cancer Center, New York, NY.)

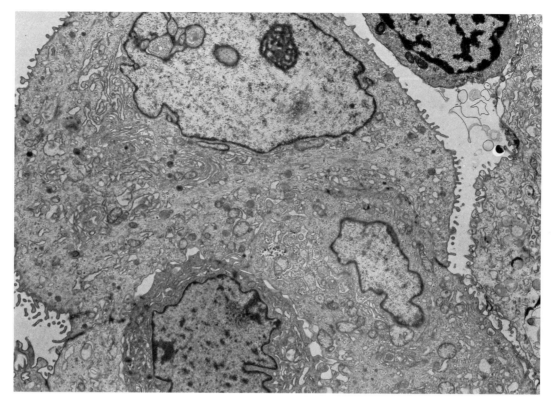

Figure 82
PAPILLARY CARCINOMA
This tumor was metastatic to a supraclavicular lymph node. Ultrastructurally, the nucleus of a tumor cell shows cytoplasmic invaginations. Microvillous differentiation is seen at the surface. X6156. (Courtesy of Dr. Robert Erlandson, Memorial Sloan-Kettering Cancer Center, New York, NY.)

of high molecular weight, in keeping with the tumor tendency to undergo squamous metaplasia (pl. X-B). Because the latter type of keratins is usually not encountered in the normal thyroid gland or in benign or malignant follicular neoplasms, it has been suggested that their presence may be useful in the differential diagnosis (100). However, the injured follicular epithelium of Hashimoto thyroiditis also expresses high–molecular-weight keratins (54). Another interesting parallel between the cells of papillary carcinoma and those of Hashimoto thyroiditis is their frequent strong immunoreactivity for S-100 protein (55a).

As far as conventional special stains are concerned, Chan and Tse (20) have shown that, contrary to general belief, stains for mucin can be positive in a considerable number of papillary carcinomas, whether in the colloid, luminal border, or cytoplasm.

Other Special Techniques. Biochemical studies of the thyroglobulin secreted by papillary (and follicular) carcinomas suggest that, at least in some cases, there are structural differences from the thyroglobulin secreted by the normal gland. These include a lesser degree of iodination, lesser degree of binding to some monoclonal antibodies, lesser degree of absorption in affinity chromatography on a concanavalin A–sepharose column, decrease in high-mannose–type oligosaccharides with corresponding increase of other neutral oligosaccharides, and replacement of sialylated oligosaccharides for phosphorylated oligosaccharides (112,113). A set of monoclonal antibodies raised against the thyroglobulin of a papillary carcinoma and thought to recognize iodine-related (hormonogenic) epitopes was found to stain preferentially the colloid but not the cytoplasm in normal or hyperplastic glands. It exhibited an inverse pattern in

PLATE X
PAPILLARY CARCINOMA

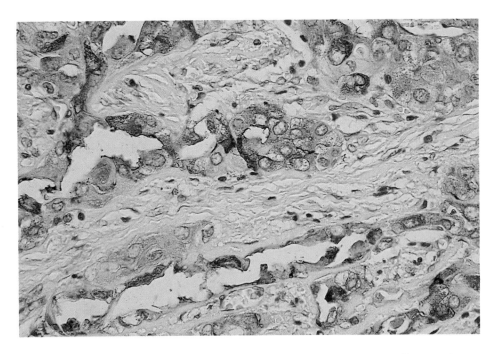

A. Immunohistochemical positivity for thyroglobulin is evident in this papillary carcinoma. Most of the tumor cells show cytoplasmic reactivity that ranges from moderate to strong.

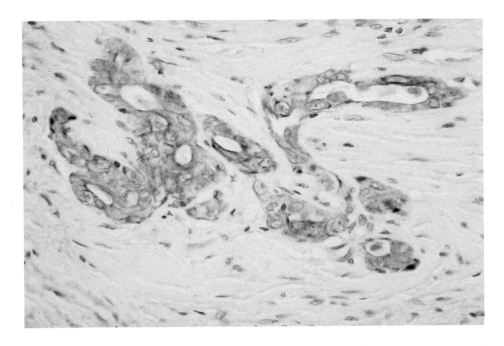

B. Immunocytochemical positivity for keratin can be seen in the invasive component of the tumor, which is surrounded by a prominent desmoplastic reaction. Keratin reactivity is particularly prominent in these invasive foci.

papillary carcinoma, in which the intraluminal colloid was negative, whereas the cytoplasm was strongly stained (usually apically but sometimes also basolaterally) (113).

Estrogen and progesterone receptor protein have been detected immunohistochemically in the nuclei of papillary carcinoma cells in a high proportion of cases, regardless of the hormonal status of the patients (31,118a). They have also been detected in follicular carcinoma (and, less frequently, in follicular adenoma) and seem to bear no relation to clinical presentation, pathologic features, or metastatic potential (118a). DNA analysis, either by static or flow-cytometric methods, has shown that most papillary carcinomas are diploid. The number of cases with an aneuploid or otherwise abnormal pattern has been reported to be approximately 20 percent. One chromosomal analysis study showed that most papillary carcinomas were characterized by normal stem lines (8). In another study, clonal karyotypical abnormalities were detected in four of seven cases, all of them involving 10q (60). In still another study, a 7:10 (q35: q21) translocation was documented (3).

In several series, most fatal cases have belonged to the aneuploid group (4,27,61,111). This is a very interesting finding, but it should be noted that nearly all of these cases would have already been identifiable as being in the high-risk group in view of the patient's age, sex, and some of the microscopic features.

Several types of oncogene alterations have been described in papillary carcinoma (38). An increase in the expression of the oncogene *ras* product (p21 antigen) was detected immunohistochemically by Mizukami and coworkers (85) in the apical surface of papillary carcinoma cells, compared with those of normal, inflamed, hyperplastic, or benign neoplastic glands, but the significance of this finding is not known. Johnson and coworkers (65) showed that p21 antigen was more strongly expressed in papillary carcinoma and other thyroid diseases than in the normal gland; however, no significant differences were found between neoplastic and non-neoplastic conditions or between benign and malignant tumors.

Wright and coworkers (128) found by transfection techniques an incidence of *ras* point mutation of 17 percent for papillary carcinoma and 53 percent for follicular carcinoma. They specu-lated that this statistically significant difference was probably related to the known differences in epidemiology, pathology, and clinical behavior between the two tumors. Interestingly, introduction of mutant *ras* genes into a subcloned rat thyroid follicular epithelial cell line induced a wide spectrum of clonal phenotypes (10a).

An Italian group studied 16 papillary carcinomas for transforming activity and detected it in 10 cases (62 percent) (9,40). This was found to be due to activation of three different oncogenes, identified in 4 cases as PTC (rearrangement), TRK (rearrangement), and N-*ras* (point mutation). The PTC (papillary thyroid carcinoma) oncogene is thought to represent a rearranged form of the *ret* proto-oncogene and has been assigned to chromosome 10 q11–q12 (32,43). Because both PTC and TRK display a tyrosine protein kinase activity, the authors proposed that the activation of this class of oncogenes is specifically involved in the pathogenesis of papillary carcinoma (9).

Wyllie and coworkers (129) could not detect any evidence of rearrangement or amplification of c-*myc* or of any other member of the nuclear oncogene family in papillary carcinoma or any of the other thyroid neoplasms they studied. Mizukami and coworkers (86) also failed to find differences in c-*myc* expression between benign and malignant thyroid tumors, including papillary carcinomas. They found instead a possible higher expression of epidermal growth factor among the papillary carcinomas that recurred compared with those that did not.

Cytologic Features. Cytologic specimens from papillary carcinoma tend to be highly cellular. Colloid is generally scant or absent. When present, it often exhibits a peculiar streaking and smearing effect ("bubble-gum" appearance). Papillary formations may be found, admixed with flat monolayers of cells (fig. 83). These may be combined with syncytium-like formations and follicles.

The individual cells may be low columnar or cuboidal. The nuclei have a fine (powdery or dusty) chromatin pattern and an irregular contour, with frequent creases and grooves (figs. 84, 85) (30a). Intranuclear pseudoinclusions representing cytoplasmic invaginations are common. They demonstrate one of the most important diagnostic features of papillary carcinoma (23), but they are not entirely pathognomonic of this tumor type (71). It should be noted that the

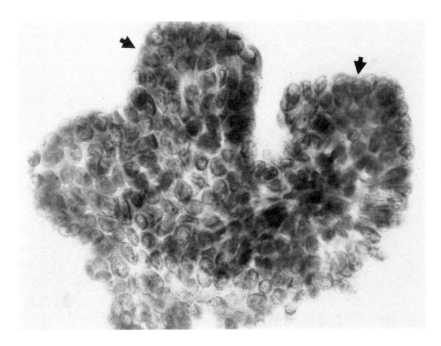

Figure 83
PAPILLARY CARCINOMA
A branching papillary tissue fragment from papillary carcinoma that shows a syncytial pattern of growth is visible in this fine-needle aspiration specimen. Note the smooth external contour and the peripheral palisading of nuclei (arrows). Papanicolaou preparation. X453. (Fig. 8.17 from Kini SR. Thyroid. In: Kline TS, ed. Guides to clinical aspiration biopsy; Vol 3. New York: Igaku-Shoin, 1987.)

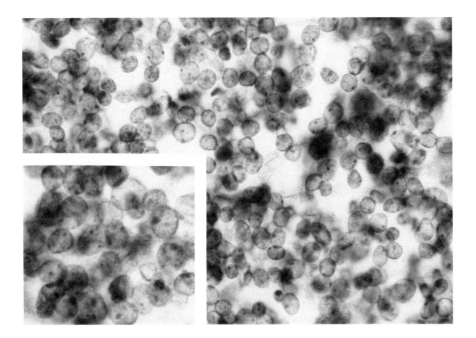

Figure 84
PAPILLARY CARCINOMA
Papillary carcinoma cells with characteristic nuclear morphology as seen in a fine-needle aspiration specimen. The nuclei are large, appear empty due to peripheral condensation of the chromatin, and contain micronucleoli, giving the typical ground-glass appearance. Papanicolaou preparation. X288. The inset shows a higher magnification. Papanicolaou preparation. X453. (Fig. 8.12 from Kini SR. Thyroid. In: Kline TS, ed. Guides to clinical aspiration biopsy; Vol 3.New York: Igaku-Shoin, 1987.)

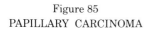

Figure 85
PAPILLARY CARCINOMA
This fine-needle aspiration specimen of papillary carcinoma shows tumor cells with characteristic nuclear grooves (arrows). Papanicolaou preparation. X453. (Fig. 8.13 from Kini SR. Thyroid. In: Kline TS, ed. Guides to clinical aspiration biopsy; Vol 3. New York: Igaku-Shoin, 1987.)

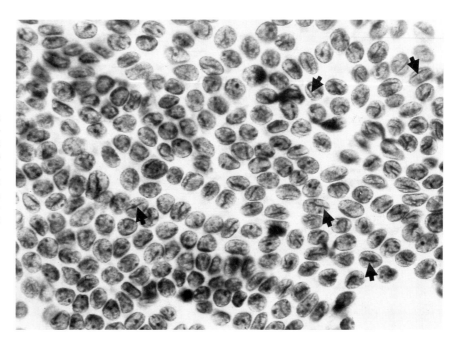

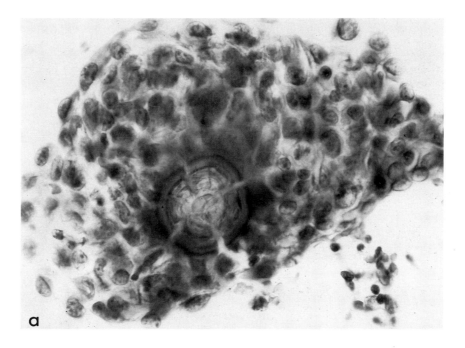

Figure 86
PSAMMOMA BODY
This psammoma body, seen in a fine-needle aspiration specimen from papillary carcinoma, shows concentric laminations and is incorporated into a syncytial-type tissue fragment. The nuclei show the typical morphology of this tumor type. Papanicolaou preparation. X453. (Fig. 8.26a from Kini SR. Thyroid. New York: Igaku-Shoin, 1987 In: Kline TS, ed. Guides to clinical aspiration biopsy; Vol 3.)

ground-glass appearance constantly seen in histologic sections is inconspicuous in cytologic preparations. Multiple small or large nucleoli are usually identified. The cytoplasm is variable in amount and tinctorial qualities; it may appear pale, foamy, vacuolated, or dense. Psammoma bodies may be identified (fig. 86) (67). A difficult problem is created by the papillary carcinomas with cystic degeneration because the aspirate may show lymphocytes, foamy macrophages, and few or no tumor cells (41).

Spread and Metastasis. One of the most notable attributes of papillary carcinoma is its tendency for multicentric involvement of the gland (fig. 87). Controversy exists as to whether this phenomenon is the result of intrathyroidal lymph vessel spread or of true multicentric transformation of the follicular epithelium. It is our impression that both mechanisms operate and that the latter is the more important, but the phenomenon is discussed in this section for convenience.

In most reported series, the incidence of multicentricity has ranged from 18 to 22 percent (14). The outstanding exception is the figure of 87.5 percent reported by Russell and coworkers (96) in a whole-mount study of 80 well-differentiated thyroid carcinomas, most of which were of the papillary type. It is obvious that the frequency of this phenomenon is directly dependent on the thoroughness of the sampling, although the liberality of the pathologist in interpreting minimal microscopic changes is probably also a factor.

Extrathyroid extension into the soft tissues of the neck has been reported to occur in 10 to 34 percent of the cases, according to the various series (12,14,25,36,107,116,127). The growth may take place along fascial planes and perineural spaces and within skeletal muscle. In advanced stages, direct extension into larynx, trachea, esophagus, or skin can be encountered (fig. 88) (44,117).

Papillary carcinoma has a great propensity to metastasize to cervical lymph nodes (pl. XI-A; figs. 89–91). Thirty-five percent of the patients have clinically evident lymphadenopathy at the time of presentation (14). Even in cases thought to be negative on palpation, microscopic examination reveals metastatic tumor in approximately 50 percent (39). The deposits are usually on the same side as the tumor, but bilateral involvement occurs in about 10 percent of the

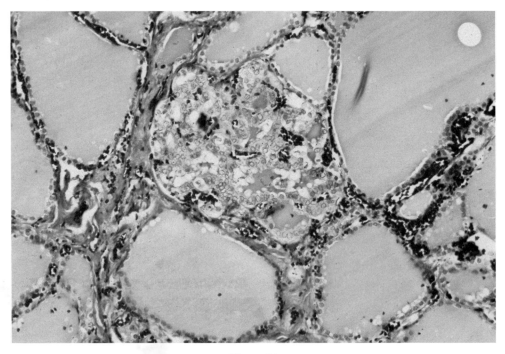

Figure 87
MULTICENTRIC FOCUS OF PAPILLARY CARCINOMA
The main tumor was in the contralateral lobe.

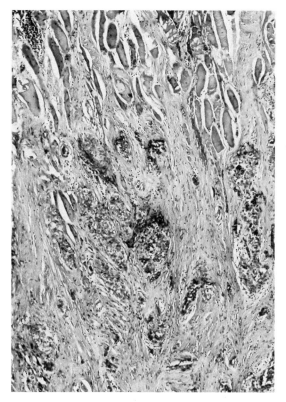

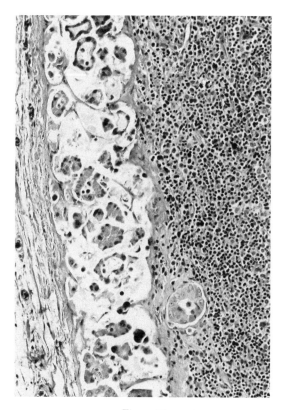

Figure 88
EXTRATHYROID SPREAD
OF PAPILLARY CARCINOMA
The extrathyroid spread of papillary carcinoma with invasion of skeletal muscle fibers is shown.

Figure 90
METASTATIC PAPILLARY CARCINOMA
Papillary carcinoma cells metastatic to the marginal sinus of a cervical lymph node.

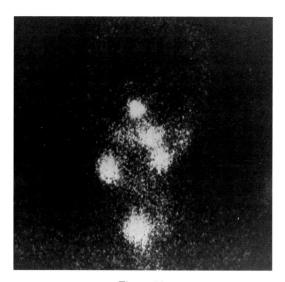

Figure 89
METASTATIC PAPILLARY CARCINOMA
Multiple cervical lymph node metastases of papillary carcinoma are shown in a radioactive iodine scan. There is also uptake in residual thyroid tissue.

cases (88). Spread to mediastinal nodes is usually secondary to extensive cervical disease.

Nodal metastases of papillary carcinoma tend to undergo cystic degeneration and/or to grow in an obvious papillary pattern, even when these features are not well developed in the primary tumor. The cystic change can be so pronounced that it may result in a misdiagnosis of branchial cleft cyst on microscopic examination (123). Presence of papillae, nuclear abnormalities, and/or psammoma bodies provides the clues for the diagnosis, which can be easily confirmed with a thyroglobulin stain.

Blood-borne metastasis also occurs, although less commonly than with most other thyroid malignant tumors. The incidence ranges from 4 to 14 percent in the various series (7,14,36,47, 58,102, 127). The lung is by far the most common site for these deposits, which can occur in the absence of cervical nodal involvement (pl. XI-B) (97). The lung metastases may have a "miliary"

PLATE XI

A. THYROID PAPILLARY CARCINOMA METASTATIC TO A LYMPH NODE

The specimen on the left shows two nodules of tumor within the gland. The two specimens on the right represent a partially cystic metastasis to a cervical lymph node. Note that the lymph node metastasis is several times larger than either of the tumor nodules within the thyroid gland. (Plate I-C from Fascicle 14, First Series.)

B. THYROID PAPILLARY CARCINOMA METASTATIC TO LUNG

The nodule grows freely inside the pulmonary parenchyma, and features an exuberance of papillary formations.

C. THYROID PAPILLARY CARCINOMA METASTATIC TO BRAIN

This solitary brain metastasis from thyroid papillary carcinoma resulted in neurologic symptoms. The thyroid primary was clinically occult. (Courtesy of Dr. Nikola Kostich, Minneapolis, MN.)

PLATE XI

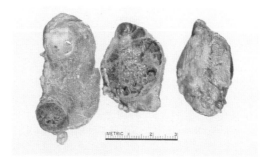

A

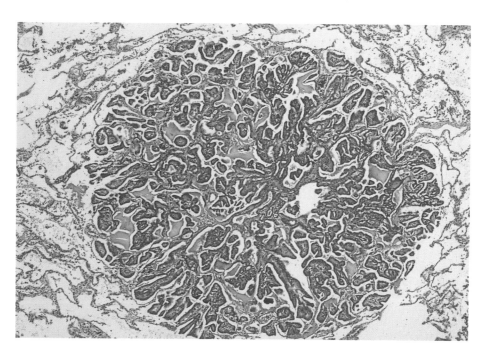

B

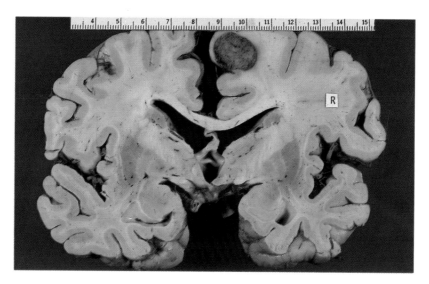

C

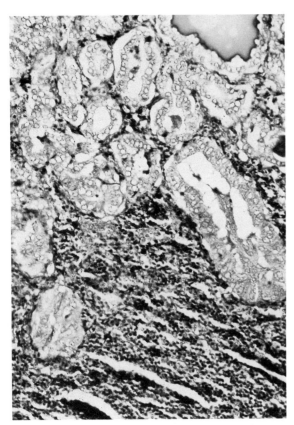

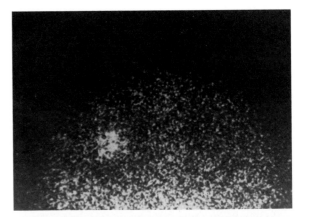

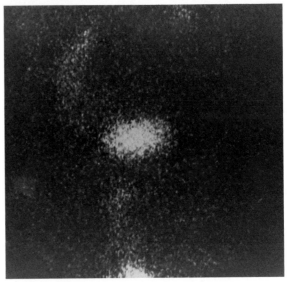

Figure 91
METASTATIC PAPILLARY CARCINOMA
This papillary carcinoma with a predominantly follicular pattern of growth was metastatic to a cervical lymph node. The large number of follicles, variation in size and shape, and characteristic ground-glass nuclei distinguish this process from ectopic thyroid tissue.

Figure 92
METASTATIC PAPILLARY CARCINOMA
This illustration shows metastasis from papillary carcinoma to skull (top) and T10 vertebra (bottom) in a radioactive iodine scan. The area of positivity seen at the lower edge of the bottom photograph represents uptake in the bladder, a normal finding.

(micronodular) appearance, may be large and rounded (macronodular), or may result in diffuse pulmonary infiltration ("snowflake") (58). Other sites include skeletal system, liver, and central nervous system (pl. XI-C; fig. 92).

Treatment. The treatment of papillary carcinoma is controversial and probably will remain so until a proper prospective study is carried out. In the past, the standard approach in many institutions has been the performance of a total thyroidectomy together with a radical lymph node dissection on the side of the tumor. The rationale for this aggressive approach has been the high frequency of intraglandular spread and/or multicentricity and of regional lymph node metastases. The performance of a formal cervical lymphadenectomy has been largely abandoned, partly because it fails

to remove many of the first-station lymph nodes but mainly because no detectable improvements in prognosis have been documented as a result of this formidable operation (45,59,89). Currently, the surgeon's approach toward these nodes is to leave them undisturbed if they appear grossly normal, and to perform a modified lymph node dissection (with preservation of the sternomastoid muscle) if they appear involved.

As far as the thyroid gland itself is concerned, some groups strongly advocate total thyroidectomy followed by the administration of radioactive iodine in an attempt to ablate any possible metastatic sites (24,46,75,77,78). Other groups regard this approach as unnecessarily radical and maintain that similarly good results can be obtained with a lesser operation followed by suppression of thyroid-stimulating hormone secretion, without the addition of radioactive iodine postoperatively (26,29,104,114,122). Our own experience (14) and the evaluation of two large series on the subject (122,130) suggest that the latter, more conservative approach is just as effective and perhaps preferable for most of the cases, i.e., those papillary carcinomas appearing clinically and scintigraphically localized to one lobe, not belonging to one of the microscopically unfavorable variants (such as diffuse sclerosing or tall and/or columnar), and occurring in low-risk patients (women under the age of 50 years or men under the age of 40 years). The specific type of operation, whether lobectomy, lobectomy with isthmusectomy, or subtotal thyroidectomy, seems to be of no great significance. We would only question the advisability of performing a nodulectomy, with the definite risk of leaving gross tumor behind and of carrying out a total thyroidectomy, with the small but ever-present risk of inducing hypoparathyroidism or recurrent laryngeal nerve injury, two potentially serious complications.

Prognosis. The overall probability of long-term survival for patients with papillary carcinoma is excellent, to the point that in some series, the figures are not significantly different from those of a normal population of similar age (28,79). The incidence of tumor deaths in most large series has been about 5 percent (14,98). The following factors are shown to be associated with a worsened prognosis:

Age. This is of paramount importance. In most series, no tumor deaths from papillary carcinoma are seen below the age of 40 years, the probability of a fatal outcome increasing exponentially with each decade (12,14,30,73,101).

Sex. In most series, women have fared better than men, but the difference has not been as striking as for age (76,101,110). Cady and co-workers (12) proposed dividing patients with well-differentiated (including papillary) carcinomas into two groups on the basis of the two factors listed above: a low-risk group (composed of men 40 years old or younger and women 50 years old or younger) and a high-risk group

(older patients). Almost all deaths from papillary carcinoma occur in the latter.

Tumor size. The probability of tumor recurrence increases when the tumor size exceeds 5 cm. The best prognosis is associated with the papillary carcinomas measuring 1.5 cm in diameter or less (see page 65) (79).

Multicentricity. We have found that tumors in which this feature is easily detectable are associated with increased chances of nodal and pulmonary metastases and a corresponding decrease in disease-free survival rates (14).

Blood vessel invasion. According to most authors, this feature is of only modest prognostic impact, barely significant at the statistical level (11,14,48,57).

Extrathyroid extension. This constitutes one of the worst morphologic prognostic signs in papillary carcinoma, being associated with an over sixfold increase in the number of tumor deaths (14). Actually, of all the pathologic features of papillary carcinoma not exhibiting dedifferentiation, it would seem that the presence of extrathyroid disease has the most significant bearing on prognosis (101,116,127).

Distant metastases. The occurrence of lung metastases is associated with a moderate but obvious deleterious effect on prognosis (particularly if macronodular rather than "miliary" or "snowflake"), whereas the development of bone metastases carries an ominous prognostic significance, even when they concentrate ^{131}I (14,58,80).

Aneuploidy. See page 87.

High microscopic grade. This rare event, which is related to the following item, is associated with a more aggressive clinical course(79).

Progression to a poorly differentiated (including insular) or undifferentiated (anaplastic) pattern. These two types of dedifferentiation, which carry an adverse prognostic significance (particularly the latter) are discussed on pages 126 and 153, respectively.

Features associated with an improved prognosis, other than those indirectly mentioned in the above paragraphs, include total encapsulation, pushing margins of growth, and cystic changes (14). These three features often coexist. It has also been claimed that papillary carcinoma featuring aggregates of S-100 protein-positive cells in the stroma fare better than the others, but independent confirmation is needed (105).

Features that are not statistically significant prognostic indicators include history of head and neck irradiation in childhood (98), relative numbers of papillae and follicles, presence and type of fibrosis, presence and amount of squamous metaplasia, presence and number of psammoma bodies, and presence or absence of cervical lymph node metastases (14). In our experience, presence of trabecular and/or solid areas did not have an adverse impact on prognosis as long as the typical nuclear features of papillary carcinoma were retained (14), but others claim otherwise (86b). Another parameter that does not carry prognostic significance in most series is the type of therapy carried out, as already mentioned (14, 26,28,29,121).

PAPILLARY CARCINOMA VARIANTS

Papillary Microcarcinoma

The WHO Committee (151) defines this variant as a papillary carcinoma measuring 1.0 cm or less in diameter and prefers for it the term papillary microcarcinoma, originally proposed by Hazard (150). It roughly corresponds to the entity classically designated *occult sclerosing carcinoma* (154), also known as *nonencapsulated sclerosing tumor* (150) and *occult papillary carcinoma* (152). It is a common finding in population-based autopsy studies and (as an incidental finding) in carefully examined thyroidectomy specimens (136,148,155,165, 175,176). The reported incidence in autopsy material has ranged in most series from 4 to 20 percent. However, Harach and coworkers (148) reported a figure of 35.6 percent in their series.

In one surgical series of papillary carcinomas, the number of microcarcinomas was 6.4 percent. Most of these were found either incidentally or because of the development of cervical lymph node metastases (138).

The term papillary microcarcinoma is preferable to the others because 1) it clearly identifies the tumor as belonging to the papillary family; 2) sclerosis may not be prominent; 3) a capsule may be present, although tumor cells are usually evident outside it; and 4) it may not be necessarily "occult," whereas sometimes a lesion larger than 1 cm is, depending on the location within the gland and the skill of the clinician. The qualifier "occult" should be used as a clinical rather than pathologic

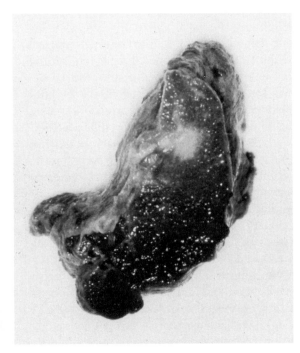

Figure 93
PAPILLARY MICROCARCINOMA
This figure shows the typical gross appearance of papillary microcarcinoma. The lesion measures only a few millimeters in diameter and has an irregular configuration, solid appearance, and white discoloration.

designation. Due to their small size, these lesions can be missed at the gross level unless a careful and systematic search for them is carried out (see page 332) (pl. XII-A; fig. 93).

Microscopically, the typical lesion has an irregular, scar-like configuration (pl. XII-B; fig. 94). The neoplastic elements predominate at the periphery of the fibrotic area, but others are seen entrapped in the center. The attributes of papillary carcinoma are present in them, including typical nuclear changes, psammoma bodies, and occasionally even well-formed papillae. In most areas, however, the tumor cells display a follicular or solid architecture, a feature to be expected of a papillary carcinoma growing in such a sclerotic milieu.

Some papillary microcarcinomas are accompanied by little or no fibrosis (fig. 95). Conversely, others are totally surrounded by an extremely thick fibrous capsule that may be focally calcified. A variant of this is represented by the case in which tumor is present both inside and outside

PLATE XII
PAPILLARY MICROCARCINOMA

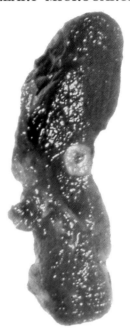

A. This tumor, which is unusually well circumscribed and focally cystic, measures less than 2 mm in diameter.

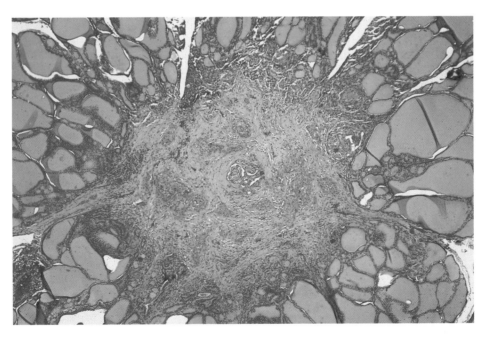

B. At low magnification, the marked fibrosis and stellate configuration characteristic of this tumor can be seen. Islands of tumor cells can be readily identified, the central one having well-formed papillary structures.

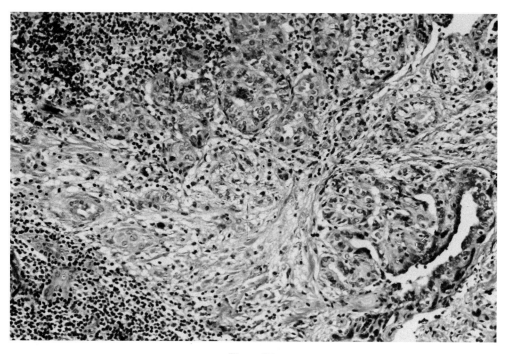

Figure 94
PAPILLARY MICROCARCINOMA
This tumor has an irregular configuration and is accompanied by marked fibrosis and mononuclear inflammatory infiltrate. Most of the neoplastic papillae and follicles are located at the periphery of the lesion.

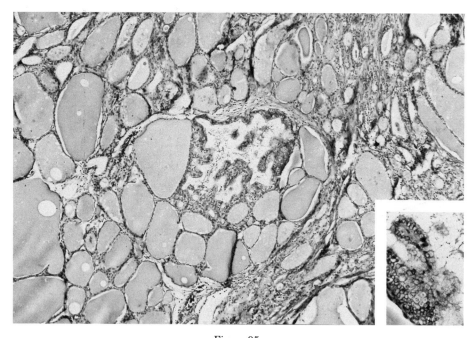

Figure 95
PAPILLARY MICROCARCINOMA WITH SCANT FIBROSIS
The architectural and cytologic features are typical of papillary carcinoma. The latter are particularly well appreciated in the inset.

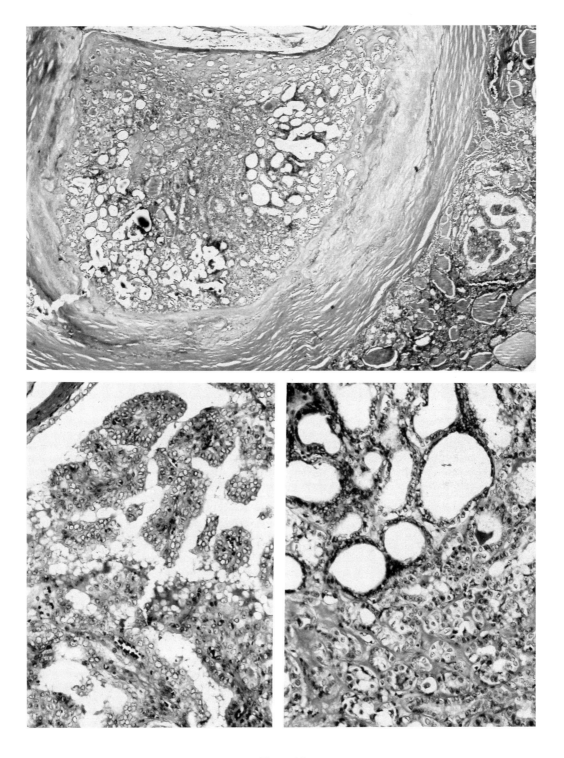

Figure 96
PAPILLARY MICROCARCINOMA
This papillary microcarcinoma shows a predominantly follicular pattern of growth inside the capsule and a predominantly papillary configuration on the outside. The bottom two photographs show higher magnifications of the papillary (left) and follicular (right) patterns.

the capsule, sometimes in roughly equivalent amounts. In such cases, the component located within the capsule tends to have a predominantly follicular configuration, whereas that on the outside is likely to feature a more conventional papillary pattern of growth (fig. 96).

The fact that these lesions are indeed malignant, has been proven by the repeated demonstration that they can metastasize to regional nodes (135,146,164). The overall prognosis is excellent: in one series, 93 percent of the patients were free of disease on follow-up, and there was not a single instance of distant metastases (138). However, rare examples of these tumors metastasizing through the bloodstream and resulting in fatalities are on record (133,162,171).

Encapsulated Variant

One of the most distinctive features of papillary carcinoma is its capacity to invade the surrounding gland. In most cases, the interface between the tumor periphery and the normal tissue is irregular and completely devoid of a capsule. In others, there is focal evidence of capsular formation, but this is associated with areas of obvious invasion. However, a type of papillary carcinoma exists that is totally surrounded by a fibrous capsule that may be intact or focally infiltrated by tumor growth (pl. XIII). This type, designated the encapsulated variant of papillary carcinoma, comprises about 10 percent of all cases of papillary carcinoma (135,138,149,167). In the past, tumors with these features were sometimes designated *papillary adenomas* (159). The fact that they have been found associated with cervical lymph node metastases in over 25 percent of the cases is enough evidence that these lesions should be regarded as malignant (135,138, 142,167). The main differential diagnosis is with follicular adenoma with papillary hyperplasia, discussed on page 40. The main point to remember is that for a lesion to qualify as encapsulated papillary carcinoma, it should have the typical architecture and, most important, the nuclear changes of this tumor type (fig. 97). When thus defined, encapsulated papillary carcinoma has an excellent prognosis. As mentioned, regional nodal metastases may be present, but blood-borne metastases are rare, and the survival rate is nearly 100 percent (142,167).

Follicular Variant

This designation is given to papillary carcinomas with an exclusively or almost exclusively follicular pattern of growth (140,156,164). This lesion represents the extreme expression of the fact that papillary carcinomas are formed by papillae and follicles and that the latter may predominate over the former (158,173). This variant shares many features with conventional papillary carcinoma: capsule formation is usually absent or incomplete, fibrous septa are common and sometimes extensive, and scattered psammoma bodies may be found in the interfollicular stroma (fig. 98). The follicles themselves offer many clues. Some are markedly elongated, resembling tubular glands, whereas others exhibit irregularities of their lining epithelium, with formations of folds, ridges, buds, and other intraluminal protrusions that probably represent rudimentary attempts to form papillae. On occasion, the neoplastic follicles are very large, the appearance thus simulating that of nodular hyperplasia (fig. 99). This has been referred to as the *macrofollicular variant* of papillary carcinoma (132). Regardless of follicle size, the nuclei of the lining cells have features analogous to those of conventional papillary carcinoma (see page 72) (figs. 100, 101). These features can also be appreciated in fine-needle aspiration specimens (fig. 102). In rare instances, the cytoplasm may exhibit oncocytic features locally (fig. 103). The colloid within the lumina of the neoplastic follicles often has a strong and homogeneous eosinophilic quality and a scalloped configuration, the latter being similar to that seen in markedly hyperplastic glands (fig. 100). We have seen a case with crystalloid material in the follicular lumina (fig. 104), and a similar finding has been reported in a case of the same tumor type developing in struma ovarii (163).

Careful search for papillae usually demonstrates a few scattered representatives. It has been suggested that if these tumors were to be exhaustively sampled, all of them would be found to contain foci of clear-cut papillary configuration. This might be true, but it is important to remember that identification of papillae is not a requisite for the diagnosis of this variant; as a matter of fact, if

PLATE XIII

ENCAPSULATED PAPILLARY CARCINOMA

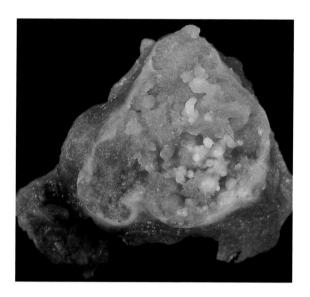

A. The tumor is surrounded by an irregular but complete fibrous capsule. The papillary formations are evident at the gross level.

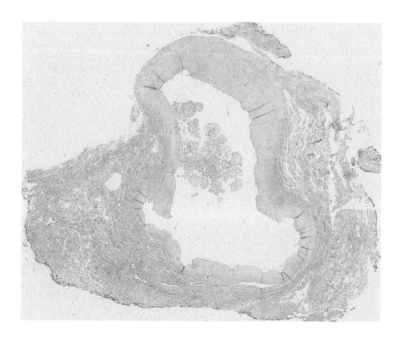

B. At low magnification, the capsule of this tumor, which is very thick, has not been violated by tumor growth. Papillary formations are present within, with most of the tumor having undergone cystic degeneration.

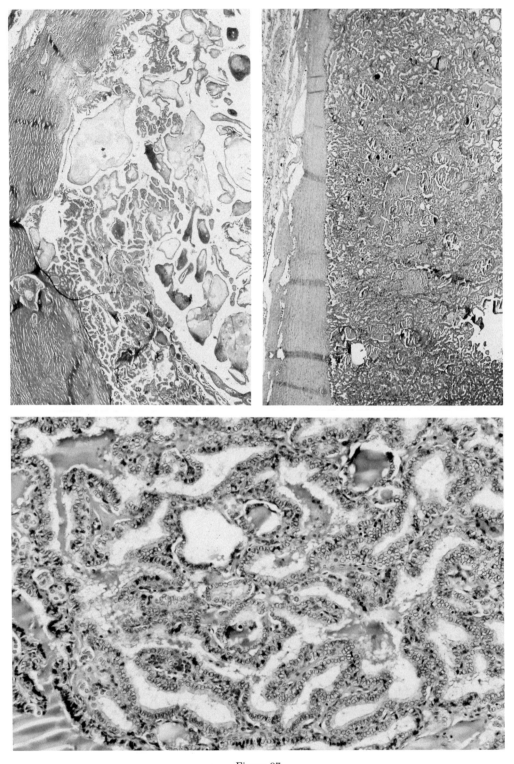

Figure 97
ENCAPSULATED PAPILLARY CARCINOMA
The tumor on the top left has a typical papillary appearance, whereas that on the right shows a combination of papillary and follicular structures, as seen on high magnification in the bottom photograph.

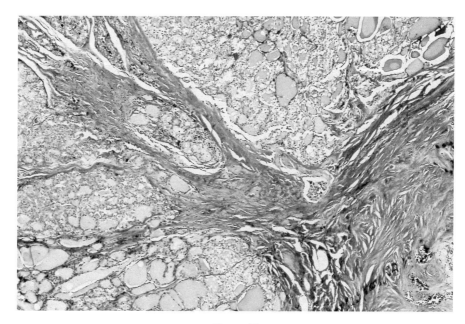

Figure 98
PAPILLARY CARCINOMA, FOLLICULAR VARIANT
The wide, fibrous bands incompletely dividing the tumor into lobules are characteristic of this tumor type.

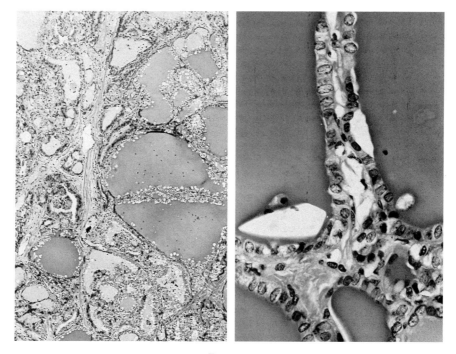

Figure 99
LARGE (MACROFOLLICULAR) FORMATIONS IN THE FOLLICULAR
VARIANT OF PAPILLARY CARCINOMA
This pattern can be easily confused with that of nodular hyperplasia. The figure on the right is a high magnification of one of the macrofollicles, showing the ground-glass nuclear features of the lining epithelium.

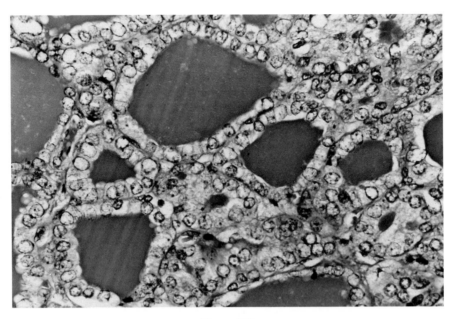

Figure 100
PAPILLARY CARCINOMA, FOLLICULAR VARIANT
The nuclei have the characteristic ground-glass overlapping quality. The cytoplasm is clear,
and the intraluminal colloid has a homogeneous acidophilic staining quality.

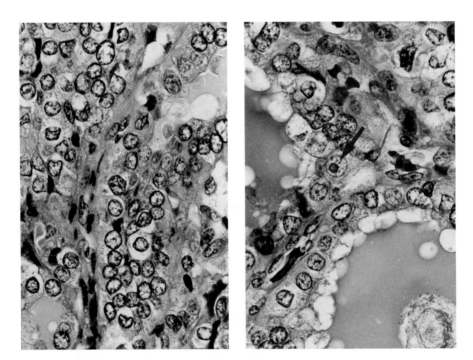

Figure 101
PAPILLARY CARCINOMA, FOLLICULAR VARIANT
The nuclear features of a cell from the follicular variant of papillary carcinoma can be seen
on high-power examination. Many of the nuclei have an empty appearance and an overlapping
quality. A nuclear pseudoinclusion is present (arrow).

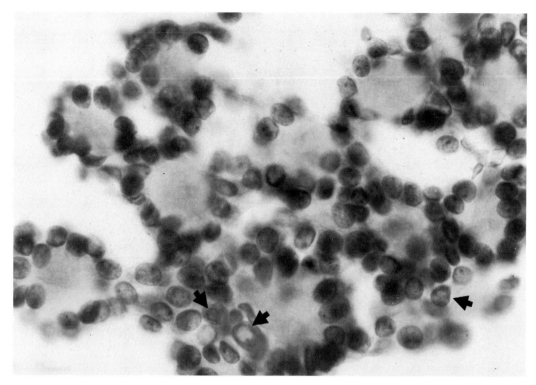

Figure 102
PAPILLARY CARCINOMA, FOLLICULAR VARIANT
The nuclei seen in this fine-needle preparation specimen have powdery chromatin and nuclear pseudoinclusions (arrows). The colloid within the follicles is dense. Papanicolaou preparation. X611. (Fig. 8.31 from Kini SR. Thyroid. In: Kline TS, ed. Guides to clinical aspiration biopsy; Vol 3.New York: Igaku-Shoin, 1987.)

papillae are easily found, the tumor should not be placed within the follicular variant.

Support for the interpretation that this tumor belongs to the papillary family of thyroid neoplasms comes from several sources. 1) Some of these tumors have multicentric foci within the thyroid that have a conventional papillary appearance (164). 2) The natural history of these tumors matches that of conventional papillary carcinoma in practically all regards, particularly in regard to the high incidence of cervical lymph node involvement (138,143). 3) These nodal metastases often have a papillary configuration (138,140). 4) The types of keratin expressed by the tumor cells match those of papillary rather than follicular carcinoma (160,174).

Sobrinho-Simões and co-workers (170) described a *diffuse form* of the follicular variant of papillary carcinoma, characterized by diffuse involvement of the whole thyroid (usually without formation of grossly discernible nodules) and

aggressive behavior, mainly manifested by distant metastases to lung and bone. This probably corresponds to the *widely invasive form* of the macrofollicular variant described by Albores-Saavedra and co-workers (132).

Encapsulated Follicular Variant and Related Lesions

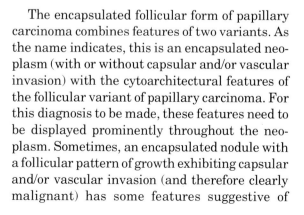

The encapsulated follicular form of papillary carcinoma combines features of two variants. As the name indicates, this is an encapsulated neoplasm (with or without capsular and/or vascular invasion) with the cytoarchitectural features of the follicular variant of papillary carcinoma. For this diagnosis to be made, these features need to be displayed prominently throughout the neoplasm. Sometimes, an encapsulated nodule with a follicular pattern of growth exhibiting capsular and/or vascular invasion (and therefore clearly malignant) has some features suggestive of

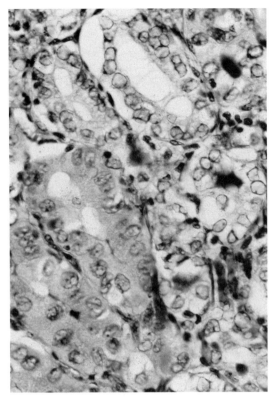

Figure 103

PAPILLARY CARCINOMA, FOLLICULAR VARIANT

Some of the neoplastic follicles are lined by granular acidophilic cells.

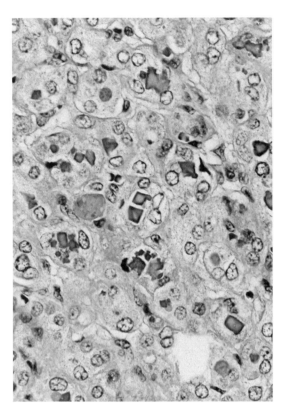

Figure 104

PAPILLARY CARCINOMA, FOLLICULAR VARIANT

Some of the intraluminal colloid in this example has a crystalloid appearance. This finding is unusual.

papillary carcinoma (e.g., vesicular nuclei or darkly staining colloid) but lacks others. In such instances, assignment to a follicular versus papillary carcinoma category becomes extremely subjective and probably unwarranted. It may be appropriate to simply designate such tumors *well-differentiated carcinoma, not otherwise specified* without trying to push them artificially into one category or another.

A related and equally difficult diagnostic dilemma arises when some of the cytologic and/or architectural features of papillary carcinoma are found *focally* within a lesion that otherwise appears to be a benign follicular lesion, i.e., a hyperplastic nodule or a follicular adenoma. Closer examination of the process may allow it to be placed into one of the following three categories:

- A focus of *typical* papillary carcinoma (usually of the follicular variant rather than the conventional type) merging with areas that greatly resemble a hyperplastic nodule but in which high magnification reveals numerous foci of transition and the presence in some of the benign-looking follicles with nuclear features similar to those in the more typical foci (figs. 105, 106). This is to be interpreted as an extreme variation of the follicular variant of papillary carcinoma, in which the tumor resembles a hyperplastic nodule (because of the large size of some follicles) more than an adenoma (132,158). As such, it is equivalent to the macrofollicular variant of follicular adenoma, as previously discussed (see page 22).

- A focus of *typical* papillary carcinoma (usually of the conventional but sometimes of the follicular variant type) within a lesion that appears otherwise benign, with no areas of transition between them. This rare phenomenon could be interpreted as a papillary carcinoma arising in either a hyperplastic nodule or a follicular adenoma (figs. 107, 108) (158).

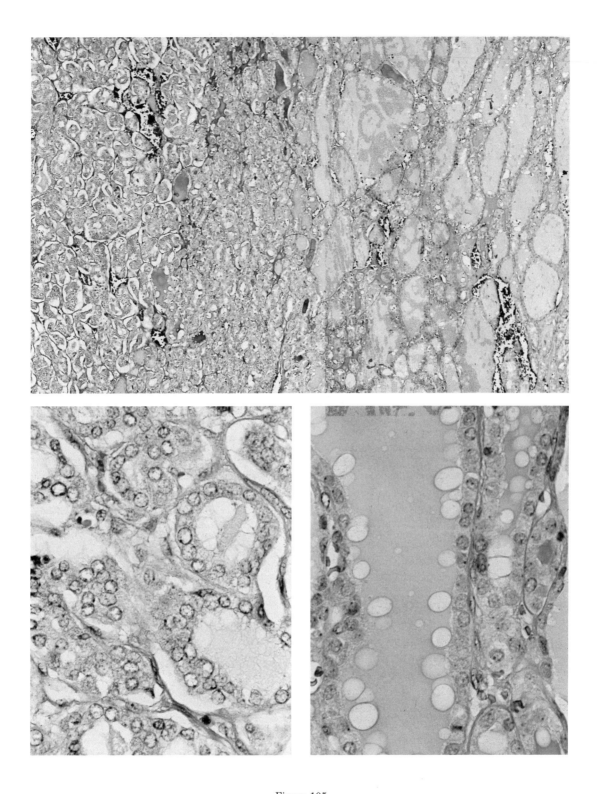

Figure 105
PAPILLARY CARCINOMA, FOLLICULAR VARIANT
This illustration shows an admixture of micro- and macrofollicular patterns in the follicular variant of papillary carcinoma. The nuclear features are similar in both components, as seen in the two bottom photographs.

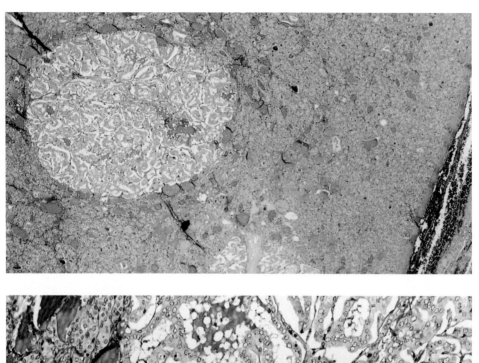

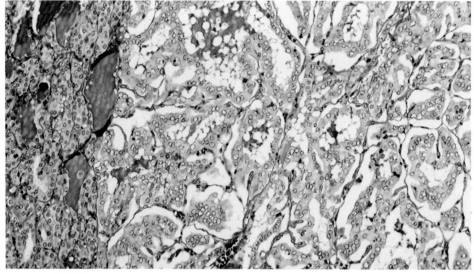

Figure 106
PAPILLARY CARCINOMA DEVELOPING IN A FOLLICULAR ADENOMA
The malignant component has a predominantly follicular appearance, as seen in the bottom
photograph, which is at the junction of the two components.

• A lesion with the features of a hyperplastic nodule or an adenoma in which occasional follicles are lined by follicular cells with vesicular nuclei, some of which may approach a ground-glass appearance. If no supporting morphologic features for papillary carcinoma exist (e.g., tubular follicles, abortive papillae, or darkly staining colloid), these nuclear changes should not be regarded as sufficient for a diagnosis of malignancy.

The distinction between these three situations (admitting that they are indeed pathogenetically distinct, which may not necessarily be the case) is not always possible. Table 1 is an attempt to enumerate the list of possibilities involving encapsulated well-differentiated thyroid lesions with a predominant or exclusively follicular pattern of growth. Fortunately, the practical implications of the differential diagnosis in this field are relatively minor, because the

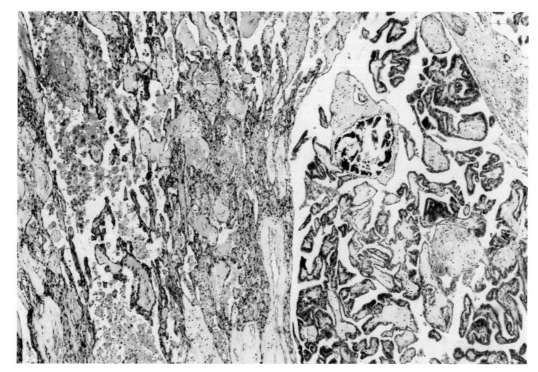

Figure 107
PAPILLARY CARCINOMA DEVELOPING IN A FOLLICULAR ADENOMA
In this instance, the malignant component has a typical papillary configuration.

outcome is likely to be favorable for all of them. Thus, a conservative diagnostic attitude and, even more important, a conservative therapeutic approach are warranted.

Solid/Trabecular Variant

It is not unusual for papillary carcinoma to exhibit foci of solid and/or trabecular growth (see fig. 68). The phenomenon seems to be more common in pediatric tumors, in the diffuse sclerosing variant, and in the papillary microcarcinoma type. The term *solid/trabecular variant* should be used when all or nearly all of a tumor not belonging to any of the other variants has a solid and/or trabecular appearance. When thus defined, this variant is rare; however, it is important to be aware of its existence to not overdiagnose it as poorly differentiated or undifferentiated. Diagnostic clues include the presence of irregular fibrous trabeculae within the tumor, an occasional psammoma body, and clusters of lymphocytes in or around the tumor. An absolute requirement for the diagnosis of this

variant is that the typical nuclear features of papillary carcinoma must be retained. When this is the case, the tumor behavior will not be significantly different from that of the conventional type of papillary carcinoma.

Diffuse Sclerosing Variant

This variant, originally proposed by Vickery and coworkers (173), is characterized by the following features: 1) diffuse involvement of one or (more commonly) both lobes; 2) numerous small papillary formations located within intrathyroidal cleft-like spaces, probably representing lymph vessels; 3) extensive squamous metaplasia; 4) a large number of psammoma bodies; 5) marked lymphocytic infiltration; and 6) prominent fibrosis (pl. XIV; figs. 109–112).

Of all these features, the widespread lymphatic permeation is the most important because it probably conditions the other morphologic findings and tumor behavior. Other features of the tumor are analogous to those of conventional papillary carcinoma. These include the presence, in

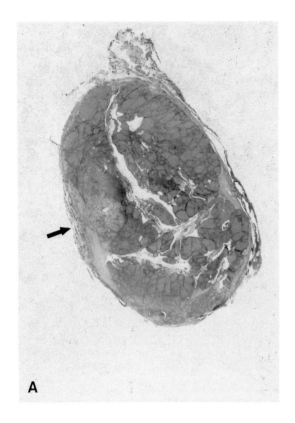

A

Figure 108

FOLLICULAR VARIANT OF PAPILLARY CARCINOMA DEVELOPING FOCALLY IN A FOLLICULAR ADENOMA

The malignant component, which is very small, is associated with marked thickening of the capsule (arrow) (A). High power view of the carcinoma in an area of capsular invasion (B). High power view of the follicular adenoma (C).

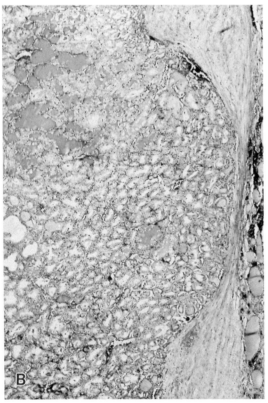

B

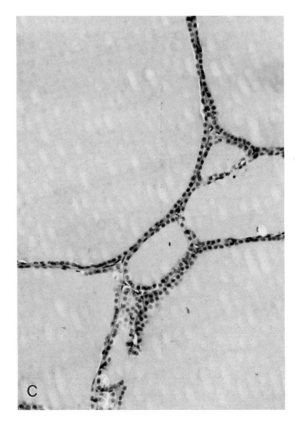

C

Table 1

DIFFERENTIAL DIAGNOSIS OF ENCAPSULATED THYROID LESIONS WITH A PREDOMINANTLY OR EXCLUSIVELY FOLLICULAR PATTERN OF GROWTH

Capsular and/or Vascular Invasion	Cytoarchitectural Features of Papillary Carcinoma, Follicular Variant		Terminology
PRESENT	Absent		Well-differentiated carcinoma, follicular type
	Imperfectly developed		Well-differentiated carcinoma, NOS
	Well developed, widespread		Well-differentiated carcinoma, papillary type (encapsulated follicular variant)
ABSENT	Absent		Follicular adenoma
	Imperfectly developed		Follicular adenoma
	Well developed, widespread		Well-differentiated carcinoma, papillary type (encapsulated follicular variant)
	Well developed, focal	Rest of nodule showing similar features on closer inspection	Well-differentiated carcinoma, papillary type (encapsulated follicular variant)
		Rest of nodule perfectly benign	Follicular adenoma with focal well-differentiated carcinoma, papillary type (follicular variant)*

*This type is exceptionally rare. A somewhat more common situation is that in which the focal carcinoma in the benign follicular nodule has a typical papillary configuration.

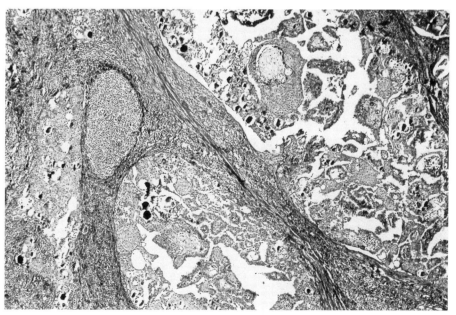

Figure 109
PAPILLARY CARCINOMA, DIFFUSE SCLEROSING VARIANT
Note the dense fibrosis, heavy lymphocytic infiltration, formation of germinal centers, and widespread growth of tumor with numerous psammoma bodies.

PLATE XIV

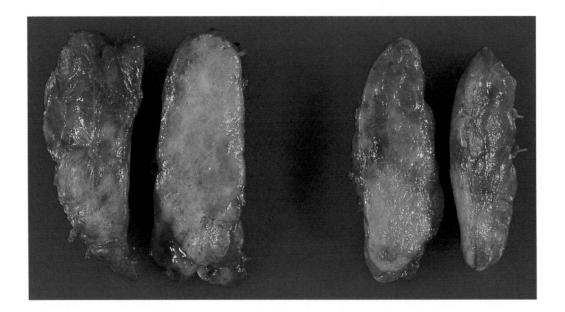

PAPILLARY CARCINOMA, DIFFUSE SCLEROSING VARIANT
The outer aspect and cut surface of both thyroid lobes in this illustration are involved by papillary carcinoma of the diffuse sclerosing variant. The diffuse pattern of growth and the fibrosing features are evident throughout.

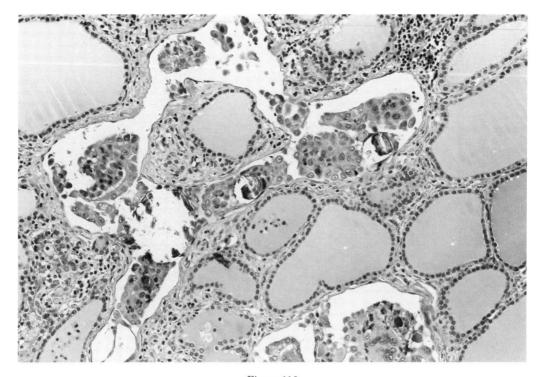

Figure 110
PAPILLARY CARCINOMA, DIFFUSE SCLEROSING VARIANT
This tumor is growing within endothelium-lined spaces and is associated with psammoma body formation and fibrosis.

Figure 111
PAPILLARY CARCINOMA, DIFFUSE
SCLEROSING VARIANT

The tumor cells, which are located within an endo-thelium-lined space, show squamoid features and psam-moma body formation. Extensive fibrosis and inflamma-tion are seen outside the tumor nest.

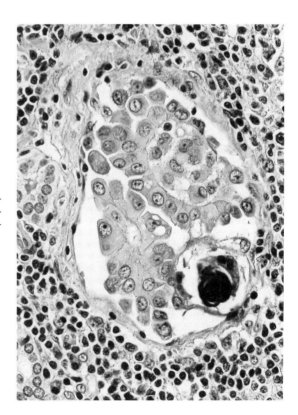

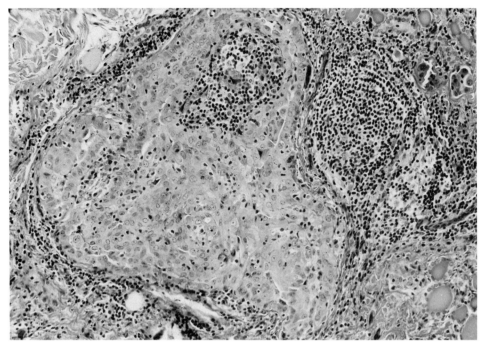

Figure 112
PAPILLARY CARCINOMA, DIFFUSE SCLEROSING VARIANT
In this area, the tumor has a predominantly solid pattern of growth and is associated with lymphocytic infiltration.

some cases, of dense accumulations of S-100 protein–positive cells in the stroma (147,166).

When compared with conventional papillary carcinoma, this variant exhibits: 1) similar prevalence in women, 2) greater incidence of cervical lymph node involvement, 3) greater incidence of pulmonary metastases, and 4) lesser probability of disease-free survival on follow-up.

An interesting clinical observation is that there is often a delay in diagnosis, probably explainable by the fact that the diffuse glandular enlargement simulates thyroiditis clinically and on thyroid scan (137). It is also interesting that, despite the high incidence of pulmonary metastases, the tumor death rate is extremely low (137,139,145,161, 166,168). It is possible that the young age of most patients with this variant counterbalances the adverse clinical significance of the other findings (145).

In one series, a "dominant" tumor nodule was found in over half of the cases (137). This finding may indicate that this variant, like its conventional counterpart, begins as a single tumor mass and that its subsequent configuration is the result of an early widespread permeation of intrathyroid lymph vessels, as originally proposed by Lindsay (156). In regard to therapy, the clinicopathologic features of this variant would seem to fully justify the performance of a total or near-total thyroidectomy followed by the administration of radioactive iodine.

Tall and Columnar Cell Variants

Hawk and Hazard (149) first proposed the existence of the tall cell variant of papillary carcinoma and found that it made up about 10 percent of all cases in their material. According to these authors, this variant tends to occur in older patients and be large (usually >5 cm). Extrathyroid extension is frequent, and there is a greater incidence of vascular invasion. The papillae, which are well formed, are covered by cells that are twice as tall as they are wide (fig. 113) (172). These cells often have a rather abundant acidophilic (pink) cytoplasm that approaches but does not attain the appearance of oncocytes (fig. 113, *inset*). Mitotic figures can be found easily (in striking contrast to conventional papillary carcinoma), and the nuclei are normo- or

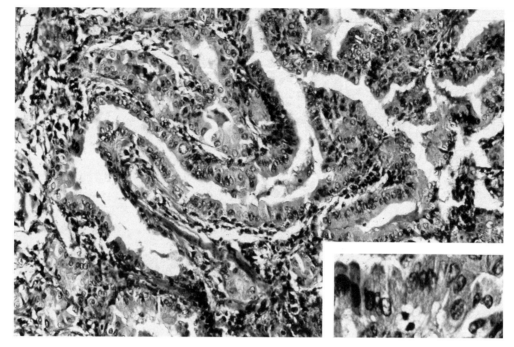

Figure 113
PAPILLARY CARCINOMA, TALL CELL VARIANT
The tumor cells are twice as tall as they are wide. Their cytoplasm is abundant, and has an acidophilic staining quality, seen better in the inset.

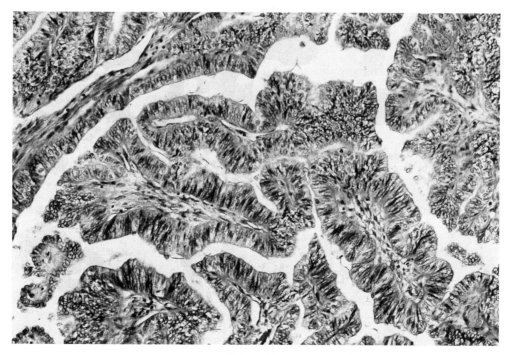

Figure 114
PAPILLARY CARCINOMA, COLUMNAR CELL VARIANT
The tumor cells have a columnar shape, and there is striking stratification of nuclei.

hyperchromatic (173). However, Flint and co-workers (144) found no difference in DNA content, chromatin texture, or nuclear size or shape between tall cell variant and conventional papillary carcinomas. The behavior of the tall cell variant of papillary carcinoma is more aggressive than that of the conventional form; the mortality rate was 25 percent in the series of Hawk and Hazard (149). Because several unfavorable features converge on this variant (e.g., advanced age, large tumor size, and mitotic activity), it is not easy to discern how much each of them contributes to this worsened outlook (153).

Columnar cell carcinoma differs from both the conventional and the tall cell forms of papillary carcinoma because of the presence of prominent nuclear stratification (fig. 114). In addition, the nuclei may lack the typical features of papillary carcinoma (141,169). LiVolsi (157) commented on the fact that the cytoplasm tends to be very clear, to the point of exhibiting subnuclear vacuolation resembling that seen in secretory endo-metrium. The few reported cases have run an aggressive clinical course. It is not clear what the relationship is between the tall and the columnar variants. However, it is interesting that a case combining features of both types has been reported (131), and we have seen similar examples.

The suggestion that P-glycoprotein (the central mediator of in vitro tumor multidrug resistance) is hyperexpressed in the tall cell variant of papillary carcinoma has been advanced by Axiotis and coworkers (134), but others have found common expression of this marker both in benign and malignant conditions (157a).

Two other variants, oncocytic papillary tumors and papillary carcinoma with clear cell changes, (the latter being an inconsequential morphologic variation of papillary carcinoma), are discussed in the chapters on Tumors with Oncocytic Features and Tumors with Clear Cell Features, respectively.

REFERENCES

Papillary Carcinoma

1. Albores-Saavedra J, Altamirano-Dimas M, Alcorta-Anguizola B, Smith M. Fine structure of human papillary thyroid carcinoma. Cancer 1971;28:763–74.
2. _____, Duràn ME. Association of thyroid carcinoma and chemodectoma. Am J Surg 1968;116: 887–90.
3. Antonini P, Venuat AM, Linares G, Caillou B, Berger R, Parmentier C. A translocation (7;10)(q35:q21) in a differentiated papillary carcinoma of the thyroid. Cancer Genet Cytogenet 1989;41:139–44.
4. Bäckdahl M. Nuclear DNA content and prognosis in papillary, follicular and medullary carcinomas of the thyroid [Dissertation]. Stockholm, Sweden: Karolinska Medical Institute, 1985.
5. Bakri K, Shimaoka K, Rao U, Tsukada Y. Adenosquamous carcinoma of the thyroid after radiotherapy for Hodgkin's disease. A case report and review. Cancer 1983;52:465–70.
6. Beaumont A, Ben Othman S, Fragu P. The fine structure of papillary carcinoma of the thyroid. Histopathology 1981;5:377–88.
7. Block MA, Miller MJ, Horn RC Jr. Carcinoma of the thyroid after external radiation to the neck in adults. Am J Surg 1969;118:764–9.
8. Bondeson L, Bengtsson A, Bondeson A-G, et al. Chromosome studies in thyroid neoplasia. Cancer 1989; 64:680–5.
9. Bongarzone I, Pierotti MA, Monzini N, et al. High frequency of activation of tyrosine kinase oncogenes in human papillary thyroid carcinoma. Oncogene 1989;4: 1457–62.
10. Buley ID, Gatter KC, Heryet A, Mason DY. Expression of intermediate filament proteins in normal and diseased thyroid glands. J Clin Pathol 1987;40:136–42.
10a. Burns JS, Shaw J, Williams ED, Wynford-Thomas D. Multiple phenotypes induced by mutant Ha-ras in thyroid epithelial cells: Correlation with level of expression. Cardiff CF4 4XN, UK: CRC Thyroid Tumor Biology Research Group, Department of Pathology, University of Wales College of Medicine, 1992.
11. Cady B, Sedgwick CE, Meissner WA, Bookwalter JR, Romagosa V, Werber J. Changing clinical, pathologic, therapeutic, and survival patterns in differentiated thyroid carcinoma. Ann Surg 1976;184:541–53.
12. _____, Sedgwick CE, Meissner WA, Wool MS, Salzman FA, Werber J. Risk factor analysis in differentiated thyroid cancer. Cancer 1979;43:810–20.
13. Calandra DB, Shah KH, Lawrence AM, Paloyan E. Total thyroidectomy in irradiated patients. A twenty-year experience in 206 patients. Ann Surg 1985;202: 356–60.
14. Carcangiu ML, Zampi G, Pupi A, Castagnoli A, Rosai J. Papillary carcinoma of the thyroid. A clinicopathologic study of 241 cases treated at the University of Florence, Italy. Cancer 1985;55:805–28.
15. _____, Zampi G, Rosai J. Papillary thyroid carcinoma: a study of its many morphologic expressions and clinical correlates. Pathol Annu 1985;20(Pt. 1):1–44.

16. Chan JK. Papillary carcinoma of thyroid: classical and variants. Histol Histopathol 1990;5:241–57.
17. _____, Carcangiu ML, Rosai J. Papillary carcinoma of thyroid with exuberant nodular fasciitis-like stroma. Report of three cases. Am J Clin Pathol 1991;95:309–14.
18. _____, Loo KT. Cribriform variant of papillary thyroid carcinoma. Arch Pathol Lab Med 1990;114:622–4.
19. _____, Saw D. The grooved nucleus. A useful diagnostic criterion of papillary carcinoma of the thyroid. Am J Surg Pathol 1986;10:672–9.
20. _____, Tse CC. Mucin production in metastatic papillary carcinoma of the thyroid. Hum Pathol 1988;19:195–200.
21. Charbord P, L'Heritier C, Cukersztein W, Lumbroso J, Tubiana M. Radioiodine treatment in differentiated thyroid carcinomas. Treatment of first local recurrences and of bone and lung metastases. Ann Radiol (Paris) 1977;20:783–6.
22. Chesky VE, Hellwig CA, Welch JW. Cancer of the thyroid associated with Hashimoto's disease: an analysis of forty-eight cases. Am Surg 1962;28:678–85.
23. Christ ML, Haja J. Intranuclear cytoplasmic inclusions (invaginations) in thyroid aspirations. Frequency and specificity. Acta Cytol 1979;23:327–31.
24. Clark OH. Total thyroidectomy: the treatment of choice for patients with differentiated thyroid cancer. Ann Surg 1982;196:361–70.
25. Cody HS III, Shah JP. Locally invasive, well-differentiated thyroid cancer. 22 years' experience at Memorial Sloan-Kettering Cancer Center. Am J Surg 1981;142:480–3.
26. Cohn KH, Bäckdahl M, Forsslund G, et al. Biologic considerations and operative strategy in papillary thyroid carcinoma: arguments against the routine performance of total thyroidectomy. Surgery 1984;96:957–71.
27. _____, Bäckdahl M, Forsslund G, et al. Prognostic value of nuclear DNA content in papillary thyroid carcinoma. World J Surg 1984;8:474–80.
28. Crile G Jr. Changing end results in patients with papillary carcinoma of the thyroid. Surg Gynecol Obstet 1971;132:460–8.
29. _____, Antunez AR, Esselstyn CB Jr, Hawk WA, Skillern PG. The advantages of subtotal thyroidectomy and suppression of TSH in the primary treatment of papillary carcinoma of the thyroid. Cancer 1985;55:2691–7.
30. Crile G, Hazard JB. Relationship of the age of the patient to the natural history and prognosis of carcinoma of the thyroid. Ann Surg 1953;138:33–8.
30a. Deligeorgi-Politi H. Nuclear crease as a cytodiagnostic feature of papillary thyroid carcinoma in fine-needle aspiration biopsies. Diagn Cytopathol 1987;3:307–10.
31. Diaz NM, Mazoujian G, Wick MR. Estrogen-receptor protein in thyroid neoplasms: An immunohistochemical analysis of papillary carcinoma, follicular carcinoma, and follicular adenoma. Arch Pathol Lab Med 1991;115:1203–7.
32. Donghi R, Sozzi G, Pierotti MA, et al. The oncogene associated with human papillary thyroid carcinoma (PTC) is assigned to chromosome 10 q11-q12 in the same region as multiple endocrine neoplasia type 2A (MEN2A). Oncogene 1989;4:521–3.
33. Doniach I. Aetiologic consideration of thyroid carcinoma. In: Smithers DW, ed. Tumours of the thyroid gland. Edinburgh: Churchill Livingstone, 1970:66–7.
34. Farbota LM, Calandra DB, Lawrence AM, Paloyan E. Thyroid carcinoma in Graves' disease. Surgery 1985;98:1148–52.
35. Filetti S, Belfiore A, Amir SM, et al. The role of thyroid-stimulating antibodies of Graves' disease in differentiated thyroid cancer. N Engl J Med 1988;318:753–9.
36. Franssila KO. Is the differentiation between papillary and follicular thyroid carcinoma valid? Cancer 1973;32:853–64.
37. Frauenhoffer CM, Patchefsky AS, Cobanoglu A. Thyroid carcinoma: a clinical and pathologic study of 125 cases. Cancer 1979;43:2414–21.
38. Frauman AG, Moses AC. Oncogenes and growth factors in thyroid carcinogenesis. Endocrinol Metab Clin North Am 1990;19:479–93.
39. Frazell EL, Foote FW Jr. Papillary thyroid carcinoma. Pathological findings in cases with and without clinical evidence of cervical node involvement. Cancer 1955;8:1165–6.
40. Fusco A, Grieco M, Santoro M, et al. A new oncogene in human thyroid papillary carcinomas and their lymphnodal metastases. Nature 1987;328:170–2.
41. Goellner JR, Johnson DA. Cytology of cystic papillary carcinoma of the thyroid. Acta Cytol 1982;26:797–9.
42. Gray A, Doniach I. Morphology of the nuclei of papillary carcinoma of the thyroid. Br J Cancer 1969;23:49–51.
43. Grieco M, Santoro M, Berlingieri MT, et al. PTC is a novel rearranged form of the *ret* proto-oncogene and is frequently detected in vivo in human thyroid papillary carcinomas. Cell 1990;60:557–63.
44. Hale RJ, Merchant W, Hasleton PS. Polypoidal intra-oesophageal thyroid carcinoma: a rare cause of dysphagia. Histopathology 1990;17:475–6.
45. Hamming JF, van de Velde CJ, Goslings BM, et al. Preoperative diagnosis and treatment of metastases to the regional lymph nodes in papillary carcinoma of the thyroid gland. Surg Gynecol Obstet 1989;169:107–14.
46. Harness JK, Thompson NW, McLeod MK, Eckhauser FE, Lloyd RV. Follicular carcinoma of the thyroid gland: trends and treatment. Surgery 1984;96:972–80.
47. _____, Thompson NW, Sisson JC, Beierwaltes WH. Differentiated thyroid carcinomas. Treatment of distant metastases. Arch Surg 1974;108:410–9.
48. Hawk WA, Hazard JB. The many appearances of papillary carcinoma of the thyroid. Cleve Clin Q 1976;43:207–16.
49. Hawkins MM, Kingston JE. Malignant thyroid tumours following childhood cancer [Letter]. Lancet 1988;2:804.
50. Hay ID. Nodal metastases from papillary thyroid carcinoma [Letter]. Lancet 1986;2:1283.
51. _____, Papillary thyroid carcinoma. Endocrinol Metab Clin North Am 1990;19:545–76.
52. Hedman I, Tisell L-E. Associated hyperparathyroidism and nonmedullary thyroid carcinoma. The etiologic role of radiation. Surgery 1984;95:392–7.
53. Hempelmann LH, Hall WJ, Phillips M, Cooper RA, Ames WR. Neoplasms in persons treated with x-rays in infancy: fourth survey in 20 years. J Natl Cancer Inst 1975;55:519–30.

54. Henzen-Logmans SC, Mullink H, Ramaekers FC, Tadema T, Meijer CJ. Expression of cytokeratins and vimentin in epithelial cells of normal and pathologic thyroid tissue. Virchows Arch [A] 1987;410:347–54.

55. Hernandez OL, Albores-Saavedra J, Benavides G, Krause LG, Merizaldi JC, Ginzo A. Multiple endocrine neoplasia. Am J Clin Pathol 1982;78:527–32.

55a. Hoda S. Personal communication, 1992.

56. Hofstädter F. Frequency and morphology of malignant tumors of the thyroid before and after the introduction of iodine-prophylaxis. Virchows Arch [A] 1980;385: 263–70.

57. _____, Unterkircher S. Histologische Kriterien zur Prognose der Struma maligna. Pathologe 1980; 1:79–85.

58. Hoie J, Stenwig AE, Kullmann G, Lindegaard M. Distant metastases in papillary thyroid cancer. A review of 91 patients. Cancer 1988;61:1–6.

59. Hutter RV, Frazell EL, Foote FW Jr. Elective radical neck dissection: an assessment of its use in the management of papillary thyroid cancer. Cancer 1970;20:87–93.

60. Jenkins RB, Hay ID, Herath JF, et al. Frequent occurrence of cytogenetic abnormalities in sporadic nonmedullary thyroid carcinoma. Cancer 1990;66:1213–20.

61. Joensuu H, Klemi P, Eerola E, Tuominen J. Influence of cellular DNA content on survival in differentiated thyroid cancer. Cancer 1986;58:2462–7.

62. Johannessen JV, Gould VE, Jao W. The fine structure of human thyroid cancer. Hum Pathol 1978;9:385–400.

63. _____, Sobrinho-Simões M. The origin and significance of thyroid psammoma bodies. Lab Invest 1980;43:287–96.

64. _____, Sobrinho-Simões M, Finseth I, Pilström L. Papillary carcinomas of the thyroid have pore-deficient nuclei. Int J Cancer 1982;30:409–11.

65. Johnson TL, Lloyd RV, Thor A. Expression of *ras* oncogene p21 antigen in normal and proliferative thyroid tissues. Am J Pathol 1987;127:60–5.

66. Kamma H, Fujii K, Ogata T. Lymphocytic infiltration in juvenile thyroid carcinoma. Cancer 1988;62:1988–93.

67. Kini SR. Thyroid. In: Kline TS, ed. Guides to clinical aspiration biopsy; Vol 3. New York: Igaku-Shoin, 1987: 121–87.

68. Klinck GH, Winship T. Psammoma bodies and thyroid cancer. Cancer 1959;12:656–62.

69. Lee T-K, Myers RT, Marshall RB, Bond MG, Kardon B. The significance of mitotic rate: a retrospective study of 127 thyroid carcinomas. Hum Pathol 1985;16:1042–6.

70. Lever EG, Refetoff S, Straus FH II, Nguyen M, Kaplan EL. Coexisting thyroid and parathyroid disease—are they related? Surgery 1983;94:893–900.

71. Lew W, Orell S, Henderson DW. Intranuclear vacuoles in nonpapillary carcinoma of the thyroid. A report of three cases. Acta Cytol 1984;28:581–6.

72. Lieberman PH, Foote FW Jr, Schottenfeld D. A study of the pathology of thyroid cancer, 1930-1960. Clin Bull (MSKCC) 1972;2:7–12.

73. Lindsay S. Carcinoma of the thyroid gland. A clinical and pathologic study of 293 patients at the University of California Hospital. Springfield, IL: Charles C. Thomas, 1960.

73a. LiVolsi V. Papillary neoplasms of the thyroid. Pathologic and prognostic features. Am J Clin Pathol 1992;97:426–34.

74. Lote K, Andersen K, Nordal E, Brennhovd IO. Familial occurrence of papillary thyroid carcinoma. Cancer 1980;46:1291–7.

75. Maheshwari YK, Hill CS Jr, Haynie TP III, Hickey RC, Samaan NA. I-131 therapy in differentiated thyroid carcinoma: M.D. Anderson Hospital experience. Cancer 1981;47:664–71.

76. Mazzaferri EL. Papillary thyroid carcinoma: factors influencing prognosis and current therapy. Semin Oncol 1987;14:315–32.

77. _____, Young RL. Papillary thyroid carcinoma: a 10 year follow-up report of the impact of therapy in 576 patients. Am J Med 1981;70: 511–8.

78. _____, Young RL, Oertel JE, Kemmerer WT, Page CP. Papillary thyroid carcinoma: the impact of therapy in 576 patients. Medicine (Baltimore) 1977;56:171–96.

79. McConahey WM, Hay ID, Woolner LB, van Heerden JA, Taylor WF. Papillary thyroid cancer treated at the Mayo Clinic, 1946 through 1970: initial manifestations, pathologic findings, therapy, and outcome. Mayo Clin Proc 1986;61:978–96.

80. McCormack KR. Bone metastases from thyroid carcinoma. Cancer 1966;19:181–4.

81. McDougall IR. Coleman CN, Burke JS, Saunders W, Kaplan HS. Thyroid carcinoma after high-dose external radiotherapy for Hodgkin's disease: report of three cases. Cancer 1980;45:2056–60.

82. Meissner WA, Adler A. Papillary carcinoma of the thyroid: a study of the pathology of two hundred twenty-six cases. Arch Pathol 1958;66:518–25.

83. Miller M, Chodos RB, Olen E, Klinck GH. Thyroid carcinoma occurring in Graves' disease. Arch Intern Med 1966;117:432–5.

84. Mills SE, Allen MS Jr. Congenital occult papillary carcinoma of the thyroid gland. Hum Pathol 1986;17: 1179–81.

85. Mizukami Y, Nonomura A, Hashimoto T, et al. Immunohistochemical demonstration of ras p21 oncogene product in normal, benign, and malignant human thyroid tissues. Cancer 1988;61:873–80.

86. _____, Nonomura A, Hashimoto T, et al. Immunohistochemical demonstration of epidermal growth factor and c-myc oncogene product in normal, benign, and malignant thyroid tissues. Histopathology 1991; 18:11–8.

86a. _____, Nonomura A, Matsubara F, Michigishi T, Ohmura K, Hashimoto T. Papillary carcinoma of the thyroid gland with fibromatosis-like stroma. Histopathology 1992;20:355–7.

86b. _____, Noguchi M, , Michigishi T, et al. Papillary thyroid carcinoma in Kanazawa, Japan: prognostic significance of histological subtypes. Histopathology 1992;20:243–50.

87. Narita T, Takagi K. Ataxia-telangiectasia with dysgerminoma of right ovary, papillary carcinoma of thyroid, and adenocarcinoma of pancreas. Cancer 1984;54:1113–6.

88. Noguchi M, Kumaki T, Taniya T, Miyazaki I. Bilateral cervical lymph node metastases in well-differentiated thyroid cancer. Arch Surg 1990;125:804–6.

89. Noguchi S, Murakami N. The value of lymph-node dissection in patients with differentiated thyroid cancer. Surg Clin North Am 1987;67:251–61.

90. Ostrowski MA, Asa SL, Chamberlain D, Moffat FL, Rotstein LE. Myxomatous change in papillary carcinoma of the thyroid. Surg Pathol 1989;2:249–56.

91. Ott RA, Calandra DB, McCall A, Shah KH, Lawrence AM, Paloyan E. The incidence of thyroid carcinoma in patients with Hashimoto's thyroiditis and solitary cold nodules. Surgery 1985;98:1202–6.

92. Patchefsky AS, Hoch WS. Psammoma bodies in diffuse toxic goiter. Am J Clin Pathol 1972;57:551–6.

93. Permanetter W, Nathrath WB, Löhrs U. Immunohistochemical analysis of thyroglobulin and keratin in benign and malignant thyroid tumours. Virchows Arch [A] 1982;398:221–8.

94. Plail RO, Bussey HJ, Glazer G, Thomson JP. Adenomatous polyposis: an association with carcinoma of the thyroid. Br J Surg 1987;74:377–80.

95. Rieger R, Pimpl W, Money S, Rettenbacher L, Galvan G. Hyperthyroidism and concurrent thyroid malignancies. Surgery 1989;106:6–10.

96. Russell WO, Ibanez ML, Clark RL, White EC. Thyroid carcinoma. Classification, intraglandular dissemination and clinicopathological study based upon whole organ sections of 80 glands. Cancer 1963;16:1425–60.

97. Samaan NA, Schultz PN, Haynie TP, Ordonez NG. Pulmonary metastasis of differentiated thyroid carcinoma: treatment results in 101 patients. J Clin Endocrinol Metab 1985;60:376–80.

98. _____, Schultz PN, Ordonez NG, Hickey RC, Johnston DA. A comparison of thyroid carcinoma in those who have and have not had head and neck irradiation in childhood. J Clin Endocrinol Metab 1987; 64:219–23.

99. Satoh Y, Sakamoto A, Yamada K, Kasai N. Psammoma bodies in metastatic carcinoma to the thyroid. Mod Pathol 1990;3:267–70.

100. Schelfhout LJ, Van Muijen GN, Fleuren GJ. Expression of keratin 19 distinguishes papillary thyroid carcinoma from follicular carcinomas and follicular thyroid adenoma. Am J Clin Pathol 1989;92:654–8.

101. Schindler A-M, van Melle G, Evequoz B, Scazziga B. Prognostic factors in papillary carcinoma of the thyroid. Cancer 1991;68:324–30.

102. Schlumberger M, Tubiana M, De Vathaire F, et al. Long-term results of treatment of 283 patients with lung and bone metastases from differentiated thyroid carcinoma. J Clin Endocrinol Metab 1986;63: 960–7.

103. Schneider AB, Pinsky S, Bekerman C, Ryo UY. Characteristics of 108 thyroid cancers detected by screening in a population with a history of head and neck irradiation. Cancer 1980;46:1218–27.

104. Schroder DM, Chambors A, France CJ. Operative strategy for thyroid cancer. Is total thyroidectomy worth the price? Cancer 1986;58:2320–8.

105. Schröder S, Schwarz W, Rehpenning W, Löning T, Böcker W. Dendritic/Langerhans cells and prognosis in patients with papillary thyroid carcinomas. Immunocytochemical study of 106 thyroid neoplasms correlated to follow-up data. Am J Clin Pathol 1988;89:295–300.

106. Segal K, Ben-Bassat M, Avraham A, Har-El G, Sidi J. Hashimoto's thyroiditis and carcinoma of the thyroid gland. Int Surg 1985;70:205–9.

107. Selzer G, Kahn LB, Albertyn L. Primary malignant tumors of the thyroid gland: a clinicopathologic study of 254 cases. Cancer 1977;40:1501–10.

108. Shapiro SJ, Friedman NB, Perzik SL, Catz B. Incidence of thyroid carcinoma in Graves' disease. Cancer 1970; 26:1261–70.

109. Sierk A, Askin FB, Reddick RL, Thomas CG Jr. Pediatric thyroid cancer. Pediatr Pathol 1990;10:877–93.

110. Simpson WJ, McKinney SE, Carruthers JS, Gospodarowicz MK, Sutcliffe SB, Panzarella T. Papillary and follicular thyroid cancer. Prognostic factors in 1,578 patients. Am J Med 1987;83:479–88.

111. Smith SA, Hay ID, Goellner JR, Ryan JJ, McConahey WM. Mortality from papillary thyroid carcinoma. A case-control study of 56 lethal cases. Cancer 1988; 62:1381–8.

112. Stanta G, Carcangiu ML, Rosai J. The biochemical and immunohistochemical profile of thyroid neoplasia. Pathol Annu 1988;23(Pt. 1):129–57.

113. _____, Carcangiu ML, Rosai J, Marchesi VT. Monoclonal antibodies reveal different thyroglobulin compartmentalization in non-neoplastic thyroid and papillary thyroid carcinoma. (Submitted for publication).

114. Starnes HF, Brooks DC, Pinkus GS, Brooks JR. Surgery for thyroid carcinoma. Cancer 1985;55:1376–81.

115. Tang TT, Holcenberg JS, Duck SC, Hodach AE, Oechler HW, Camitta BM. Thyroid carcinoma following treatment for acute lymphoblastic leukemia. Cancer 1980; 46:1572–6.

116. Tscholl-Ducommun J, Hedinger CE. Papillary thyroid carcinomas. Morphology and prognosis. Virchows Arch [A] 1982;396:19–39.

117. Tsumori T, Nakao K, Miyata M, et al. Clinicopathologic study of thyroid carcinoma infiltrating the trachea. Cancer 1985;56:2843–8.

118. Vane D, King DR, Boles ET Jr. Secondary thyroid neoplasms in pediatric cancer patients: increased risk with improved survival. J Pediatr Surg 1984;19:855–60.

118a. Van Hoeven KH, Menendez-Botet CJ, Strong EW, Huvos AG. Estrogen and progesterone receptor content in human thyroid disease. Am J Clin Pathol (in press).

119. Vestfrid MA. Papillary carcinoma of the thyroid gland with lipomatous stroma: report of a peculiar histological type of thyroid tumour. Histopathology 1986;10:97–100.

120. Viale G, Dell'Orto P, Coggi G, Gambacorta M. Co-expression of cytokeratins and vimentin in normal and diseased thyroid glands. Lack of diagnostic utility of vimentin immunostaining. Am J Surg Pathol 1989; 13:1034–40.

121. Vickery AL Jr. Thyroid papillary carcinoma. Pathological and philosophical controversies. Am J Surg Pathol 1983;7:797–807.

122. _____, Wang C-A, Walker AM. Treatment of intrathyroidal papillary carcinoma of the thyroid. Cancer 1987;60:2587–95.

123. Wallace MP, Betsill WL. Papillary carcinoma of the thyroid gland seen as lateral neck cyst. Arch Otolaryngol 1984;110:408–11.

124. Williams ED, Doniach I, Bjarnason O, Michie W. Thyroid cancer in an iodine rich area: a histopathological study. Cancer 1977;39:215–22.

125. Wilson NW, Pambakian H, Richardson TC, Stokoe MR, Makin CA, Heyderman E. Epithelial markers in thyroid carcinoma: an immunoperoxidase study. Histopathology 1986;10:815–29.

126. Wilson SD, Komorowski R, Cerletty J, Majewski JT, Hooper M. Radiation-associated thyroid tumors: extent of operation and pathology technique influence the apparent incidence of carcinoma. Surgery 1983;94:663–9.

127. Woolner LB, Beahrs OH, Black BM, McConahey WM, Keating FR Jr. Classification and prognosis of thyroid carcinoma: a study of 885 cases observed in a thirty year period. Am J Surg 1961;102:354–87.

128. Wright PA, Lemoine NR, Mayall ES, et al. Papillary and follicular thyroid carcinomas show a different pattern of ras oncogene mutation. Br J Cancer 1989;60:576–7.

129. Wyllie FS, Lemoine NR, Williams ED, Wynford-Thomas D. Structure and expression of nuclear oncogenes in multi-stage thyroid tumorigenesis. Br J Cancer 1989;60:561–5.

129a. Yoshida A, Kamma H, Asaga T, Masuzawa C, Kawahara S, Mimura T, Ito K. Proliferative activity in thyroid tumors. Cancer 1992;69:2548–52.

130. Zimmerman D, Hay ID, Gough IR, et al. Papillary thyroid carcinoma in children and adults: long-term follow-up of 1039 patients conservatively treated at one institution during three decades. Surgery 1988;104: 1157–66.

Papillary Carcinoma Variants

131. Akslen LA, Varhaug JE. Thyroid carcinoma with mixed tall-cell and columnar-cell features. Am J Clin Pathol 1990;94:442–5.

132. Albores-Saavedra J, Gould E, Vardaman C, Vuitch F. The macrofollicular variant of papillary thyroid carcinoma. A study of 17 cases. Human Pathol 1991;22:1195–205.

133. Allo MD, Christianson W, Koivunen D. Not all "occult" papillary carcinomas are "minimal." Surgery 1988; 104:971–6.

134. Axiotis C, Merino MJ, Campo E, LaPorte N, Neumann R. P-glycoprotein is expressed in thyroid carcinomas but not in benign conditions [Abstract]. Lab Invest 1991;64:31A.

135. Böcker W, Schröder S, Dralle H. Minimal thyroid neoplasia. Recent Results Cancer Res 1988;106:131–8.

136. Bondeson L, Ljungberg O. Occult papillary thyroid carcinoma in the young and the aged. Cancer 1984;53: 1790–2.

137. Carcangiu ML, Bianchi S. Diffuse sclerosing variant of papillary thyroid carcinoma. Clinicopathologic study of 15 cases. Am J Surg Pathol 1989;13:1041–9.

138. _____, Zampi G, Pupi A, Castagnoli A, Rosai J. Papillary carcinoma of the thyroid. A clinicopathologic study of 241 cases treated at the University of Florence, Italy. Cancer 1985;55:805–28.

139. Chan JK, Tsui MS, Tse CH. Diffuse sclerosing variant of papillary carcinoma of the thyroid: a histological and immunohistochemical study of three cases. Histopathology 1987;11:191–201.

140. Chen KT, Rosai J. Follicular variant of thyroid papillary carcinoma: a clinicopathologic study of six cases. Am J Surg Pathol 1977;1:123–30.

141. Evans HL. Columnar-cell carcinoma of the thyroid. A report of two cases of an aggressive variant of thyroid carcinoma. Am J Clin Pathol 1986;85:77–80.

142. _____. Encapsulated papillary neoplasms of the thyroid. A study of 14 cases followed for a minimum of 10 years. Am J Surg Pathol 1987;11:592–7.

143. _____. Follicular neoplasms of the thyroid. A study of 44 cases followed for a minimum of 10 years, with emphasis on differential diagnosis. Cancer 1984;54:533–40.

144. Flint A, Davenport RD, Lloyd RV. The tall cell variant of papillary carcinoma of the thyroid gland. Comparison with the common form of papillary carcinoma by DNA and morphometric analysis. Arch Pathol Lab Med 1991;115:169–71.

145. Fujimoto Y, Obara T, Ito Y, Kodama T, Aiba M, Yamaguchi K. Diffuse sclerosing variant of papillary carcinoma of the thyroid. Cancer 1990;66:2306–12.

146. Gikas PW, Labow SS, DiGiulio W, Finger JE. Occult metastasis from occult papillary carcinoma of the thyroid. Cancer 1967;20:2100–4.

147. Gómez-Morales M, Alvaro T, Muñoz M, et al. Diffuse sclerosing papillary carcinoma of the thyroid gland: immunohistochemical analysis of the local host immune response. Histopathology 1991;18:427–33.

148. Harach HR, Franssila KO, Wasenius V-M. Occult papillary carcinoma of the thyroid. A "normal" finding in Finland. A systematic autopsy study. Cancer 1985;56:531–8.

149. Hawk WA, Hazard JB. The many appearances of papillary carcinoma of the thyroid. Comparison with the common form of papillary carcinoma by DNA and morphometric analysis. Cleve Clin Q 1976;43:207–15.

150. Hazard JB. Small papillary carcinoma of the thyroid. A study with special reference to so-called nonencapsulated sclerosing tumor. Lab Invest 1960;9:86–97.

151. Hedinger CE, Williams ED, Sobin LH. Histological typing of thyroid tumors. In: Hedinger CE, ed. International histological classification of tumours; Vol 11. Berlin: Springer-Verlag, 1988.

152. Hubert JP Jr, Keirnan PD, Beahrs OH, McConahey WM, Woolner LB. Occult papillary carcinoma of the thyroid. Arch Surg 1980;115:394–8.

153. Johnson TL, Lloyd RV, Thompson NW, Beierwaltes WH, Sisson JC. Prognostic implications of the tall cell variant of papillary thyroid carcinoma. Am J Surg Pathol 1988;12:22–7.

154. Klinck GH, Winship T. Occult sclerosing carcinoma of the thyroid. Cancer 1955;8:701–6.

155. Lang W, Borrusch H, Bauer L. Occult carcinomas of the thyroid. Evaluation of 1,020 sequential autopsies. Am J Clin Pathol 1988;90:72–6.

156. Lindsay S. Carcinoma of the thyroid gland. A clinical and pathologic study of 293 patients at the University of California Hospital. Springfield, IL: Charles C Thomas, 1960.

157. LiVolsi VA. Surgical pathology of the thyroid. In: Bennington JL ed. Major problems in pathology; Vol 22. Philadelphia: WB Saunders, 1990.

157a. Loy TS, Gelven PL, Mullins D, Diaz-Arias AA. Methods in pathology. Immunostaining for P-glycoprotein in the diagnosis of thyroid carcinomas. Modern Pathol 1992;2:200–4.

158. Mazzaferri EL, Oertel JE. The pathology and prognosis of thyroid cancer. In: Kaplan EL, ed. Surgery of the thyroid and parathyroid glands, Vol. 6, Clinical surgery international. Edinburgh: Churchill Livingstone, 1983:22–3.

159. Meissner WA, Warren S. Tumors of the thyroid gland. Atlas of Tumor Pathology, 2nd Series, Fascicle 4. Washington, D.C.: Armed Forces Institute of Pathology, 1969:50–2.

160. Miettinen M, Franssila K, Lehto VP, Paasivuo R, Virtanen I. Expression of intermediate filament proteins in thyroid gland and thyroid tumors. Lab Invest 1984;50:262–70.

161. Mizukami Y, Nonomura A, Michigishi T, et al. Diffuse sclerosing variant of papillary carcinoma of the thyroid. Report of three cases. Acta Pathol Jpn 1990;40:676–82.

162. Patchefsky AS, Keller IB, Mansfield CM. Solitary vertebral column metastasis from occult sclerosing carcinoma of the thyroid gland: report of a case. Am J Clin Pathol 1970;53:596–601.

163. Ro JY, Sahin AA, el-Naggar AK, et al. Intraluminal crystalloids in struma ovarii. Immunohistochemical, DNA flow cytometric, and ultrastructural study. Arch Pathol Lab Med 1991;115:145–9.

164. Rosai J, Zampi G, Carcangiu ML. Papillary carcinoma of the thyroid. A discussion of its several morphologic expressions, with particular emphasis on the follicular variant. Am J Surg Pathol 1983;7:809–17.

165. Sampson RJ, Oka H, Key CR, Buncher CR, Iijima S. Metastases from occult thyroid carcinoma. An autopsy study from Hiroshima and Nagasaki, Japan. Cancer 1970;25:803–11.

166. Schröder S, Bay V, Dumke K, et al. Diffuse sclerosing variant of papillary thyroid carcinoma. S-100 protein immunocytochemistry and prognosis. Virchows Arch [A] 1990;416:367–71.

167. _____, Böcker W, Dralle H, Kortman K-B, Stern C. The encapsulated papillary carcinoma of the thyroid. A morphologic subtype of the papillary thyroid carcinoma. Cancer 1984;54:90–3.

168. Soares J, Limbert E, Sobrinho-Simões M. Diffuse sclerosing variant of papillary thyroid carcinoma. A clinicopathologic study of 10 cases. Pathol Res Pract 1989;185:200–6.

169. Sobrinho-Simões M, Nesland JM, Johannessen JV. Columnar-cell carcinoma. Another variant of poorly differentiated carcinoma of the thyroid. Am J Clin Pathol 1988;89:264–7.

170. _____, Soares J, Carneiro F, Limbert E. Diffuse follicular variant of papillary carcinoma of the thyroid: report of eight cases of a distinct aggressive type of thyroid tumor. Surg Pathol 1990;3:189–203.

171. Strate SM, Lee EL, Childers JH. Occult papillary carcinoma of the thyroid with distant metastases. Cancer 1984;54:1093–100.

172. Tscholl-Ducommun J, Hedinger CE. Papillary thyroid carcinomas. Morphology and prognosis. Virchows Arch [A] 1982;396:19–39.

173. Vickery AL Jr, Carcangiu ML, Johannessen JV, Sobrinho-Simões M. Papillary carcinoma. Semin Diagn Pathol 1985;2:90–100.

174. Yagi Y, Yagi S, Saku T. Localization of cytoskeletal proteins and thyroglobulin in thyroid microcarcinoma versus clinically manifested thyroid carcinoma. Cancer 1985;56:1967–71.

175. Yamamoto Y, Maeda T, Izumi K, Otsuka H. Occult papillary carcinoma of the thyroid. A study of 408 autopsy cases. Cancer 1990;65:1173–9.

176. Yamashita H, Nakayama I, Noguchi S, et al. Minute carcinoma of the thyroid and its development to advanced carcinoma. Acta Pathol Jpn 1985;35:377–83.

✧✧✧

POORLY DIFFERENTIATED CARCINOMA

Some carcinomas that arise from follicular cells do not fit easily into any of the categories described elsewhere in this Fascicle. Our impression is that some of these occupy both morphologically and behaviorally an intermediate place between the well-differentiated follicular and papillary carcinomas and the undifferentiated (anaplastic) carcinomas. It is arguable whether they represent independent tumor entities or simply a higher grade of existing ones. We favor the latter interpretation and therefore fully understand that, by incorporating them into this scheme, we are introducing grading criteria into a classification scheme that is largely based on other parameters (see page 19). However, we believe that this approach is justifiable not only because of the reasonably distinctive morphologic appearance of its prototypic representative, which we have designated *insular carcinoma*, but also because of the important prognostic connotations of this concept.

INSULAR CARCINOMA

Insular carcinoma is the term we have proposed for a morphologically distinctive form of poorly differentiated carcinoma arising from follicular cells (1). It is probably equivalent to the tumor described by Langhans (5) in 1907 as *wuchernde struma* (fig. 115).

General and Clinical Features. Insular carcinoma seems to be more common in some countries than in others. The cases we originally reported were from central Italy, where they constituted approximately 4 percent of all the thyroid carcinomas seen at one institution (1). In Paraguay, carcinomas with an insular pattern comprise an even higher percentage of all thyroid malignancies (Rolon A, personal communication, 1990). By contrast, in the United States, this tumor seems to be extremely rare; however, we have seen many indisputable cases (2). The disease is slightly more common in women, and the mean age at the time of the initial diagnosis is 55 years (1).

Gross Features. The tumor is solid and grayish white and often exhibits foci of necrosis (pl. XV-A). Most are over 5 cm in diameter at the time of diagnosis and show an invasive type of margin. Extrathyroid extension may be observed.

Microscopic Features. The most distinctive histologic feature of insular carcinoma is the presence of well-defined nests (insulae) of round or oval shape, composed of a monotonous population of small cells with round nuclei and scant cytoplasm (figs. 116, 117). The predominant pattern of growth is solid, but microfollicles are also commonly encountered, some of which contain dense colloid (fig. 118). Mitoses are always present but in variable number (fig. 119). The pattern of growth is characteristically infiltrative, and blood vessel invasion is common. Foci of necrosis are frequent. The small

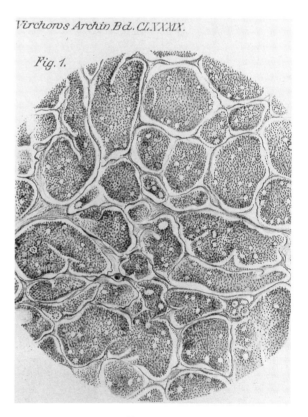

Figure 115
LANGHANS WUCHERNDE STRUMA

The insular appearance resulting from artifactual retraction from the stroma, the predominantly solid appearance of the insulae, and the scattered microfollicles can be clearly seen in this drawing. (Fig. 1 from Langhans T. Über die epithelialen formen der malignen struma. Virchows Arch 1907;189:69–188.)

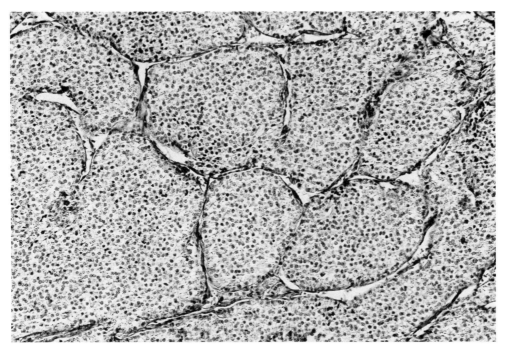

Figure 116
POORLY DIFFERENTIATED (INSULAR) CARCINOMA
Typical low-power appearance of poorly differentiated (insular) carcinoma. Well-defined nests (insulae) of tumor cells are present throughout.

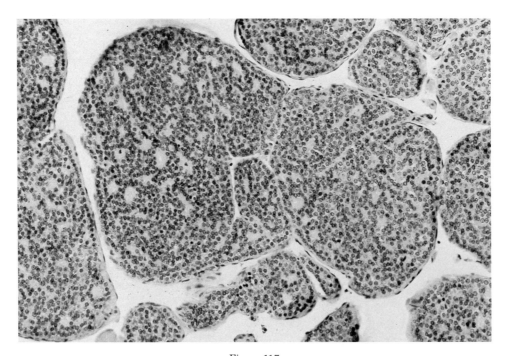

Figure 117
POORLY DIFFERENTIATED (INSULAR) CARCINOMA
The insulae are composed of small monotonous tumor cells and are separated from each other by a scant, loose connective tissue stroma.

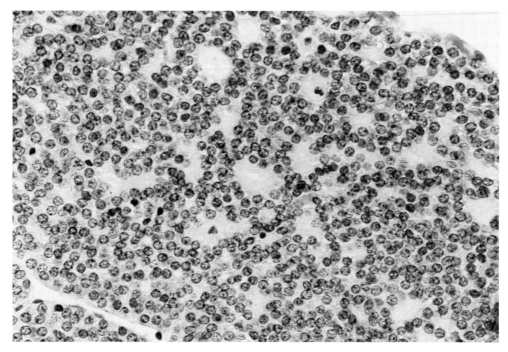

Figure 118
POORLY DIFFERENTIATED (INSULAR) CARCINOMA
At high magnification, the tumor cells have small round nuclei and scant cytoplasm. The pattern of growth is predominantly solid, but there are also abortive follicles with small lumina that contain colloid.

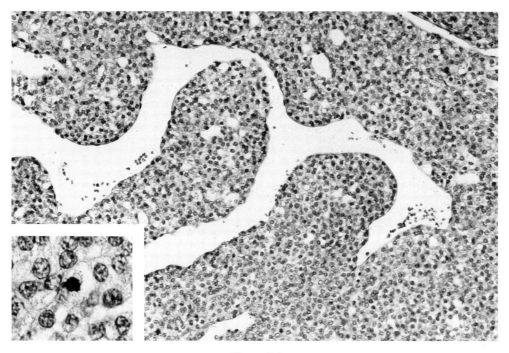

Figure 119
POORLY DIFFERENTIATED (INSULAR) CARCINOMA
This tumor exhibits an almost entirely solid pattern of growth and prominent vascularization. The inset illustrates the small size of the tumor cells and the presence of mitotic activity. This tumor was often designated in the past as the *compact* variant of small cell undifferentiated carcinoma.

foci tend to be located in the center of the insulae, whereas the larger ones are seen to spare the insulae situated around blood vessels, thus leading to a peritheliomatous appearance (fig. 120).

Immunohistochemical Features. The tumor cells are positive for keratin and thyroglobulin and negative for calcitonin (pl. XV-B). Focal reactivity for somatostatin has been described in a few instances (1).

Differential Diagnosis. This tumor can be confused with medullary carcinoma and other neuroendocrine neoplasms because of its carcinoid-like insular configuration, and it may be misdiagnosed as undifferentiated (anaplastic) carcinoma when the pattern of growth is solid throughout. It is our impression that many of the thyroid neoplasms formerly designated as the *compact subtype* of anaplastic carcinoma belong to this category (6,8).

Cytologic Features. The cytologic appearance of insular carcinoma as revealed by fine-needle aspiration has been described by Pietribiasi and coworkers (7). The main features were high cellularity and necrotic background; trabeculae and/or clusters, sometimes associated with microfollicles; poorly defined cytoplasm, occasionally vacuolated; mild to moderate nuclear atypia; and occasional nuclear pseudoinclusions and grooves.

Spread and Metastasis; Prognosis. Insular carcinoma is an aggressive and often lethal tumor. Metastases are common, both to regional lymph nodes and to distant sites (particularly lung and bone) (pl. XV-C; fig. 121). In the series of Carcangiu and coworkers (1), 14 of 25 patients had died as the result of the tumor, and 7 were alive but with persistent or recurrent disease at the time of the last follow-up.

Nosologic Considerations. Insular carcinoma is viewed by the WHO Committee as a morphologic variant of follicular carcinoma (3). This interpretation may be correct for most but not necessarily all cases of this entity. In some instances, we have seen it coexisting with or

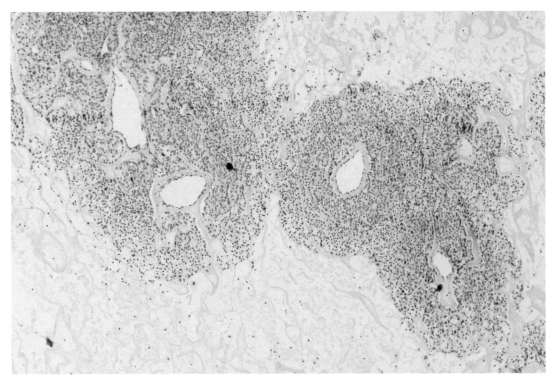

Figure 120
POORLY DIFFERENTIATED (INSULAR) CARCINOMA
Peritheliomatous appearance resulting from necrosis, associated with preservation of the tumor cells located around large blood vessels.

126

PLATE XV
POORLY DIFFERENTIATED (INSULAR) CARCINOMA

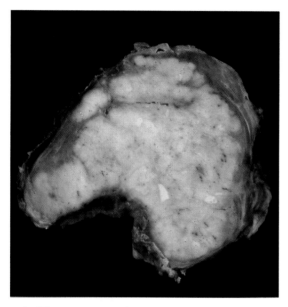

A. The tumor is replacing most of the thyroid and shows an invasive pattern of growth. There are multiple foci of necrosis.

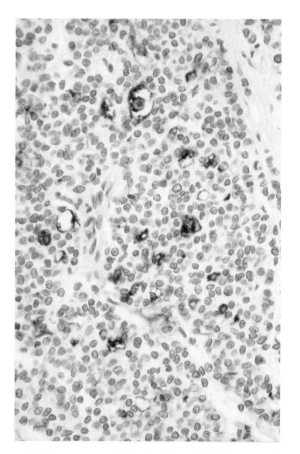

B. Immunoreactivity for thyroglobulin in poorly differentiated (insular) carcinoma. Most of the positivity is intraluminal.

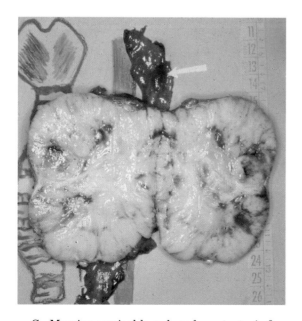

C. Massive cervical lymph node metastasis from poorly differentiated (insular) carcinoma. (Courtesy of Dr. Pedro Rolon, Asuncion, Paraguay.)

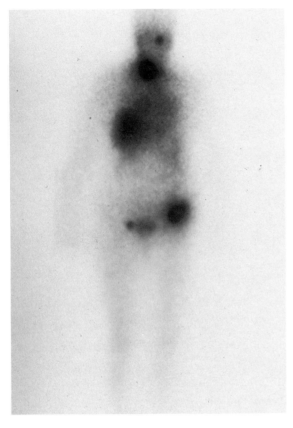

Figure 121
POORLY DIFFERENTIATED
(INSULAR) CARCINOMA
This poorly differentiated (insular) thyroid carcinoma
has metastasized to lung and pelvic bone.

pointed out that the insular pattern may be seen focally in what is otherwise a typical follicular (or, less commonly, papillary) carcinoma (figs. 123, 124). There is some suggestion that such a finding may carry prognostic significance. Johnson and coworkers (4) retrospectively identified five such cases. Four tumors were greater than 7 cm; three of these showed extrathyroid extension with lung and/or bone metastasis at presentation, and the fourth developed lung metastasis 3 years after initial diagnosis.

OTHER POORLY DIFFERENTIATED CARCINOMAS

Some thyroid carcinomas share with insular carcinoma the presence of well-defined nests, predominantly solid pattern, mitotic activity, and necrosis but are composed of larger cells, both in terms of nuclear size and cytoplasmic volume. The group is heterogeneous in the sense that some members have nuclear features similar to those of papillary carcinoma, others have an architectural configuration consistent with a follicular carcinoma, and still others have oncocytic cytoplasmic features. On occasion, a remarkably complex appearance results from the intimate admixture within the same tumor of follicular, papillary, oncocytic, and clear cell foci, some of which exhibit prominent nesting (fig. 125). As for the case of the insular carcinoma, we feel that it is more important to emphasize their poorly differentiated nature (hence anticipating a more aggressive behavior) than to make the difficult and sometimes futile attempt to place them into one conventional category or another. Other authors have attempted a grading system but within the confines of the papillary or follicular categories, and/or by using criteria somewhat different from the ones we are advocating (9,11–17). The message, however, is similar: in this particular situation, the tumor grading overrides considerations based on standard classification schemes for prognostic and therapeutic purposes. It is our strong suspicion that a high proportion of the tumors classified as either papillary or follicular carcinomas that behave in an unexpectedly aggressive fashion, even though they occurred in low-risk populations (patients under 40 years), belong to this category (10,14).

developing after a typical papillary carcinoma of either the conventional or the follicular variant type. In other instances, we have found that the architectural progression from a typical papillary to an insular pattern was paralleled by a gradual change in the nuclear appearance from the typical ground-glass nuclei of papillary carcinoma to the smaller and hyperchromatic forms that are characteristic of the insular tumor (fig. 122).

From a prognostic standpoint, we believe that it is much more important to identify the tumor as being poorly differentiated than to try to decide whether it belongs to the follicular or papillary group, a task that in some instances may be impossible. Along these lines, it should be

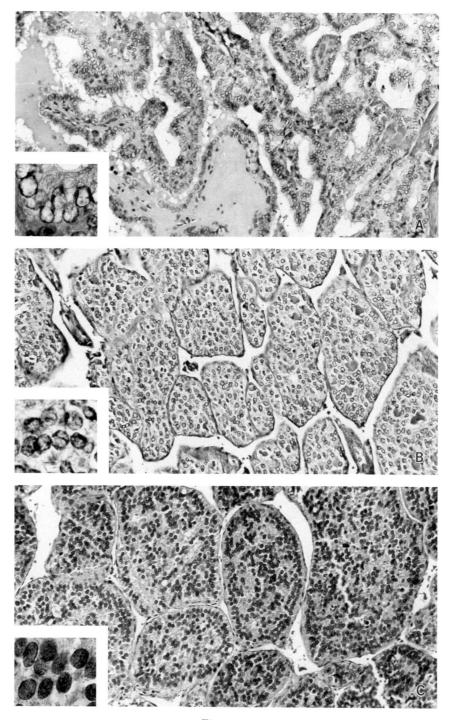

Figure 122
PROGRESSIVE TRANSFORMATION OF PAPILLARY CARCINOMA
INTO POORLY DIFFERENTIATED (INSULAR) CARCINOMA

Typical papillary carcinoma, as seen in the original excision performed in 1975 (A). In the local recurrence in 1984, the papillary pattern is replaced by an insular pattern (B). In a further local recurrence from 1987, the insular pattern is fully developed (C). These architectural changes are paralleled by similarly notable changes in the nuclear appearance (insets). (Courtesy of Dr. Aidan Carney, Mayo Clinic, Rochester, MN.)

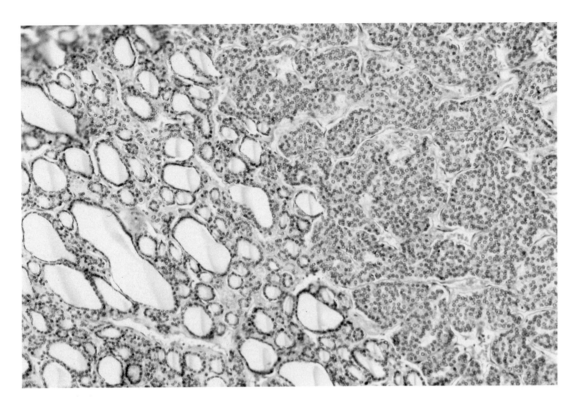

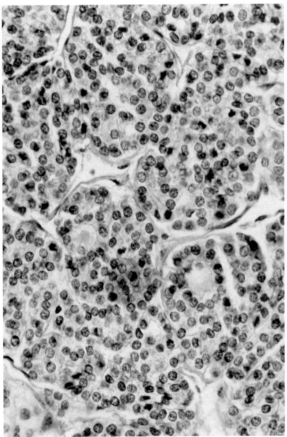

Figure 123
FOLLICULAR CARCINOMA WITH
FOCAL INSULAR PATTERN
The top photograph shows the interface between the two components. The bottom photograph shows the characteristic high-power appearance of the insular component, with well-defined tumor nests that contain minute follicles.

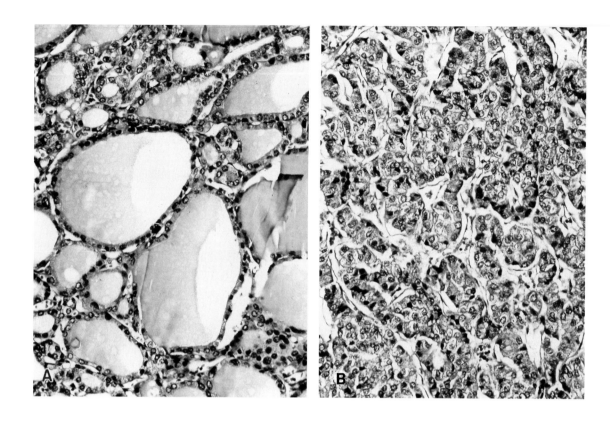

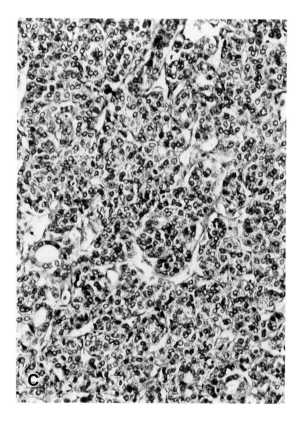

Figure 124
COMBINATION OF PATTERNS
IN THYROID CARCINOMA
Follicular (A), trabecular (B), and insular (C) patterns are illustrated in this figure. The admixture of insular and trabecular patterns is not unusual.

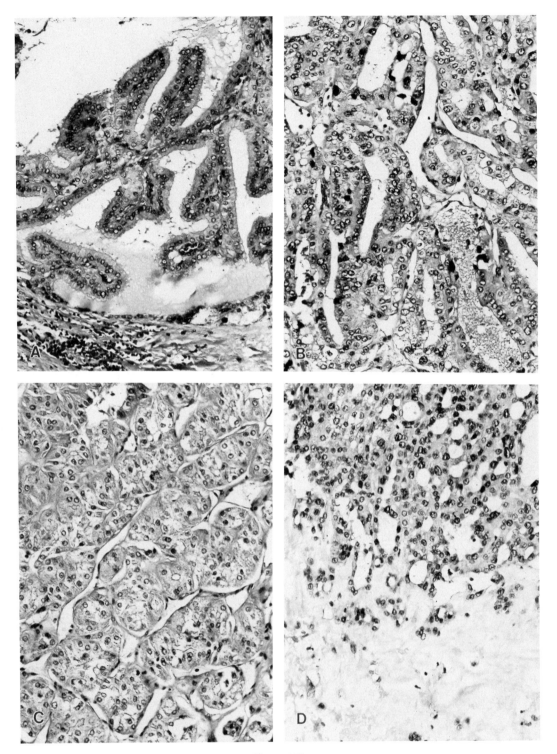

Figure 125
COMBINATION OF PATTERNS IN THYROID CARCINOMA
This thyroid carcinoma exhibited the following bewildering combination of patterns: typical papillary architecture (A), a pattern suggestive of follicular variant of papillary carcinoma (B), a trabecular arrangement and focal oncocytic change (C), and a poorly differentiated pattern with large foci of hyalinization, probably replacing areas of necrosis (D).

REFERENCES

Insular Carcinoma

1. Carcangiu ML, Zampi G, Rosai J. Poorly differentiated ("insular") thyroid carcinoma. A reinterpretation of Langhans' "wuchernde Struma." Am J Surg Pathol 1984;8:655–68.
2. Flynn SD, Forman BH, Stewart AF, Kinder BK. Poorly differentiated ("insular") carcinoma of the thyroid gland: an aggressive subset of differentiated thyroid neoplasms. Surgery 1988;104:963–70.
3. Hedinger CE, Williams ED, Sobin LH. Histological typing of thyroid tumors. In: Hedinger CE, ed. International histological classification of tumours; Vol 11. Berlin: Springer-Verlag, 1988.
4. Johnson MW, Hunnicutt JW, Bilbao JE, Bassion S. Poorly differentiated thyroid carcinoma with focal 'insular' pattern [Abstract]. Am J Clin Pathol 1990;94:497–8A.
5. Langhans T. Über die epithelialen formen der malignen struma. Virchows Arch [A] 1907;189:69–188.
6. Meissner WA, Warren S. Tumors of the thyroid gland. Atlas of Tumor Pathology, 2nd Series, Fascicle 4. Washington, D.C.: Armed Forces Institute of Pathology, 1969.
7. Pietribiasi F, Sapino A, Papotti M, Bussolati G. Cytologic features of poorly differentiated "insular" carcinoma of the thyroid, as revealed by fine-needle aspiration biopsy. Am J Clin Pathol 1990;94:687–92.
8. Rosai J, Saxén EA, Woolner L. Undifferentiated and poorly differentiated carcinoma. Semin Diagn Pathol 1985;2:123–36.

Other Poorly Differentiated Carcinomas

9. Cabanne F, Gérard-Marchant R, Heimann R, Williams ED. Tumeurs malignes du corps thyroïde. Problèmes de diagnostic histopathologique. A propos de 692 lésions recueillies par le groupe coopérateur des cancers du corps thyroïde de l'OERTC. Ann Anat Pathol (Paris) 1974;19:129–48.
10. Cohn K, Bäckdahl M, Forsslund G, et al. Prognostic value of nuclear DNA content in papillary thyroid carcinoma. World J Surg 1984;8:474–80.
11. Harach HR, Franssila KO. Thyroglobulin immunostaining in follicular thyroid carcinoma: relationship to the degree of differentiation and cell type. Histopathology 1988;13:43–54.
12. McConahey WM, Hay ID, Woolner LB, van Heerden JA, Taylor WF. Papillary thyroid cancer treated at the Mayo Clinic, 1946 through 1970: initial manifestations, pathologic findings, therapy, and outcome. Mayo Clin Proc 1986;61:978–96.
13. Mueller-Gaertner H-W, Brzac HT, Rehpenning W. Prognostic indices for tumor relapse and tumor mortality in follicular thyroid carcinoma. Cancer 1991;67:1903–11.
14. Rosen IB, Bowden J, Luk SC, Simpson JA. Aggressive thyroid cancer in low-risk age population. Surgery 1987;102:1075–80.
15. Sakamoto A, Kasai N, Sugano H. Poorly differentiated carcinoma of the thyroid. A clinicopathologic entity for a high-risk group of papillary and follicular carcinomas. Cancer 1983;52:1849–55.
16. Simpson WJ, McKinney SE, Carruthers JS, Gospodarowicz MK, Sutcliffe SB, Panzarella T. Papillary and follicular thyroid cancer. Prognostic factors in 1,578 patients. Am J Med 1987;83:479–88.
17. Tscholl-Ducommun J, Hedinger CE. Papillary thyroid carcinomas. Morphology and prognosis. Virchows Arch [A] 1982;396:19–39.

UNDIFFERENTIATED (ANAPLASTIC) CARCINOMA

Definition. A highly malignant tumor that appears partially or totally undifferentiated with standard light-microscopic techniques but in which some evidence of epithelial differentiation is found on morphologic, immunohistochemical, or ultrastructural grounds. Other terms that have been used to designate this tumor and related entities include *pleomorphic carcinoma*, *sarcomatoid carcinoma*, *metaplastic carcinoma*, and *carcinosarcoma*.

Clinical Features. Undifferentiated thyroid carcinoma is characteristically a tumor of elderly individuals. In most series, the mean age at the time of the initial diagnosis is between 60 and 65 years. Few patients present below the age of 50 years, and such a diagnosis should therefore be suspect whenever made in a young patient. However, exceptions do occur. Carcangiu and coworkers (9) reported a case in a 37-year-old patient, Schoumacher and coworkers (46) saw another in a 30-year-old patient, and Albores-Saavedra and coworkers (2) have the youngest patient on record, diagnosed at the age of 22 years.

As with most other thyroid tumors, undifferentiated carcinoma is most common in women. Most reported series quote a ratio of men to women of 1:3 to 1:4.

The clinical presentation is remarkably constant, with few cases departing from the classic description of a rapidly enlarging neck mass in the thyroid region. This is associated in about half of the cases with compression signs, such as dyspnea, dysphagia, and hoarseness. The duration is characteristically short, ranging from a few weeks to a few months. Occasionally, patients first present with symptoms or signs related to distant metastatic involvement, such as skin (5), bowel (42), or bone (personal observation), but even in these patients, there is usually clinical evidence of a thyroid mass. One case has been reported as presenting with hyperthyroidism, presumably as a result of necrosis of normal thyroid with release of thyroid hormone (40). A history of preexistent nodular or diffuse enlargement of the thyroid is given in some cases because undifferentiated thyroid carcinoma nearly always engrafts itself on an abnormal gland (see page 153).

Physical examination reveals nodular thyroid enlargement in almost every case, and this is usually of considerable magnitude. In about half of the cases, there is clinical evidence of extension beyond the thyroid gland, and in approximately one third, there is cervical lymph node enlargement resulting from metastatic disease.

Undifferentiated carcinoma is invariably cold on radioactive iodine scan, both in the primary site and in the metastatic foci, and remains so even after the residual non-neoplastic thyroid gland has been removed. Areas of uptake in the metastatic deposits are indicative of the presence of a better differentiated component. Euthyroidism is the rule in patients with undifferentiated carcinoma, even when most of the gland has been destroyed by tumor.

Gross Features. Undifferentiated carcinoma is usually large and widely invasive on gross inspection (fig. 126). The consistency is highly variable and the appearance variegated, reflecting the common presence of necrotic and hemorrhagic foci. In most instances, the tumor is found to replace most of the thyroid gland and, in many instances, to have violated the thyroid capsule, spreading into the soft tissues of the neck. One should search for areas with a granular appearance and firm consistency and those suggesting the residue of a capsule because they may provide the evidence for a preexisting papillary or follicular carcinoma, respectively. Occasionally, metaplastic cartilage or bone can be seen at the gross level (pl. XVI).

Microscopic Features. The microscopic appearance of undifferentiated carcinoma shows considerable variation from case to case and sometimes even within the same case. Three distinct morphologic patterns exist, allowing for the fact that transitions and intermediate forms among them often occur. These patterns are descriptively designated *squamoid*, *spindle cell*, and *giant cell* (9).

The squamoid (or malpighian) pattern is so named because of its morphologic similarity to nonkeratinizing squamous cell carcinoma of other organs, such as lung or cervix. The appearance in these areas is unmistakably epithelial because of the formation of distinct tumor nests

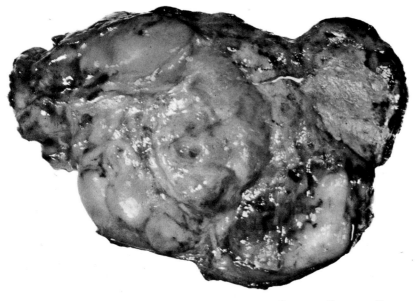

Figure 126
UNDIFFERENTIATED CARCINOMA
There is massive replacement of the gland by a large multinodular tumor with extensive foci of necrosis. (Fig. 108 from Fascicle 4, Second Series.)

of irregular configuration (fig. 127). Pleomorphism is moderate, and giant cells are generally absent. The cytoplasm is abundant and acidophilic. In rare instances, squamous pearls are seen in the center of the islands. In these cases, the appearance is epidermoid (squamous) rather than merely squamoid. Small foci of mucin accumulation can sometimes be demonstrated in these areas by the use of Mayer mucicarmine or other mucin stains.

The spindle cell pattern is best described as sarcoma-like, in the sense that, on purely morphologic grounds, it is indistinguishable from a true sarcoma. Sometimes the appearance is reminiscent of fibrosarcoma, by virtue of a fascicular arrangement and heavy deposition of collagen fibers (fig. 128). In most instances, however, the marked degree of nuclear pleomorphism, scattered giant tumor cells, storiform pattern of growth, and inflammatory infiltrate give the tumor an appearance similar to that exhibited by the usual (storiform-pleomorphic) form of malignant fibrous histiocytoma (fig. 129). These cellular areas alternate with extensive areas of necrosis and sclerohyaline deposition. The ne-

crotic foci tend to have sharply angulated outlines and to be surrounded by a palisading of tumor cells, resulting in an appearance similar to that seen in some malignant tumors of the central and peripheral nervous system, notably glioblas-toma multiforme. Areas of myxoid change can be present; when abundant, there is a resemblance to the "myxoid variant" of malignant fibrous histiocytoma (fig. 130).

Vascularization is generally prominent. Sometimes the vessels are branching, with a "staghorn" or antler-like appearance similar to that seen in hemangiopericytoma (fig. 131). In other instances, the appearance of angiosarcoma (malignant hemangioendothelioma) is simulated by the formation of freely connecting spaces lined by tumor cells. A characteristic formation often seen in the spindle cell areas is caused by the permeation of the wall of large-sized vessels by neoplastic cells, sometimes resulting in a polypoid subendothelial growth (fig. 132). Some of these structures stand out in a sea of necrotic or hyalinized tissue.

The giant cell pattern is characterized by a degree of pleomorphism that is substantially higher than that seen in association with the

PLATE XVI

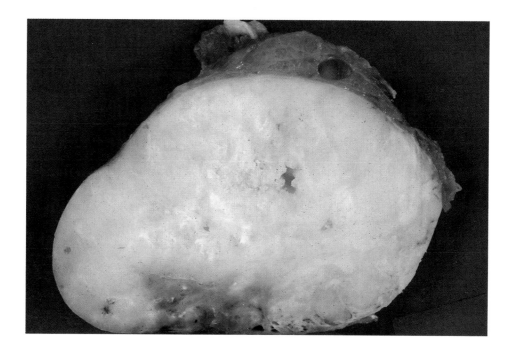

UNDIFFERENTIATED CARCINOMA

There are foci of necrosis and hemorrhage in the lower edge of the figure. A portion of residual thyroid is visible at the upper pole. The whitish area near the center represents neoplastic cartilage.

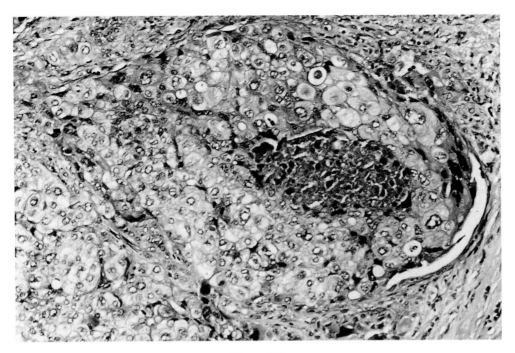

Figure 127
UNDIFFERENTIATED CARCINOMA, SQUAMOID PATTERN
This undifferentiated carcinoma shows a clearly epithelial pattern of growth, here referred to as *squamoid*. Necrosis is present in the center of this field.

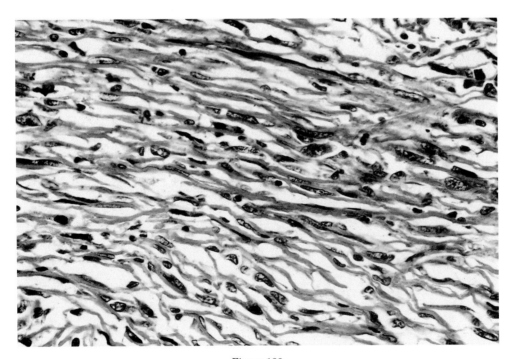

Figure 128
UNDIFFERENTIATED CARCINOMA, SPINDLE CELL PATTERN
The tumor cells are extremely elongated and are separated from each other by dense collagen bands. The appearance closely simulates that of a sarcoma.

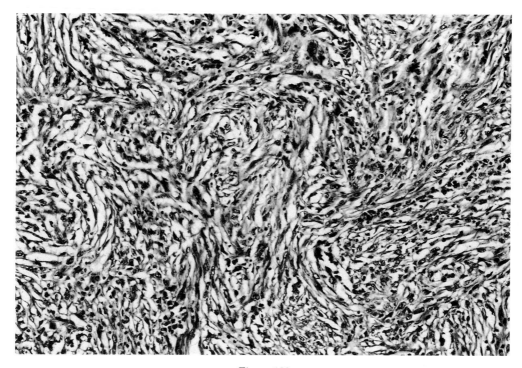

Figure 129
UNDIFFERENTIATED CARCINOMA, SPINDLE CELL PATTERN
The well-developed storiform appearance results in a striking resemblance to malignant fibrous
histiocytoma.

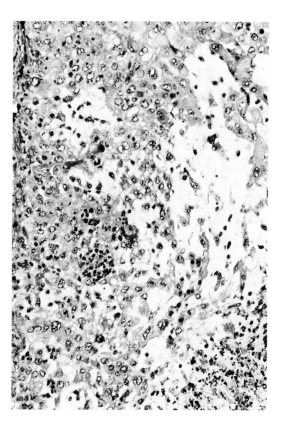

Figure 130
UNDIFFERENTIATED CARCINOMA
A focally prominent myxoid pattern and extensive secondary inflammatory infiltrate are illustrated.

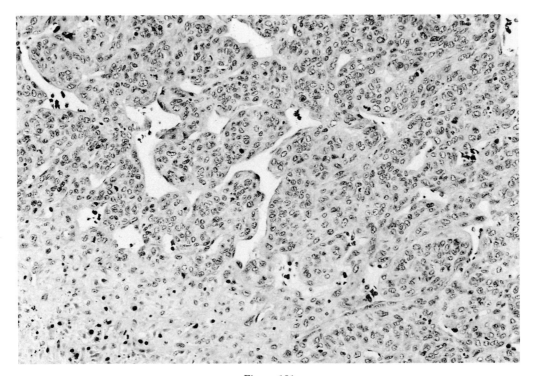

Figure 131
UNDIFFERENTIATED CARCINOMA
This tumor has a hemangiopericytoma-like pattern of growth.

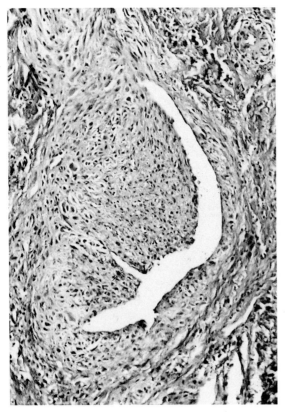

Figure 132
UNDIFFERENTIATED CARCINOMA
The wall of a vein is invaded by undifferentiated carcinoma, resulting in a polypoid projection into the lumen, which is still partially patent.

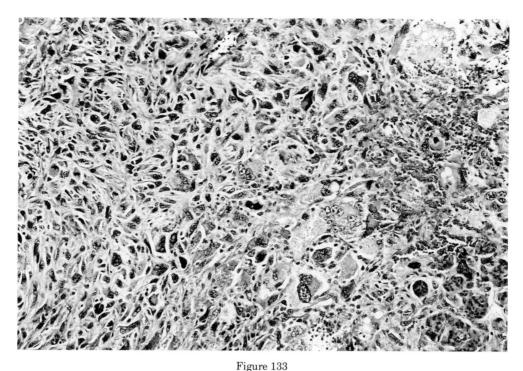

Figure 133
UNDIFFERENTIATED CARCINOMA, GIANT CELL PATTERN
There are numerous giant cells, some of which contain multiple nuclei. They are seen in a background
of spindle sarcomatoid elements.

other patterns (fig. 133). This is due to the presence of numerous tumor giant cells with bizarre (sometimes multiple) hyperchromatic nuclei, abundant amphophilic and somewhat granular cytoplasm, and a plump (round or oval) shape (fig. 134). Variations on this theme include giant cells with a homogeneous (nongranular), deeply acidophilic cytoplasm and others with variously sized, round, acidophilic, intracytoplasmic hyaline globules. The tumor giant cells may be the only element present, but more often they are seen interspersed with smaller mononuclear tumor cells that have otherwise similar morphologic features. The pattern of growth in these areas is usually solid, but on occasion an artifactual separation of the cells leads to the formation of alveolar (pseudoglandular) or pseudovascular structures. The latter are particularly notable in areas where the highly vascular nature of the tumor has led to the accumulation of red blood cells within these cavities.

A scattering of inflammatory cells is often present among the tumor cells, especially in the giant cell and squamoid patterns. When it is heavy and rich in neutrophils, the tumor resembles the "inflammatory variant" of malignant fibrous histiocytoma. In these areas, the giant tumor cells may be seen to contain numerous (possibly phagocytosed) neutrophils in their cytoplasm, further heightening the resemblance with inflammatory malignant fibrous histiocytoma.

Features common to all three patterns are high mitotic activity, large foci of necrosis, and a marked degree of invasiveness, both within the gland and in the extrathyroid structures. Malignant cells may grow between residual follicles or destroy them in their path. They invade adipose tissue and skeletal muscle and sometimes even ulcerate through the skin (fig. 135). On occasion, they penetrate inside skeletal muscle fibers, in a manner analogous to that seen more commonly in carcinoma of the breast (49). Blood vessel invasion in the form of tumor thrombi (as opposed to the infiltration of the vessel wall described above) is a common finding (figs. 136, 137).

As already mentioned, transitions and admixtures between the three major patterns are often seen. The most common is between the spindle cell

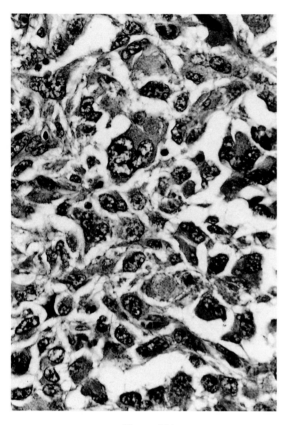

Figure 134
UNDIFFERENTIATED CARCINOMA
Bizarre multinucleated tumor giant cells are present.

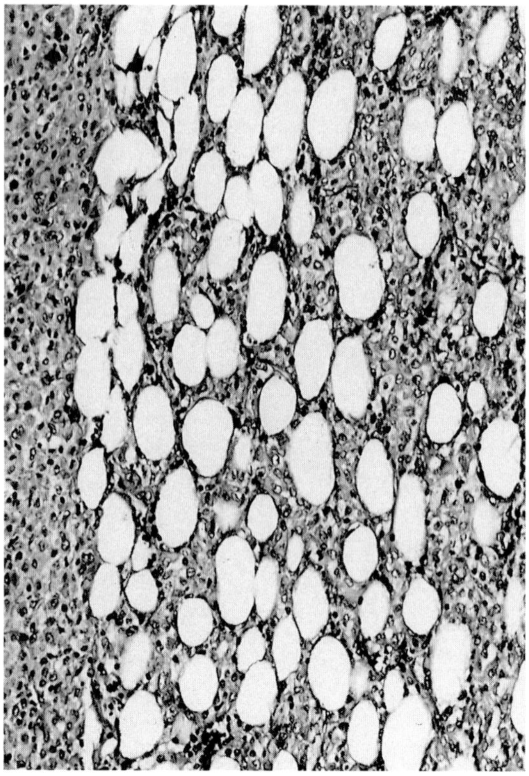

Figure 135
UNDIFFERENTIATED CARCINOMA
Diffuse infiltration of the perithyroidal fat, the pattern simulating that of malignant lymphoma.

and the giant cell patterns, but sometimes foci indistinguishable from sarcomas blend with those that have a clear-cut epithelial configuration.

Multinucleated cells with an appearance indistinguishable from osteoclasts (and therefore substantially different from the previously described tumor giant cells) are seen scattered among the neoplastic elements in about 10 percent of the cases (19,48). These cells have numerous (up to 100 or more) nuclei devoid of atypical features and are never seen undergoing mitotic division (fig. 138). Ultrastructurally and immunohistochemically, they lack epithelial features. Instead, they have been shown to express markers characteristic of cells of monocytic and/or histiocytic lineage (17). This finding suggests that these osteoclast-like elements are non-neoplastic, derived from blood-borne or indigenous monocytes and/or histiocytes, and formed as a result of cellular fusion. The phenomenon is analogous to that sometimes seen in carcinoma of breast and other organs (1) and may result in an appearance simulating aneurysmal bone cyst (17).

In a small number of cases of undifferentiated carcinoma (≤5 percent), the mesenchymal-like component of the tumor exhibits heterologous features, such as neoplastic cartilage or bone (fig. 139). This may occur in association with any of the major basic patterns but is more common with the spindle cell type. Some authors use the term *carcinosarcoma* for this particular occurrence (14), but we do not believe that a sharp separation from the larger group of undifferentiated carcinomas is warranted on either clinical or histogenetic grounds.

The microscopic appearance of the metastases generally recapitulates that of the primary tumor. No microscopic grading of undifferentiated carcinoma has been attempted or seems feasible. By definition, all representatives of this tumor type belong to the highest category of any grading system.

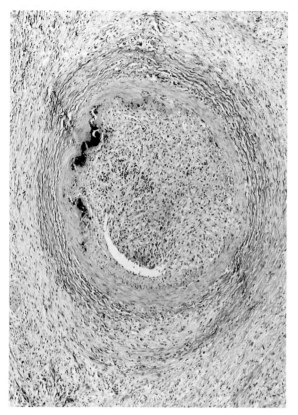

Figure 136
UNDIFFERENTIATED CARCINOMA
A tumor thrombus in a partially calcified artery is illustrated.

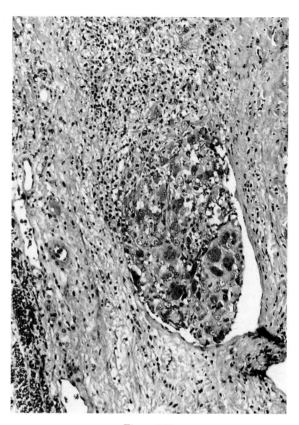

Figure 137
UNDIFFERENTIATED CARCINOMA
This figure shows an intravascular tumor thrombus. There is a scattering of osteoclast-like giant cells and an extensive inflammatory reaction around the vessel.

Immunohistochemical Features. The immunohistochemical profile of undifferentiated carcinoma is somewhat related to the pattern of growth. In the squamoid and other epithelial-appearing foci, there is strong and consistent expression of both high– and low–molecular-weight keratins. Spindle and giant cell foci generally lack high–molecular-weight keratins but show reactivity for the low–molecular-weight forms of this marker in a variable number of cases (pl. XVII-A). The incidence of positivity has ranged from 47 percent to 100 percent in the reported series (9,22,35,41,51,52). The positivity is often in the form of individual cells or cell clusters (30). Many of the tumor cells coexpress vimentin, especially in the spindle cell areas (35,51).

Staining for epithelial membrane antigen (EMA) recapitulates the pattern described for high–molecular-weight keratin in the sense that the more epithelial-looking tumors are the only ones likely to exhibit positivity. Thus, the diagnostic utility of this marker is limited (12a,41).

CEA positivity has been found in some of the more squamoid examples of undifferentiated carcinoma. This is usually limited to the center of the tumor nests (pl. XVII-B) (9,41).

Intense positivity for laminin (a component of basal lamina) has been found by Miettinen and Virtanen (36) in scattered tumor cells; however, neoplasms lacking a distinct compartmentalization of tumor cells also lacked pericellular laminin.

Conflicting results were obtained when staining these tumors for thyroglobulin and other thyroid hormone-related markers, such as thyroxine and triiodothyronine. Carcangiu and coworkers (9) did not encounter convincing positivity for thyroglobulin in any of the tumors they examined. Other authors reported reactivity ranging from 9 to 71 percent (3,6,8,22,27,32,47). In most cases,

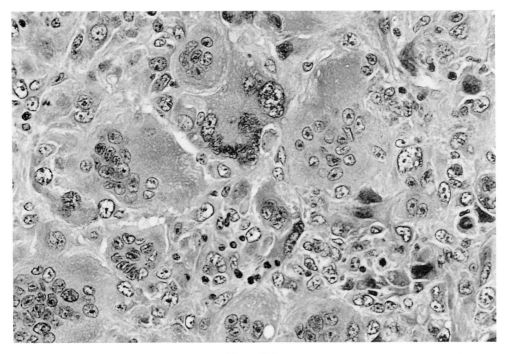

Figure 138
UNDIFFERENTIATED CARCINOMA
WITH NUMEROUS OSTEOCLAST-LIKE GIANT CELLS
Notice the marked difference in nuclear morphology between the mono- and multinuclear neoplastic cells and the osteoclast-like giant cells.

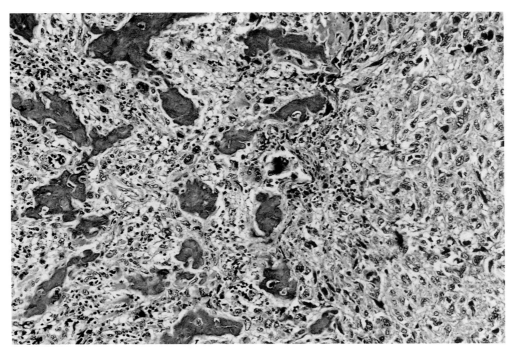

Figure 139
UNDIFFERENTIATED CARCINOMA
This figure illustrates bone formation in this tumor.

PLATE XVII
UNDIFFERENTIATED CARCINOMA

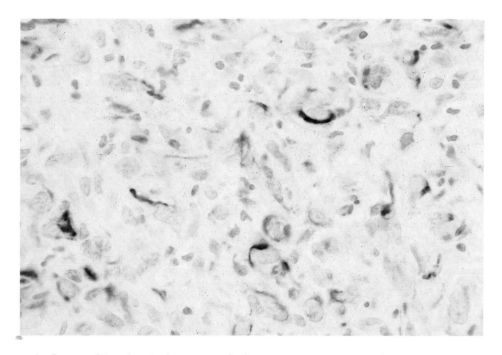

A. Immunohistochemical positivity for keratin is seen in many of the mesenchymal-like tumor cells.

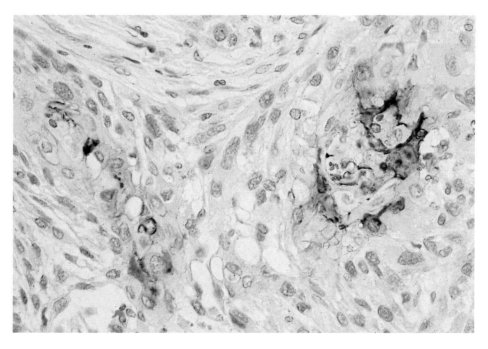

B. Focal immunoreactivity for CEA is evident in the necrotic and inflamed areas of an undifferentiated carcinoma with a squamoid pattern of growth.

however, the reaction was described as weak, focal, and restricted to a few tumor cells. The interpretation of this stain is subject to two important pitfalls: 1) entrapment of non-neoplastic follicles and isolated follicular cells and 2) release of thyroglobulin from the entrapped follicles, with secondary diffusion into the cytoplasm of the tumor cells, a phenomenon analogous to that seen in other sites (pl. XVIII) (15,31). In our experience and that of others (31,44), thyroglobulin has been found to be of little use in the evaluation of undifferentiated carcinoma. In the few instances in which we have found convincing tumor positivity, this was restricted to the residual better differentiated components, which were already clearly identifiable on morphologic grounds. Perhaps the use of monoclonal antibodies will provide better and more consistent results (13).

Another controversial marker in this context is calcitonin. Occasional examples of undifferentiated carcinoma have been found to be immunohistochemically reactive for this hormone, but we believe that most of them are recognizable as anaplastic variants of medullary carcinoma on morphologic grounds. Our own findings (9) and those of others (31,41,53) have failed to support the surprising claim (39) that most of undifferentiated carcinomas are calcitonin-positive and therefore related to medullary carcinoma. It seems to us that all the available evidence concerning undifferentiated carcinoma indicates otherwise.

All things considered, we would conclude that low–molecular-weight keratin is the most useful marker for the evaluation of undifferentiated carcinoma. It may not indicate the follicular origin of the tumor and is not even entirely pathognomonic of its epithelial nature (see page 260), but if it is present in a substantial number of tumor cells in the absence of vascular markers, it constitutes strong supporting evidence for the diagnosis, probably the strongest that can be marshaled with available techniques.

Ultrastructural Features. Evidence suggesting epithelial differentiation in the form of specialized cell functions of zonula adherens type and arrays of microvilli projecting into intercellular spaces has been described in the cells of undifferentiated carcinoma by several authors (figs. 140, 141) (9,16,20,24,38). However, such features may not necessarily be present, pre-

sumably because of total dedifferentiation of the neoplasm. In the series of Carcangiu and coworkers (9), they were detected in only four of seven cases.

The nuclei are large, with clumped chromatin and prominent nucleoli. The cytoplasm is abundant. Usually it has a primitive appearance, being mostly occupied by ribosomes, scattered mitochondria, and vesicles of granular endoplasmic reticulum. Randomly distributed cytoplasmic filaments of intermediate thickness (11 nm) can be found in some cases. Judging from the immunohistochemical results, we assume that some of these filaments are composed of vimentin and others of keratin. Occasionally, they form huge cytoplasmic whorls that fill most of the cytoplasm. These correspond to the cells determined by light microscopy as having a homogeneous, deeply acidophilic cytoplasm.

Membrane-bound, highly electron-dense cytoplasmic granules are frequently present. Their irregular size and shape is in keeping with a lysosomal nature. Granules clearly identifiable as secretory, neuroendocrine or otherwise, are consistently absent. Basal lamina deposition may be detected focally.

Other Special Techniques. DNA aneuploidy by flow-cytometric techniques has been found in most of the cases of undifferentiated carcinoma so far investigated, and it is likely to be present in all cases (18,29). In one series, all 7 patients with a DNA index greater than 1.30 died within 7 months, whereas 5 of the 11 patients with tumors that had an index of less than 1.30 survived longer than 1 year after the diagnosis (29).

Johnson and coworkers (25) examined four undifferentiated carcinomas for expression of *ras* oncogene p21 antigen by immunohistochemistry and found much less intense staining than in most other carcinoma types arising from follicular cells.

Microscopic Types. Traditionally, undifferentiated carcinomas have been divided into three types: spindle cell, giant cell or pleomorphic, and small cell. The first two have been amply discussed in the section on Microscopic Features but not as separate types. We view them instead as two morphologic manifestations of the same tumor that can be seen singly or in combination. We have added a squamoid pattern, which we believe to be as distinctive, albeit not as common, as

PLATE XVIII

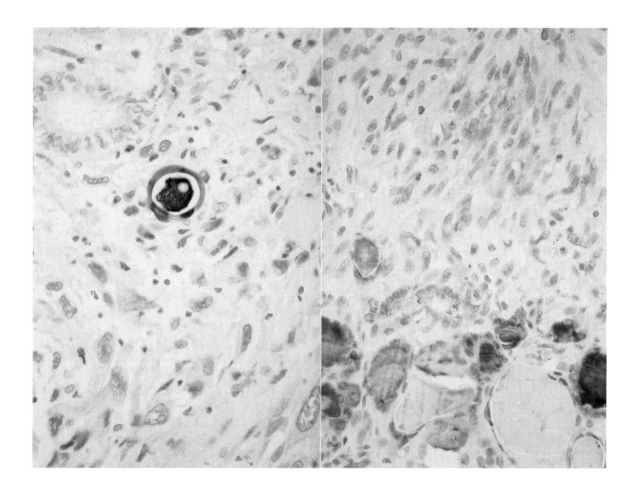

THYROGLOBULIN IMMUNOREACTIVITY IN UNDIFFERENTIATED CARCINOMA
In this field, an entrapped thyroglobulin-positive non-neoplastic follicle is surrounded by unreactive tumor cells (left). Apparent focal positivity for thyroglobulin is evident in the malignant tumor cells surrounding entrapped follicles (right). This is probably the result of thyroglobulin release from the latter followed by nonspecific absorption by the tumor cells.

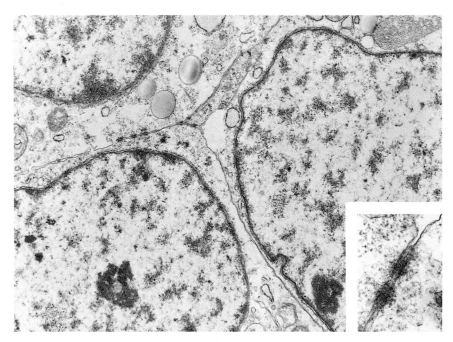

Figure 140
UNDIFFERENTIATED CARCINOMA
Ultrastructurally, the tumor cells appear extremely primitive, but a few specialized cell junctions are present, as highlighted in the inset. X9580; inset X38,250. (Courtesy of Dr. Robert Erlandson, Memorial Sloan-Kettering Cancer Center, New York, NY.)

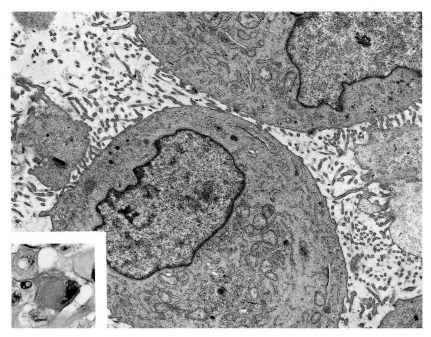

Figure 141
UNDIFFERENTIATED CARCINOMA
This electron micrograph shows retention of microvilli and an abundance of intracytoplasmic intermediate filaments in tumor cells. X5875. The latter result in a hyaline appearance at the light-microscopic level (inset). (Courtesy of Dr. Robert Erlandson, Memorial Sloan-Kettering Cancer Center, New York, NY.)

the others, and which, although undifferentiated, has an unmistakable epithelial appearance at the morphologic, immunohistochemical, and ultrastructural levels (9).

The wisdom of grouping the latter pattern with the other two could be questioned, especially because, in other organs in which this situation occurs, this practice is not followed. In the lung, for instance, undifferentiated but clearly epithelial tumors are designated *large cell undifferentiated carcinomas*; tumors with a predominant component of tumor giant cells are known as *giant cell carcinomas*; and carcinomas that are mostly composed of spindle cells and/or contain heterologous mesenchymal tissues are variously designated *spindle cell*, *sarcomatoid*, or *metaplastic*. Perhaps the best argument for keeping the thyroid tumors under discussion in a single category is the commonly observed merging of patterns and their essentially identical natural history.

The issue raised by undifferentiated small cell carcinoma is very different. Traditionally, it has been regarded as a distinctive form of undifferentiated carcinoma, and even subdivided into diffuse and compact subtypes (33). Currently, it is accepted that nearly all thyroid tumors reported in the old literature as diffuse small cell undifferentiated carcinomas represent malignant lymphomas instead (7,12,21,43,45).

As far as the compact subtype is concerned, they are a heterogeneous group. Some, probably most, are varieties of medullary carcinoma with a prominent nesting pattern, predominance of small cells, and scanty or no amyloid (see page 231). Others are examples of poorly differentiated (insular) carcinoma in which follicles are scanty or absent (see page 123) (10). Still others are analogous in all respects to small cell (oat cell) carcinoma of the lung and, as such, exhibit evidence of neuroendocrine differentiation (see page 231).

It could be argued that, because the aforementioned malignant tumors are epithelial, mostly undifferentiated (at least by conventional techniques), and composed of small cells, it is not inaccurate to call them small cell carcinoma. However, it is obvious that their natural histories and associations are so different from those of bona fide undifferentiated carcinoma that placing them into the same category would be highly misleading. Thus, we believe that the use of the term *undiffer-*

entiated small cell carcinoma without a qualifier should be avoided.

Differential Diagnosis. The differential diagnosis of undifferentiated carcinoma includes a relatively long list of tumors, depending on the pattern of growth they may exhibit.

True sarcoma. This can be primary in the thyroid or can reach the gland through direct invasion or metastatic spread from a soft tissue site. As already indicated, undifferentiated carcinoma may simulate a variety of soft tissue sarcomas, including fibrosarcoma, malignant fibrous histiocytoma (conventional, myxoid, and inflammatory); malignant hemangiopericytoma; and angiosarcoma (malignant hemangioendothelioma). Features favoring the diagnosis of carcinoma are the presence of recognizable epithelial foci, immunohistochemical positivity for keratin, and ultrastructural presence of desmosomes and microvilli. In general, the diagnosis of undifferentiated carcinoma should be favored in the presence of any pleomorphic malignant tumor that seems to arise in the thyroid, especially if the patient is elderly and if there is evidence of a residual better differentiated epithelial neoplasm in the gland, even if no clear-cut evidence of epithelial differentiation is found by any technique. Under these circumstances, the diagnosis of *undifferentiated malignant tumor, consistent with carcinoma* is justified. The only possible exception to this rule is angiosarcoma, a tumor discussed on page 259.

Solid variant of papillary carcinoma. The cells of this neoplasm retain the nuclear features of the more conventional types of papillary carcinoma, mitotic activity is minimal, and pleomorphism is not pronounced.

Poorly differentiated (insular) carcinoma. The nesting arrangement, uniformity in size and shape of the small, round tumor cells, focal microfollicular differentiation, and immunohistochemical positivity for thyroglobulin should result in an easy distinction.

Medullary carcinoma. Diagnostic confusion is more likely to arise in the spindle cell and pleomorphic variants of this tumor (26,34). The latter is particularly prone to misinterpretation because of the presence of bizarre cellular forms with monstrous nuclei (see page 232). In most instances, however, these features are accompanied by areas with a more conventional appearance. Stains for calcitonin and chromogranin should be performed in problem cases. If necessary, this can be supplemented by an electron-microscopic examination.

Malignant lymphoma. This entity still constitutes the most common source of diagnostic error. As a rule, the cells of malignant lymphoma are more evenly distributed, smaller, more uniform in size, and have a rounder shape than those of undifferentiated carcinoma. Intraluminal packing of entrapped follicles by tumor cells is a common feature (12). Stains for leukocyte-common antigen are generally positive, whereas keratin is invariably negative. The adjacent thyroid is likely to exhibit changes of Hashimoto thyroiditis.

Metastatic tumor. Multiple nodules are usually present, and their margins are likely to be sharper. Most of them exhibit a lesser degree of pleomorphism than undifferentiated thyroid carcinoma.

Cytologic Features. The tumor cells are pleomorphic, round, oval, or spindle shaped, and appear either isolated or in tissue fragments. The nuclei are bizarre and have clumped chromatin with excessive parachromatic clearing (figs. 142, 143). The nucleoli are large, multiple, and irregular. Intranuclear in-

clusions are frequent. Mitoses may be present. The abundant cytoplasm may be pale, vacuolated, dense, and sometimes keratinized.

Spread and Metastasis. There are very few tumors in the human body that tend to spread through all routes as quickly as undifferentiated thyroid carcinoma. Extrathyroid extension is the rule at the time of initial diagnosis. The tumor grows luxuriantly in the soft tissues of the neck, surrounds and invades the major vessels and nerves of the region, and spreads into the larynx, trachea, and esophagus (pl. XIX-A) (37). Metastases to regional lymph nodes are also common, although they are usually overshadowed by the massiveness of the primary growth; in contrast to other types of thyroid malignancy, they rarely are the first clinical manifestation of the disease. Blood-borne distant metastases are also frequent, the most common sites being adrenal glands, lung, and digestive tract (pl. XIX-B and C; fig. 144).

Treatment. Surgical excision is the first line of therapy, although in most cases, the tumor is so widespread that total removal is impossible.

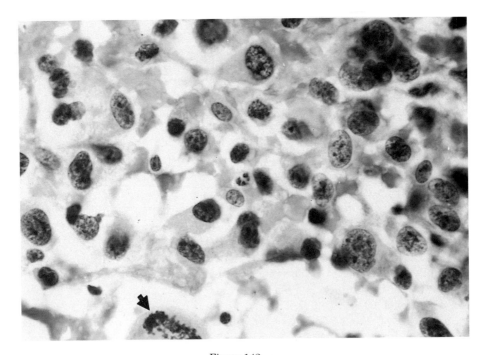

Figure 142
UNDIFFERENTIATED CARCINOMA
Pleomorphic tumor cells with bizarre nuclei and a mitotic figure (arrow) are seen in this cytologic specimen. Papanicolaou preparation. X504. (Fig. 9.7 from Kini SR. Thyroid. In: Kline TS, ed. Guides to clinical aspiration biopsy; Vol 13.New York, Igaku-Shoin 1987.)

It is more likely to be effective for the small undifferentiated tumors found incidentally in an otherwise well-differentiated neoplasm, but unfortunately this is a rare event. Suppression of thyroid function and administration of ^{131}I are of no value. Postoperative radiation therapy is generally administered but has proved ineffective in most cases. Many chemotherapeutic agents have been tried, singly or in combination. Initial tumor regression can be obtained with some regularity, and this may render a previously inoperable tumor amenable to surgical excision; however, in nearly all cases the tumor will quickly recur and kill the patient. Currently, it would seem that the best chances for cure, however slim, are obtained with a combination of surgery, radiation therapy, and multidrug chemotherapy (4,28).

Prognosis. Undifferentiated thyroid carcinoma is fatal in most cases. In the series of Carcangiu and coworkers (9), all patients died as

a result of tumor in a matter of weeks or months, the longest survival time being 2.5 years. In the series of Venkatesh and coworkers (52), the mean survival was 7.2 ±10 months.

Unrestrained tumor growth in the neck is most often the cause of death, with widespread distant metastatic involvement accounting for the others. Casterline and coworkers (11) reviewed 10 series of undifferentiated carcinoma in a search for patients who had survived for 2 or more years after initial diagnosis. Only 14 were found among 420, i.e., 3.3 percent of the total. The real percentage is probably even lower, because some of these series are probably contaminated with malignant lymphomas and other tumor types (10). However, indisputable cases of long-term cure of clinically obvious undifferentiated thyroid carcinoma exist. We have seen a case in which the patient was alive and well 8 years after the removal of an undifferentiated carcinoma that had spread to the soft tissues of the neck and

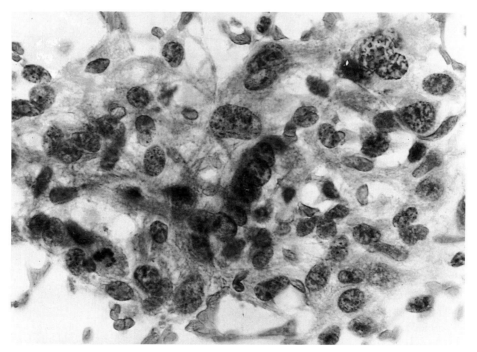

Figure 143
UNDIFFERENTIATED CARCINOMA
This fine-needle aspiration specimen shows a mixture of giant and spindle cells with pleomorphic nuclei and dense, abundant cytoplasm. Note the amorphous debris in the background. Papanicolaou preparation. X504. (Fig. 9.11 from Kini SR. Thyroid. Kline TS, ed. Guides to clinical aspiration biopsy; Vol 13.New York, Igaku-Shoin 1987.)

PLATE XIX
METASTATIC UNDIFFERENTIATED CARCINOMA

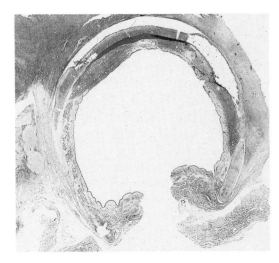

A. This autopsy specimen shows direct invasion of the trachea by undifferentiated thyroid carcinoma.

B. Multiple metastases of undifferentiated thyroid carcinoma in the stomach. Most of them show an ulcerated center. (Courtesy of Dr. Cleo Siderides, Stamford, CT.)

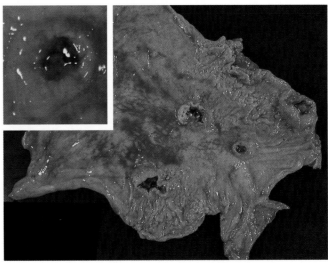

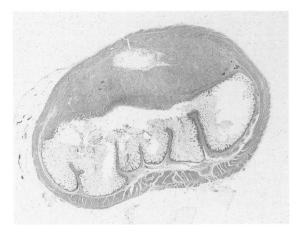

C. Metastasis of undifferentiated thyroid carcinoma in the wall of the large bowel. (Courtesy of Dr. Cleo Siderides, Stamford, CT.)

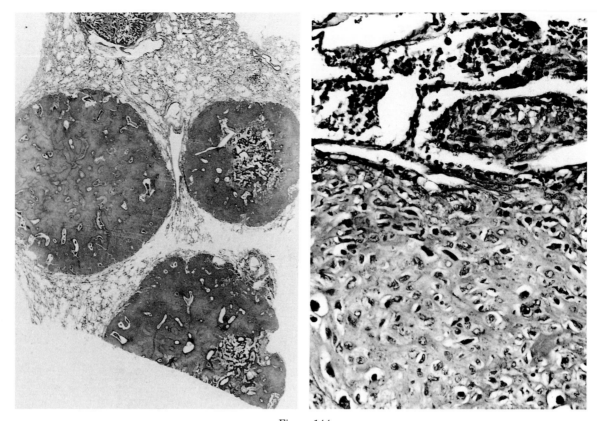

Figure 144

METASTATIC UNDIFFERENTIATED THYROID CARCINOMA

This figure shows low (left) and high (right) magnifications of metastatic undifferentiated thyroid carcinoma to lung.
The tumor nodules have a prominent cartilaginous component.

metastasized to the lung. The best available survival figures are those reported by Aldinger and coworkers (4), with 4 survivors among 14 patients who had a combination of surgery, radiation therapy, and chemotherapy. The follow-up was short, however, and in most cases, the undifferentiated carcinoma was small. Indeed, small tumor size is said to be a relatively favorable sign (37). It has also been claimed that the prognosis is better when evidence of a residual well-differentiated tumor is found, but in most series, no significant difference has been noted (23,50,54).

Antecedent Diseases. A significant number of undifferentiated carcinomas are topographically and probably causally associated with a preexisting well-differentiated thyroid tumor (fig. 145) (59,61,63,68). The admixture can be seen in the initial pathologic specimen, or the undifferentiated tumor may develop months or years after the removal of a well-differentiated neoplasm (fig.

146). The incidence of this occurrence in undifferentiated carcinoma varies from 8.5 percent (71) to 80 percent (67). The lower figures probably represent underestimates, either because the sampling was not thorough or because the undifferentiated component was so extensive that it totally obscured the other. It may be that all undifferentiated carcinomas arise against a background of a well-differentiated tumor, as some authors have suggested (67). Occasionally, well-differentiated and undifferentiated patterns coexist in metastatic foci. Even more rarely, the anaplastic transformation supervenes only in a local recurrence or metastasis of a well-differentiated tumor.

All major types of thyroid carcinoma of follicular cell derivation are susceptible to this change (figs. 131, 145, 147, 148). In some series, the follicular tumors greatly predominate (67), whereas in others, there is a preponderance of

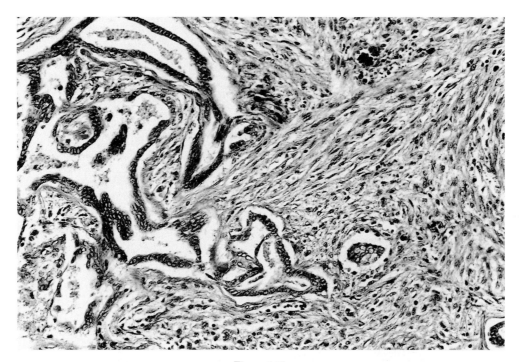

Figure 145
UNDIFFERENTIATED CARCINOMA WITH RESIDUAL PAPILLARY CARCINOMA
A sharp segregation of the two components can be seen in this field. The undifferentiated carcinoma is of the spindle cell type.

papillary carcinomas (55,70). It is not clear whether this represents a true difference, perhaps geographically based, or is simply the result of variations in diagnostic criteria. There is no relationship between the type of well-differentiated carcinoma and the pattern of undifferentiated carcinoma that it may give rise to, except between papillary carcinoma and the squamoid or squamous type of undifferentiated carcinoma (66) and specifically between the tall cell variant of papillary carcinoma and the spindle cell form of squamous cell carcinoma (57a). Fortunately, the probability of an anaplastic transformation occurring in any of the well-differentiated thyroid neoplasms is very low, probably not higher than 1 or 2 percent.

It has been suggested that the anaplastic transformation may be induced in these tumors by the administration of radioactive iodine (57,58) or external irradiation therapy. Kapp and coworkers (65) found 60 cases of this association. Regardless of whether the radiation is related causally to the transformation, the event is so rare that it should not interfere with the admin-istration of radiation therapy if this is necessary to control unresectable, locally recurrent, or metastatic well-differentiated thyroid carcinomas (65). On the other hand, this potential danger should be kept in mind when considering prophylactic administration of ^{131}I after surgical removal of a papillary thyroid carcinoma, especially because the benefit of this approach is far from proven.

Another antecedent mentioned in some series of undifferentiated carcinoma is a history of long-standing goiter. The incidence quoted is around 40 percent in most series (56,64) but substantially higher in others (67). Perhaps related to this is the observation that undifferentiated carcinoma has a higher incidence in areas of endemic goiter and that its frequency in those areas has decreased with the introduction of iodine prophylaxis (62).

An interesting model for human undifferentiated thyroid carcinoma is represented by a thyroid tumor induced in mice by sustained stimulation of the gland with endogenous thyrotropic hormone–secreting tumors. One such tumor, originally thyrotropic hormone dependent, able

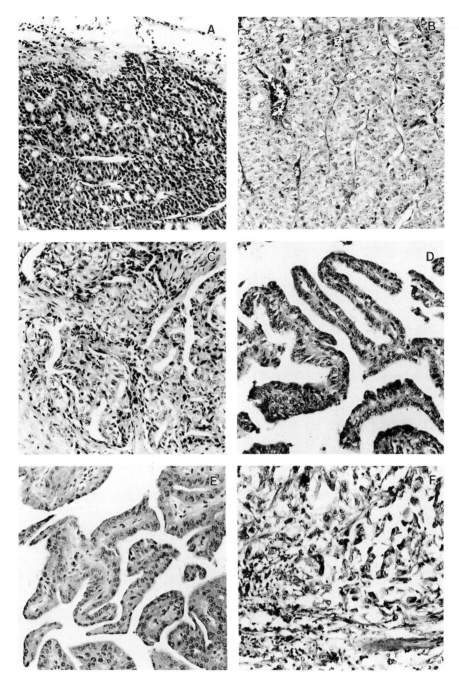

Figure 146
SEQUENTIAL MORPHOLOGIC VARIATIONS OF THYROID CARCINOMA
WITH EVENTUAL TRANSFORMATION TO UNDIFFERENTIATED CARCINOMA

The initial presentation was in 1974 in the form of a lung metastasis. The pattern of growth is microfollicular (A). The primary thyroid tumor was first detected in 1977. The pattern of growth is trabecular (B). The tumor recurred locally in the thyroid in 1979. The predominant pattern of growth is follicular, but there is a suggestion of papillary formations (C). The tumor further recurred in 1979. It now exhibits a typical papillary structure (D). The tumor recurred in soft tissue in 1980. The tumor has a papillary pattern of growth and vaguely oncocytic cytologic appearance (E). In 1983, the tumor underwent transformation to undifferentiated carcinoma (F). The patient died a few months later.

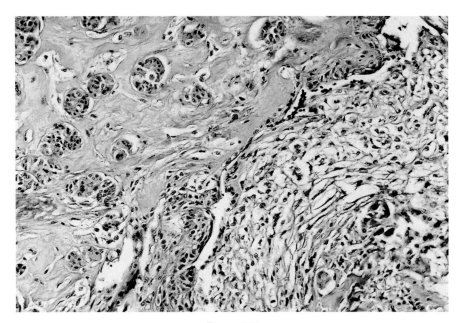

Figure 147
FOLLICULAR CARCINOMA WITH AN UNDIFFERENTIATED COMPONENT
This illustration shows follicular carcinoma (left) with marked hyalinization of the stroma and transformation to an undifferentiated sarcomatoid pattern (right).

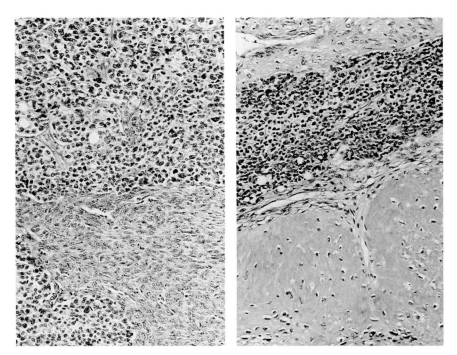

Figure 148
POORLY DIFFERENTIATED (INSULAR) CARCINOMA
WITH AN UNDIFFERENTIATED COMPONENT
In the photograph on the left, the appearance of the undifferentiated component is predominantly spindle, whereas in the photograph on the right, it has acquired well-developed cartilaginous features.

to trap ^{131}I and composed of papillary and/or follicular structures, became transformed after 7 years of serial transplantation into a pure sarcomatoid growth, one line with and the other without osteoclast-like giant cells (69).

Another animal model that is relevant to the issue of histogenesis of undifferentiated thyroid carcinoma is that described by Greenburg and Hay (60). The authors showed that follicular epithelium from normal rat thyroid growing in tridimensional collagen gels moved into the matrix, acquired mesenchymal-like morphologic and immunohistochemical features, and lost immunoreactivity for thyroglobulin.

REFERENCES

Undifferentiated (Anaplastic) Carcinoma

1. Agnantis NT, Rosen PP. Mammary carcinoma with osteoclast-like giant cells. A study of eight cases with follow-up data. Am J Clin Pathol 1979;72:383–9.

2. Albores-Saavedra J, Alcantara-Vazquez A, Meza Chavez L, de la Garza T, Rodriguez Martinez EA. Carcinoma anaplasico de celulas fusiformes y gigantes del tiroides: estudio de 63 casos. Prensa Med Mex 1972;37:421–6.

3. _____, Nadji M, Civantos F, Morales AR. Thyroglobulin in carcinoma of the thyroid: an immunohistochemical study. Hum Pathol 1983;14:62–6.

4. Aldinger KA, Samaan NA, Ibanez M, Hill CS Jr. Anaplastic carcinoma of the thyroid: a review of 84 cases of spindle and giant cell carcinoma of the thyroid. Cancer 1978;41:2267–75.

5. Barr R, Dann F. Anaplastic thyroid carcinoma metastatic to skin. J Cutan Pathol 1974;1:201–6.

6. Böcher W, Dralle H, Husselmann H, Bay B, Brassow M. Immunohistochemical analysis of thyroglobulin synthesis in thyroid carcinomas. Virchows Arch [A] 1980;385:187–200.

7. Burke JS, Butler JJ, Fuller LM. Malignant lymphomas of the thyroid: a clinical pathologic study of 35 patients including ultrastructural observations. Cancer 1977;39:1587–602.

8. Burt A, Goudie RB. Diagnosis of primary thyroid carcinoma by immunohistological demonstration of thyroglobulin. Histopathology 1979;3:279–86.

9. Carcangiu ML, Steeper T, Zampi G, Rosai J. Anaplastic thyroid carcinoma. A study of 70 cases. Am J Clin Pathol 1985;83:135–58.

10. _____, Zampi G, Rosai J. Poorly differentiated ("insular") thyroid carcinoma. A reinterpretation of Langhans' "wuchernde Struma." Am J Surg Pathol 1984;8:655–68.

11. Casterline PF, Jaques DA, Blom H, Wartofsky L. Anaplastic giant cell and spindle-cell carcinoma of the thyroid: a different therapeutic approach. Cancer 1980;45:1689–92.

12. Compagno J, Oertel JE. Malignant lymphoma and other lymphoproliferative disorders of the thyroid gland. A clinicopathologic study of 245 cases. Am J Clin Pathol 1980;74:1–11.

12a. Cuevas-Alvarez E, Forteza-Vila J. Carcinoma anaplásico de tiroides. Estudio inmunohistoquímico de 15 casos. Patología 1991;24:287–95.

13. De Micco C, Ruf J, Carayon P, Chrestian M-A, Henry J-F, Toga M. Immunohistochemical study of thyroglobulin in thyroid carcinomas with monoclonal antibodies. Cancer 1987;59:471–6.

14. Donnell CA, Pollock WJ, Sybers WA. Thyroid carcinosarcoma. Arch Pathol Lab Med 1987;111:1169–72.

15. Eusebi V, Bondi A, Rosai J. Immunohistochemical localization of myoglobin in nonmuscular cells. Am J Surg Pathol 1984;8:51–5.

16. Fisher ER, Gregorio R, Shoemaker R, Horvat B, Hubay C. The derivation of so-called "giant-cell" and "spindle-cell" undifferentiated thyroidal neoplasms. Am J Clin Pathol 1974;61:680–9.

17. Gaffey MJ, Lack EE, Christ ML, Weiss LM. Anaplastic thyroid carcinoma with osteoclast-like giant cells. A clinicopathologic, immunohistochemical, and ultrastructural study. Am J Surg Pathol 1991;15:160–8.

18. Galera-Davidson H, Bibbo M, Dytch HE, Gonzalez-Campora R, Fernandez A, Wied GL. Nuclear DNA in anaplastic thyroid carcinoma with a differentiated component. Histopathology 1987;11:715–22.

19. Hashimoto H, Koga S, Watanabe H, Enjoji M. Undifferentiated carcinoma of the thyroid gland with osteoclast-like giant cells. Acta Pathol Jpn 1980;30:323–34.

20. Hayashi Y, Tokuoka S. Anaplastic carcinoma of the thyroid gland. An ultrastructural study of four cases. Acta Pathol Jpn 1979;29:119–33.

21. Heimann R, Vannineuse A, De Sloover C, Dor P. Malignant lymphomas and undifferentiated small cell carcinoma of the thyroid: a clinicopathological review in the light of the Kiel classification for malignant lymphomas. Histopathology 1978;2:201–13.

22. Hurlimann J, Gardiol D, Scazziga B. Immunohistology of anaplastic thyroid carcinoma. A study of 43 cases. Histopathology 1987;11:567–80.

23. Hutter RV, Tollefsen HR, De Cosse JJ, Foote FW Jr, Frazell EL. Spindle and giant cell metaplasia in papillary carcinoma of the thyroid. Am J Surg 1965;110:660–8.

24. Jao W, Gould VE. Ultrastructure of anaplastic (spindle and giant cell) carcinoma of the thyroid. Cancer 1975;35:1280–92.

25. Johnson TL, Lloyd RV, Thor A. Expression of *ras* oncogene p21 antigen in normal and proliferative thyroid tissues. Am J Pathol 1987;127:60–5.

26. Kakudo K, Miyauchi A, Ogihara T, et al. Medullary carcinoma of the thyroid. Giant cell type. Arch Pathol Lab Med 1978;102:445–7.

27. Kawaoi A, Okano T, Nemoto N, Shiina T, Shikata T. Simultaneous detection of thyroglobulin (Tg), thyroxine (T4), and triiodothyronine (T3) in nontoxic thyroid tumors by the immunoperoxidase method. Am J Pathol 1982;108:39–49.

28. Kim JH, Leeper RD. Treatment of anaplastic giant and spindle cell carcinoma of the thyroid gland with combination Adriamycin and radiation therapy. A new approach. Cancer 1983;52:954–7.

29. Klemi PJ, Joensuu H, Eerola E. DNA aneuploidy in anaplastic carcinoma of the thyroid gland. Am J Clin Pathol 1988;89:154–9.

30. Kobayashi S, Yamadori I, Ohmori M, Kurokawa T, Umeda M. Anaplastic carcinoma of the thyroid with osteoclast-like giant cells. An ultrastructural and immunohistochemical study. Acta Pathol Jpn 1987;37:807–15.

31. LiVolsi VA, Brooks JJ, Arendash-Durand B. Anaplastic thyroid tumors. Immunohistology. Am J Clin Pathol 1987;87:434–42.

32. LoGerfo P, LiVolsi V, Colacchio D, Feind C. Thyroglobulin production by thyroid cancers. J Surg Res 1978;24:1–6.

33. Meissner WA, Phillips MJ. Diffuse small-cell carcinoma of the thyroid. Arch Pathol 1962;74:291–7.

34. Mendelsohn G, Baylin SB, Bigner SH, Wells SA Jr, Eggleston JC. Anaplastic variants of medullary thyroid carcinoma: a light microscopic and immunohistochemical study. Am J Surg Pathol 1980; 4:333–41.

35. Miettinen M, Franssila K, Lehto V-P, Paasivuo R, Virtanen I. Expression of intermediate filament proteins in thyroid gland and thyroid tumors. Lab Invest 1984;50:262–70.

36. _____, Virtanen I. Expression of laminin in thyroid gland and thyroid tumors: an immunohistologic study. Int J Cancer 1984;34:27–30.

37. Nel CJ, van Heerden JA, Goellner JR, et al. Anaplastic carcinoma of the thyroid: a clinicopathologic study of 82 cases. Mayo Clin Proc 1985;60:51–8.

38. Newland JR, Mackay B, Hill CS Jr, Hickey RC. Anaplastic thyroid carcinoma: an ultrastructural study of 10 cases. Ultrastruct Pathol 1981;2:121–9.

39. Nieuwenhuijzen Kruseman AC, Bosman FT, van Bergen Henegouw JC, Cramer-Knijnenburg G, de la Riviere GB. Medullary differentiation of anaplastic thyroid carcinoma. Am J Clin Pathol 1982;77:541–7.

40. Oppenheim A, Miller M, Anderson GH Jr, Davis B, Slagle T. Anaplastic thyroid cancer presenting with hyperthyroidism. Am J Med 1983;75:702–4.

41. Ordóñez NG, el-Naggar AK, Hickey RC, Samaan NA. Anaplastic thyroid carcinoma. Immunocytochemical study of 32 cases. Am J Clin Pathol 1991;96:15–24.

42. Phillips DL, Benner KG, Keeffe EB, Traweek ST. Isolated metastasis to small bowel from anaplastic thyroid carcinoma. With a review of extra-abdominal malignancies that spread to the bowel. J Clin Gastroenterol 1987;9:563–7.

43. Rayfield EJ, Nishiyama RH, Sisson JG. Small cell tumors of the thyroid. Cancer 1971;28:1023–30.

44. Ryff-de Leche A, Staub JJ, Kohler-Faden R, Müller-Brand J, Heitz PU. Thyroglobulin production by malignant thyroid tumors. An immunocytochemical and radioimmunoassay study. Cancer 1986;57:1145–53.

45. Schmid KW, Kroll M, Hofstadter F, Ladurner D. Small cell carcinoma of the thyroid. A reclassification of cases originally diagnosed as small cell carcinomas of the thyroid. Pathol Res Pract 1986;181:540–3.

46. Shoumacher P, Metz R, Bey P, Chesneau AM. Anaplastic carcinoma of the thyroid gland. Eur J Cancer 1977; 13:381–3.

47. Shvero J, Gal R, Avidor I, Hadar T, Kessler E. Anaplastic thyroid carcinoma. A clinical, histologic and immunohistochemical study. Cancer 1988;62:319–25.

48. Silverberg SH, DeGiorgi LS. Osteoclastoma-like giant cell tumor of the thyroid. Report of a case with prolonged survival following partial excision and radiotherapy. Cancer 1973;31:621–5.

49. Slatkin DN, Pearson J. Intramyofiber metastases in skeletal muscle. Hum Pathol 1976;7:347–9.

50. Tallroth E, Wallin G, Lundell G, Lowhagen T, Einhorn J. Multimodality treatment in anaplastic giant cell thyroid carcinoma. Cancer 1987;60:1428–31.

51. Tötsch M, Dobler G, Feichtinger H, Sandbichler P, Ladurner D, Schmid KW. Malignant hemangioendothelioma of the thyroid. Its immunohistochemical discrimination from undifferentiated thyroid carcinoma. Am J Surg Pathol 1990;14:69–74.

52. Venkatesh YS, Ordóñez NG, Schultz PN, Hickey RC, Goepfert H, Samaan NA. Anaplastic carcinoma of the thyroid. A clinicopathologic study of 121 cases. Cancer 1990;66:321–30.

53. Wilson NW, Pambakian H, Richardson TC, Stokoe MR, Makin CA, Heyderman E. Epithelial markers in thyroid carcinoma: an immunoperoxidase study. Histopathology 1986;10:815–29.

54. Wychulis AR, Beahrs OH, Woolner LB. Papillary carcinoma with associated anaplastic carcinoma in the thyroid gland. Surg Gynecol Obstet 1965;120:28–34.

Antecedent Diseases

55. Albores-Saavedra J, Alcantara-Vazquez A, Meza Chavez L, de la Garza T, Rodriguez Martinez EA. Carcinoma anaplasico de celulas fusiformes y gigantes del tiroides: estudio de 63 casos. Prensa Med Mex 1972;37:421–6.

56. Aldinger KA, Samaan NA, Ibanez M, Hill CS Jr. Anaplastic carcinoma of the thyroid: a review of 84 cases of spindle and giant cell carcinoma of the thyroid. Cancer 1978;41:2267–75.

57. Baker HW. Anaplastic thyroid cancer twelve years after radioiodine therapy. Cancer 1969;23:885–90.

57a. Bronner MP, LiVolsi VA. Spindle cell squamous carcinoma of the thyroid: An unusual anaplastic tumor associated with tall cell papillary cancer. Mod Pathol 1991;4:637–43.

58. Crile G Jr, Wilson DH. Transformation of low grade papillary carcinoma of the thyroid to an anaplastic carcinoma after treatment with radioiodine. Surg Gynecol Obstet 1959;108:355–60.

59. Fisher ER, Gregorio R, Shoemaker R, Horvat B, Hubay C. The derivation of so-called "giant-cell" and "spindle-cell" undifferentiated thyroidal neoplasms. Am J Clin Pathol 1974;61:680–9.
60. Greenburg G, Hay ED. Cytoskeleton and thyroglobulin expression change during transformation of thyroid epithelium to mesenchyme-like cells. Development 1988;102:605–22.
61. Harada T, Ito K, Shimaoka K, Hosoda Y, Yakumaru K. Fatal thyroid carcinoma. Anaplastic transformation of adenocarcinoma. Cancer 1977;39:2588–96.
62. Hofstadter F. Frequency and morphology of malignant tumours of the thyroid before and after the introduction of iodine prophylaxis. Virchows Arch [A] 1980;385:263–70.
63. Hutter RV, Tollefsen HR, De Cosse JJ, Foote FW Jr, Frazell EL. Spindle and giant cell metaplasia in papillary carcinoma of the thyroid. Am J Surg 1965;110:660–8.
64. Jereb B, Stjernswärd J, Lowhagen T. Anaplastic giant-cell carcinoma of the thyroid. A study of treatment and prognosis. Cancer 1975;35:1293–5.
65. Kapp DS, LiVolsi VA, Sanders MM. Anaplastic carcinoma following well-differentiated thyroid cancer: etiological considerations. Yale J Biol Med 1982;55:521–8.
66. Katoh R, Sakamoto A, Kasai N, Yagawa K. Squamous differentiation in thyroid carcinoma with special reference to histogenesis of squamous cell carcinoma of the thyroid. Acta Pathol Jpn 1989;39:306–12.
67. Nishiyama RH, Dunn EL, Thompson NW. Anaplastic spindle-cell and giant-cell tumors of the thyroid gland. Cancer 1972;30:113–27.
68. Spires JR, Schwartz MR, Miller RH. Anaplastic thyroid carcinoma. Association with differentiated thyroid cancer. Arch Otolaryngol Head Neck Surg 1988;114:40–4.
69. Ueda G, Furth J. Sarcomatoid transformation of transplanted thyroid carcinoma. Similarity to anaplastic human thyroid carcinoma. Arch Pathol 1967;83:3–12.
70. Woolner LB, Beahrs OH, Black BM, McConahey WM, Keating FR Jr. Classification and prognosis of thyroid carcinomas. Am J Surg 1961;102:354–87.
71. Wychulis AR, Beahrs OH, Woolner LB. Papillary carcinoma with associated anaplastic carcinoma in the thyroid gland. Surg Gynecol Obstet 1965;120:28–34.

TUMORS WITH ONCOCYTIC FEATURES
(HÜRTHLE CELL TUMORS)

Definition. Oncocytic tumors are thyroid neoplasms composed exclusively or predominantly (over 75 percent) of follicular cells exhibiting oncocytic features. In practice, one rarely has to make a precise quantitative evaluation because most thyroid neoplasms are either composed entirely of oncocytes or feature them in small, inconspicuous clusters.

General Considerations. The subject of thyroid neoplasms composed of oncocytes is one of the most controversial in thyroid pathology. This controversy involves several related issues that need to be discussed individually.

Terminology. The follicular cells crowded with mitochondria that characterize the tumors described in this section have been variously designated *Hürthle cells, Askanazy cells, oxyphilic cells, large cells,* and *oncocytes* (2,3,6). It has been repeatedly pointed out that Hürthle cell is a misnomer. The cells that Hürthle described in the thyroid of dogs were probably C cells (3,4), whereas Askanazy provided a very accurate and pictorially beautiful demonstration of the cells discussed in this chapter. The term *oxyphilic cell* suffers from lack of specificity. It has the same meaning as acidophilic cell, and therefore it could be applied to many cell types in addition to those that are the subject of this section. It is also obvious that the designation *large cell* is too general. The term *oncocyte* is probably the most appropriate. Although etymologically oncocyte simply means "swollen cell," its use has been restricted in the thyroid and other sites to the cell under discussion. We have therefore chosen to use it in this section, with due mention of the fact that the WHO Committee prefers the term *oxyphilic cell* and that the designation *Hürthle cell neoplasm* is too entrenched (especially among American clinicians and surgeons) to be expunged easily.

Nature of the oncocyte. The identification of a cell as an oncocyte has been traditionally based on the presence of an abundant granular acidophilic cytoplasm. Only later did special (supravital) stains, such as Janus green, and ultrastructural studies reveal that this granularity was due to the presence of a large number of mitochondria. Further electron-microscopic studies showed that, on rare occasions, a cytoplasmic granularity of somewhat similar light-microscopic appearance could be due instead to a richness in granular endoplasmic reticulum (ergastoplasm). It was therefore suggested that granular acidophilic follicular cells (and their tumors) be divided on the basis of their ultrastructural appearance into mitochondrion rich and ergastoplasm rich and that only the former be equated with oncocytes. This seems an impractical and unnecessarily restrictive policy, and we have not followed it in this section. It should also be remembered that the acidophilia must be granular for the cell to qualify as oncocytic. Diffuse or fibrillary acidophilia is usually due to accumulation of cytoplasmic filaments and therefore represents an entirely unrelated phenomenon (5). It should also be pointed out that, although neoplastic C cells can also undergo oncocytic change (see page 233), the term *oncocyte,* when applied to the thyroid, refers to a variant of follicular cell. As such, this cell has been found to possess an intact thyroid-stimulating hormone receptor–adenylate cyclase system, even in the neoplastic state (1). Finally, some authors draw a distinction between mitochondrion-rich cells and oncocytes, stating that in the latter the mitochondria are more numerous and have structural alterations. It is doubtful whether the distinction has validity on either biologic or practical grounds.

Existence of oncocytoma as a tumor entity. Some authors have taken the view that thyroid tumors composed of oncocytes should not be placed into a special category but simply classified on the basis of their architectural features independent of the presence and degree of oncocytic transformation (4). The implication of this position is that the oncocytic change is an inconsequential event that has no effect on the natural history of the disease. We are on the side of those who have taken a somewhat different viewpoint, i.e., that the tumors made up of this cell type have gross, microscopic, behavioral, cytogenetic (and conceivably etiopathogenetic) features that set them apart from all others and justify discussing them in a separate section (6). Incidentally, a similar approach has been taken in most other organs in which this phenomenon occurs, such as salivary gland and kidney.

Malignancy of oncocytomas. It has been suggested by some workers that all thyroid oncocytic neoplasms should be regarded as malignant or potentially malignant and treated accordingly (see page 163). Most authors, ourselves included, believe in the existence of both benign and malignant forms of this neoplasm and that the former predominate over the latter (6).

ONCOCYTIC ADENOMA (HÜRTHLE CELL ADENOMA)

Definition. A benign thyroid neoplasm composed exclusively or predominantly (over 75 percent) of oncocytes. Synonyms include *follicular adenoma of oxyphilic cell type* (15), *Hürthle cell adenoma* (perhaps the most widely used), and *benign oncocytoma*.

Gross Features. The tumor is completely encapsulated, round or oval, and usually solitary. Its most distinctive feature is the brown color of the cut surface, which is directly correlated with the richness in mitochondria and perhaps due to the cytochrome present in these organelles. It tends to be homogeneously solid, although secondary changes in the form of calcification, hemorrhage, cystic change, and central scarring are just as likely to be present as in other forms of follicular adenoma. Sometimes, the entire tumor undergoes massive infarct-type necrosis, a type of complication to which oncocytomas of other organs (e.g., salivary glands) are also prone. It may develop spontaneously or be precipitated by the performance of a fine-needle biopsy (19). At the gross level, this dramatic event results in a friable, grumous, deep brown mass with a bulging cut surface (pl. XX).

Microscopic Features. This tumor shares most of the features of follicular adenoma of ordinary type, as described on page 22. The pattern of growth is usually follicular (fig. 149). It can also be trabecular or solid, but in the presence of either of these two patterns, the index of suspicion for malignancy should rise. The intrafollicular colloid tends to be basophilic.

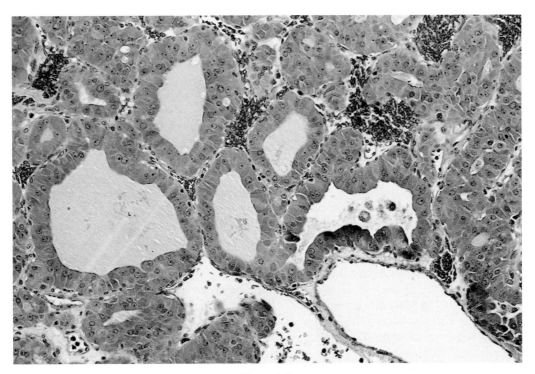

Figure 149
ONCOCYTIC ADENOMA WITH FOLLICULAR PATTERN
The cytoplasm is abundant and has a striking granular eosinophilic appearance.

It is common to find, in the center of the follicle, round calcified bodies with concentric laminations that resemble psammoma bodies (fig. 150). The main difference between these structures and true psammoma bodies as seen in papillary carcinoma lies in their intraluminal position. Under these circumstances, their presence is of no diagnostic significance. They should be disregarded even when secondary changes obscure their original intraluminal site (fig. 151).

The nuclei of the oncocytic cells are usually vesicular and uniform; however, these adenomas often feature marked nuclear atypia in the form of scattered enlarged hyperchromatic forms, sometimes reaching giant dimensions (fig. 152). This change is not indicative of malignancy per se. In fact, it can also be encountered in non-neoplastic thyroid disorders associated with oncocytic change, such as Hashimoto thyroiditis. When the tumor cells are round or polygonal, the nuclei tend to be centrally located. When the cells acquire a columnar shape, the nuclei may be centrally located or placed at the very apical

side. This results in a peg-like configuration and suggests an inversion of cell polarity (fig. 153). Variations in the cytoplasmic appearance relate to shape (round, vesicular, or columnar), size (usually larger than nononcocytic cells, but see the note under Oncocytic Carcinoma on page 173), and degree of granularity. Most commonly, this granularity is uniformly distributed throughout the cytoplasm (fig. 154). Variations in which the granularity within the cell is focal may be because either the oncocytic change itself is focal or part of it has undergone a secondary vesicular swelling of the mitochondria. The latter phenomenon, which results in progressive clearing of the originally oncocytic areas, is discussed in the section on Tumors With Clear Cell Features (see page 183). Infarct-type necrosis may be present, sometimes involving the entire neoplasm. This dramatic complication is analogous to that seen in oncocytomas of other organs (e.g., salivary glands) and is probably a reflection of the greater sensitivity to anoxia of the abnormal mitochondria that characterize the condition. It

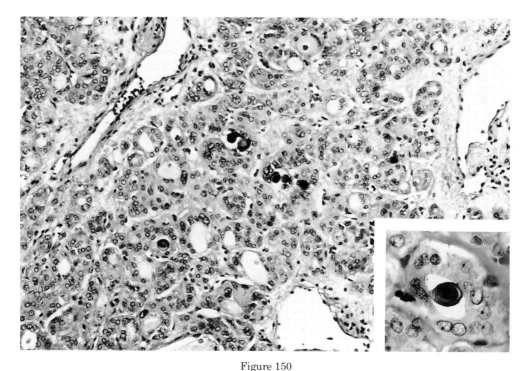

Figure 150
ONCOCYTIC ADENOMA WITH PSAMMOMA BODY–LIKE FORMATIONS
The inset shows that these formations are located within the lumina of the follicles, an important feature in the differential diagnosis with papillary carcinoma.

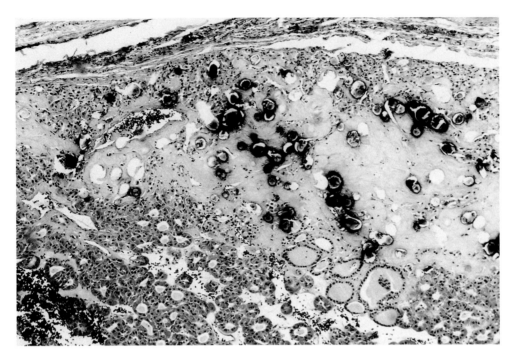

Figure 151
ONCOCYTIC ADENOMA
This tumor has a hyalinized area near the capsule that contains a large number of psammoma bodies.
These bodies probably originally had an intraluminal position.

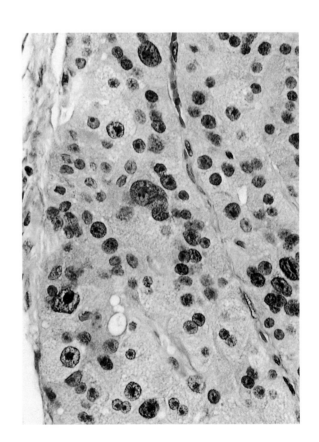

Figure 152
ONCOCYTIC ADENOMA
Large hyperchromatic nuclei and prominent
nucleoli are present in this field. This feature by itself
does not indicate malignancy.

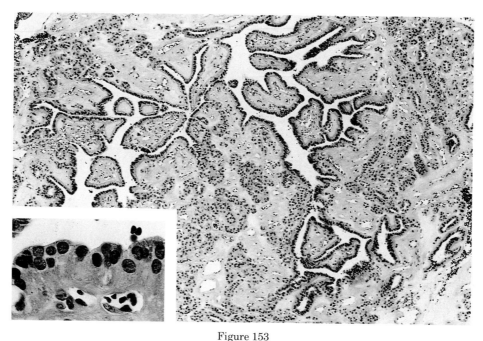

Figure 153
ONCOCYTIC ADENOMA
Note the focal papillary formations lined by columnar oncocytic epithelium. The inset shows the apical location of the nuclei.

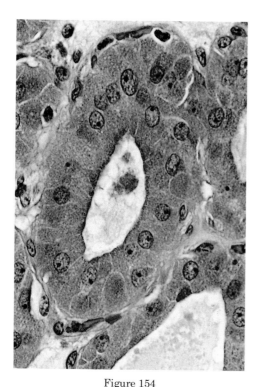

Figure 154
ONCOCYTIC ADENOMA
The fine granularity distributed homogeneously throughout the cytoplasm can be easily appreciated.

can occur spontaneously but is most commonly seen after fine-needle aspiration. The shadows of necrotic oncocytes can sometimes be identified, particularly when arranged in a follicular pattern (fig. 155). This complication is probably the result of the increased intratumoral pressure from the edema and hemorrhage induced by the procedure. Support for this interpretation was obtained by examining an oncocytic neoplasm with focal capsular invasion in which the entire tumor underwent necrosis after fine-needle aspiration except for the invasive portion, which was not subjected to the pressure increase (fig. 156). It would seem then as if this event could supervene in either benign or malignant oncocytic tumors as long as a complete or an incomplete fibrous capsule is present. Other complications from fine-needle aspiration that can cause diagnostic difficulties include the irregular growth of proliferating follicles along the needle tract through the capsule (fig. 157) and the vaguely pseudoangiosarcomatous appearance that may appear as the result of hemorrhage and thrombosis with subsequent organization (fig. 158) (7).

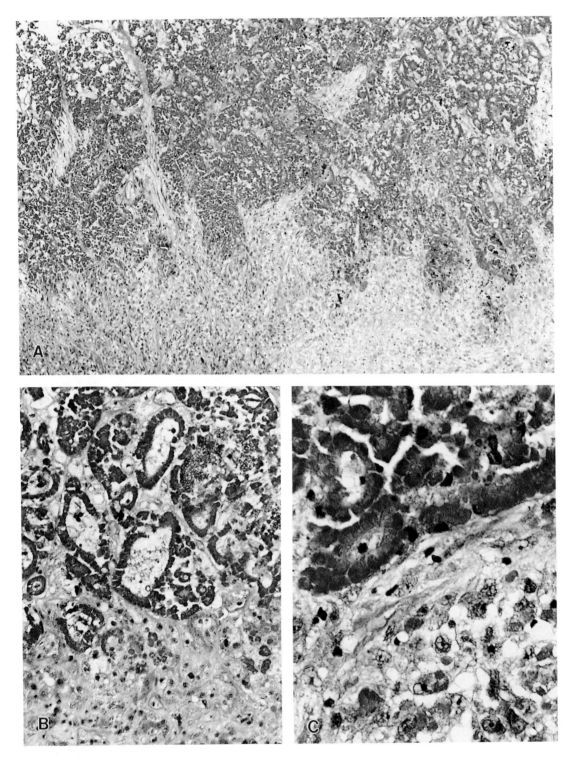

Figure 155
MASSIVE INFARCT OF ONCOCYTIC ADENOMA
At low magnification, the damage that resulted from fine-needle biopsy is visible (A). The shadows of necrotic neoplastic follicles can be appreciated (B). At high magnification, the strongly eosinophilic cytoplasm of the necrotic tumor cells is seen adjacent to reactive tissue (C).

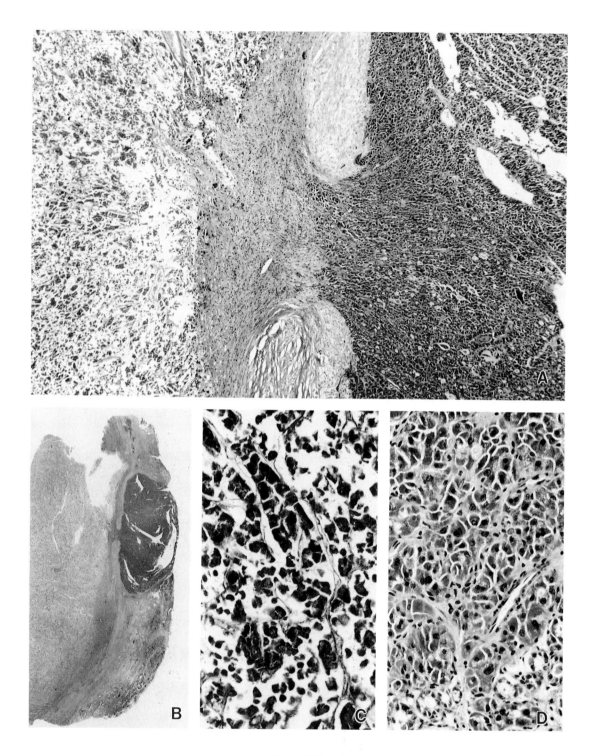

Figure 156
MINIMALLY INVASIVE ONCOCYTIC CARCINOMA WITH
FINE-NEEDLE BIOPSY–INDUCED NECROSIS
The entire tumor is necrotic except for the area beyond the capsule (A,B). High magnification shows the necrotic center of the tumor (C) and the well-preserved invasive component (D). This phenomenon suggests that the necrosis is the result of increased pressure within the encapsulated nodule.

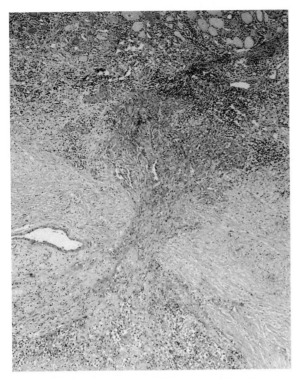

Figure 157
FOLLICULAR ADENOMA
WITH FINE-NEEDLE
BIOPSY–INDUCED CHANGES
This highly proliferating and irregularly
shaped follicular epithelium was found growing
in the capsule along the fine-needle biopsy tract
of a follicular adenoma. This should not be confused with true tumor invasion.

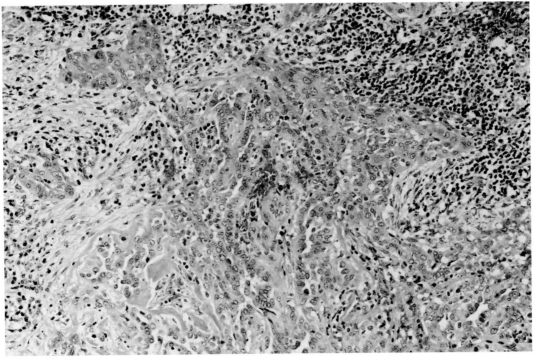

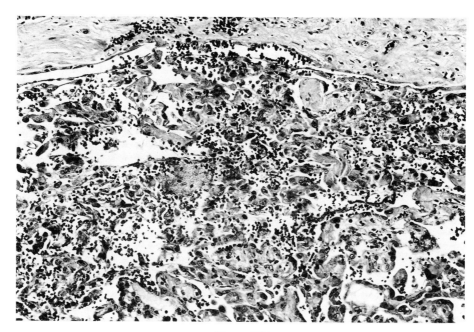

Figure 158
PSEUDOANGIOSARCOMATOUS PATTERN IN ONCOCYTIC NEOPLASM
This pattern was observed after a fine-needle aspiration procedure and resulted from extensive hemorrhage and proliferation of reactive mesenchymal elements.

Ultrastructural Features. The distinctive feature of the cells of oncocytic adenoma is the packing of the cytoplasm by mitochondria (fig. 159). In the most advanced stages of this process, few other organelles persist. Some of the mitochondria have a normal appearance; they are provided with a large number of inner membranes and a matrix of relatively high density. In most instances, however, marked abnormalities of size, shape, and content can be observed, and there may be an increase in the number, size, and pleomorphism of the intramitochondrial dense bodies (fig. 160) (23). Some mitochondria may appear dilated, with distortion and eventual disappearance of the cristae. When this secondary change becomes prominent, the organelles acquire a round vesicular shape and may no longer be recognizable as mitochondria. This is the ultrastructural equivalent of the progressive clearing of the cytoplasm seen at the light-microscopic level (see page 183). It should be pointed out that ultrastructural abnormalities of mitochondria in the thyroid gland are not restricted to oncocytomas or, for that matter, to oncocytes (21). The presence of distinct smooth-surfaced cells interspersed with cells with many microvilli is said to be a distinctive feature

of oncocytic neoplasms when examined under the scanning electron microscope (23).

Immunohistochemical Features. Immunoreactivity for thyroglobulin is present (18), but this is generally of a lesser degree than in ordinary follicular cells. Actually, the more pronounced the mitochondrial accumulation, the less intense the reactivity for thyroglobulin. Positivity for keratin is also diminished compared with that exhibited by the nononcocytic forms. Johnson and coworkers (18) found consistent expression of CEA by benign and malignant oncocytic tumors, a somewhat surprising finding that has not been confirmed in two other studies (9,23) or in our own experience.

Recently, an immunohistochemical technique for the demonstration of the mitochondria themselves was described. It is based on the use of a monoclonal antibody against cytochrome C oxidase, one of the enzymes of the mitochondrial respiratory chain (24).

Other Special Techniques. These are discussed in the section on Carcinoma, Oncocytic Type (page 173).

Cytologic Features. Cytologic specimens from oncocytic tumors are usually highly cellular, and the amount of colloid is generally

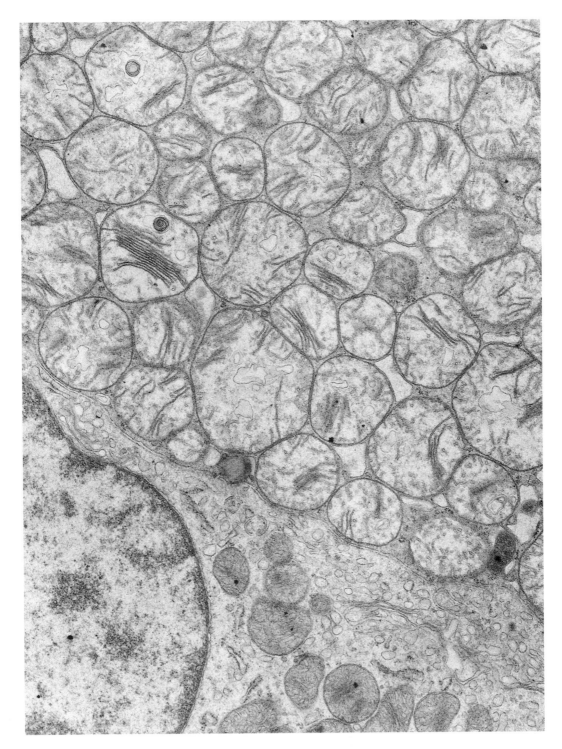

Figure 159
ONCOCYTIC ADENOMA
Ultrastructurally, the cytoplasm of a tumor cell is packed with abnormal mitochondria with very few residual organelles. Several abnormalities of these mitochondria can be observed, including the formation of myelin figures. The tumor cell present in the lower third of the photograph has mitochondria with a more normal appearance. X19,950. (Courtesy of Dr. Robert Erlandson, Memorial Sloan-Kettering Cancer Center, New York, NY.)

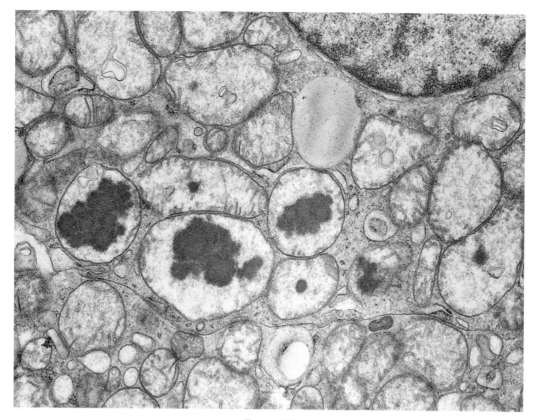

Figure 160
ONCOCYTIC ADENOMA
The mitochondria in this tumor cell are dilated and show diminution in the number of cristae; several of them have large, irregularly shaped, and pleomorphic intramitochondrial bodies. X16,000. (Courtesy of Dr. Robert Erlandson, Memorial Sloan-Kettering Cancer Center, New York, NY).

scanty. The cells have a polygonal shape, relatively large size, and a distinctly granular cytoplasm. The nuclei are large, round to oval, with generally fine chromatin and often prominent nucleoli. It is not unusual to find binucleation and marked nuclear atypia in the form of large hyperchromatic elements (fig. 161).

The aspirated cells are poorly cohesive. They may be seen as loose aggregates, as isolated cells, or (rarely) in a follicular arrangement (fig. 162).

The distinction between benign and malignant types of oncocytic neoplasms is generally not possible on cytologic grounds; however, the presence of intranuclear cytoplasmic inclusions and small oncocytic cells with altered nucleocytoplasmic ratio should be regarded as possible indicators of malignancy (20). The distinction between oncocytic neoplasms and hyperplastic oncocytic nodules may also cause difficulties.

However, aspirates from hyperplastic nodules tend to be more cohesive than those from neoplasms and often exhibit cell clusters with a honeycomb pattern. In general, the cells in these clusters have smaller nuclei and nucleoli than those featured by neoplastic cells.

Treatment. We believe that the surgical procedure for oncocytic adenoma need not be more extensive than that carried out for the conventional follicular adenoma. This seems to be the consensus, even among groups that had previously advocated a more aggressive approach (16,22).

Prognosis. In most reported series, conservative surgical excision of oncocytic adenoma has resulted in permanent cure. There were no instances of recurrence or metastasis in any of the 27 cases reported by Horn (follow-up time not specified) (17); the 34 cases reported by Bronner and

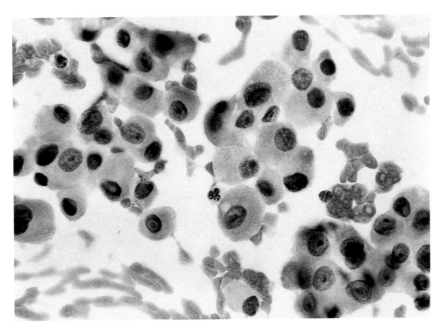

Figure 161
ONCOCYTIC ADENOMA
The cells of this oncocytic tumor are discrete, round to oval, with abundant granular cytoplasm and eccentric nuclei with prominent single macronucleoli. Papanicolaou preparation. X447. (Fig. 7.5 from Kini SR. Thyroid. In: Kline TS, ed. Guides to clinical aspiration biopsy; Vol 13.New York, Igaku-Shoin, 1987.)

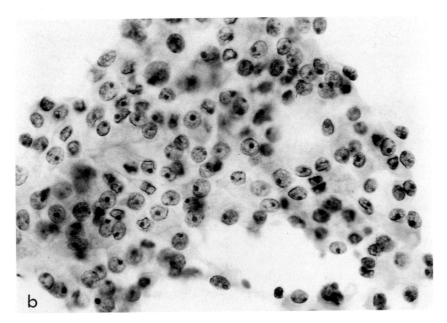

Figure 162
ONCOCYTIC ADENOMA
This field shows oncocytic cells in syncytial-type tissue fragments with crowding and overlapping of nuclei. The prominent single macronucleolus is characteristic, and the nuclear membranes are irregular. There is parachromatin clearing. Papanicolaou preparation. X447. (Fig. 7.8b from Kini SR. Thyroid. In: Kline TS, ed. Guides to clinical aspiration biopsy; Vol 13.New York, Igaku-Shoin, 1987.)

LiVolsi (mean follow-up time, 10.4 years) (9); the 34 cases reported by Bondeson and coworkers (follow-up time 2 to 20 years) (8); the 26 patients reported by Caplan and coworkers (follow-up time 2 to 22 years) (10); the 32 cases reported by Gerken and coworkers (follow-up time, 2 to 27 years) (13); the 71 patients reported by Gosain and Clark follow-up time, 675 patient years) (14); or the 90 cases reported by Carcangiu and coworkers (follow-up time 5 to 26 years) (11). However, in two other series, the results were startlingly different. The first, from Switzerland, recorded the development of recurrence in the form of carcinoma in 5 of 30 patients operated for oncocytic adenoma (25). In the second series, much more widely quoted, Thompson and coworkers (26) recorded the development of metastases in 3 of 4 cases that they had diagnosed as adenomas, this being the basis for their proposed radical approach to the treatment of oncocytic thyroid neoplasms. We have no explanation for this bizarre experience, other than that advanced by pathologists from the same institution who reviewed these cases years later; i.e., that the sampling of those tumors might have been inadequate (12). Interestingly, a subsequent report from the same group listed 23 additional cases of oncocytic adenoma, none of which gave rise to metastases (22).

ONCOCYTIC CARCINOMA (HÜRTHLE CELL CARCINOMA)

Definition. A malignant thyroid neoplasm composed exclusively or predominantly (over 75 percent) of oncocytes.

General Features. Oncocytic carcinomas account for 2 to 3 percent of all patients with thyroid carcinoma and approximately 20 percent of patients with follicular carcinoma (41). In one series, a third of the patients had associated nonmalignant thyroid diseases (41).

Clinical Features. Oncocytic carcinomas are most common in women; however, the predominance in this sex is not as pronounced as for oncocytic adenomas (ratio of women to men of 2:1 vs. 8:1), a fact to remember in the differential diagnosis (29,41). The mean age at the time of initial diagnosis is about 55 years (i.e., a decade older than for the benign oncocytic tumors) (29,41).

The clinical presentation does not differ from that of other malignant follicular tumors.

On the whole, oncocytic carcinomas do not take up radioactive iodine. They therefore appear as cold nodules on a thyroid scintigram, and the metastases may not be detectable with this technique.

Gross Features. On average, oncocytic carcinomas are larger than their benign counterparts, but the size range is wide (33,41). They share with the oncocytic adenoma the characteristic light brown color and the predominantly solid appearance (pl. XX). Multiplicity is rare. Secondary degenerative features in the form of necrosis, hemorrhage, and central scarring are more common than in the adenoma.

The boundaries of the tumor vary depending on the subtype. In the minimally invasive neoplasms, a complete capsule surrounds them so that the distinction from adenomas at the gross level becomes impossible. In the widely invasive tumors, the capsule is violated by tumor masses, or it may be altogether absent. It is characteristic for this tumor type to invade the surrounding thyroid in the form of sharply outlined nodules that connect with each other and with the main tumor mass. Sometimes these nodules are so distinct that they are misinterpreted at the gross level (and even microscopically) as separate neoplasms.

Microscopic Features. The cytologic features of oncocytic carcinomas resemble those of oncocytic adenomas in many ways, so that it becomes impossible in most cases to decide whether a given oncocytic tumor is benign or malignant on cytologic grounds alone. However, some differences exist, at least at a statistical level. In many oncocytic carcinomas, the amount of cytoplasm is less abundant than in the adenomas, resulting in an increased nuclear/cytoplasmic ratio. A greater percentage of tumor cells are tall cuboidal or columnar, as opposed to round or polygonal. The appearance of the nuclei varies a great deal. Scattered bizarre hyperchromatic forms may be seen, just as in the adenomas. More important, there is a tendency for increased mitotic activity and for all the nuclei to be more hyperchromatic than those of benign tumors.

Architecturally, most tumors have a solid/trabecular pattern of growth, as opposed to the predominantly follicular pattern of adenomas (figs. 163, 164). Sometimes the cells group in well-defined nests or insulae (fig. 165).

PLATE XX

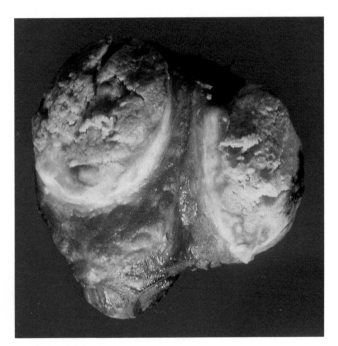

A. ONCOCYTIC ADENOMA
WITH MASSIVE INFARCT

The infarct in this tumor resulted from the performance of a fine-needle aspiration procedure. The entire tumor has a grumous appearance and is extremely friable.

B. ONCOCYTIC CARCINOMA

At the gross level, the tumor is mostly encapsulated, but several foci of invasion of the capsule can be appreciated. The cut surface has the characteristic brown color of this tumor type and exhibits foci of hemorrhage and necrosis.

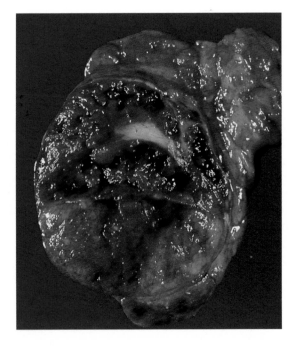

Although a careful evaluation of the cytologic and architectural features described above is important, it cannot be overemphasized that the feature that overrides all of them in terms of diagnostic importance is invasion. Its presence identifies an oncocytic neoplasm as malignant, and, if so, the degree of this invasion determines whether the carcinoma should be regarded as low grade (minimally invasive) or high grade (widely invasive). Although some degree of overlap exists, these two grades are distinct enough to be described separately.

Minimally invasive. This type is sometimes also designated *encapsulated* because it features a fibrous capsule similar to that of an adenoma. However, the capsule is invaded at one or more points by the tumor growth (fig. 166). In addition, invasion of blood vessels lying within the capsule is detected in most instances, hence the alternative designation *angioinvasive carcinoma*. The criteria used to decide whether capsular or vascular invasion exists are not different from those used in conventional follicular carcinoma (see page 50) and will therefore not be repeated here. In our experience, the phenomenon of blood vessel invasion by thyroid tumors is expressed in a more florid fashion (both in terms of number of vessels involved and degree of tumor infiltration) in oncocytic carcinoma than in follicular carcinoma of nononcocytic type (fig. 167).

Widely invasive. Whereas tumors in the previous category are wholly encapsulated and the question is whether this capsule is invaded or not, in the widely invasive types, the invasion is obvious and the difficulty (although obviously not an important one) is to determine whether there is a capsule at all. It is rare for the invasive component to be accompanied by the prominent desmoplastic reaction commonly seen with papillary carcinoma. Instead, it often presents in the form of compact nodules or cords that may be separated by residual follicles (fig. 168). Vascular permeation is more common and widespread than in the minimally invasive form.

Differential Diagnosis. The appearance of oncocytic thyroid neoplasms is so distinctive that a problem of cell type recognition seldom arises. The problem usually concerns whether the lesion

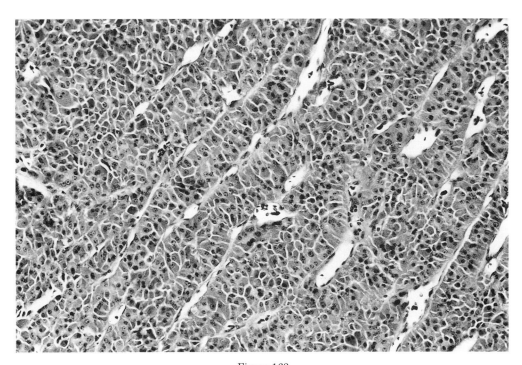

Figure 163
ONCOCYTIC CARCINOMA WITH TRABECULAR PATTERN
This configuration is more common in malignant than benign oncocytic tumors.

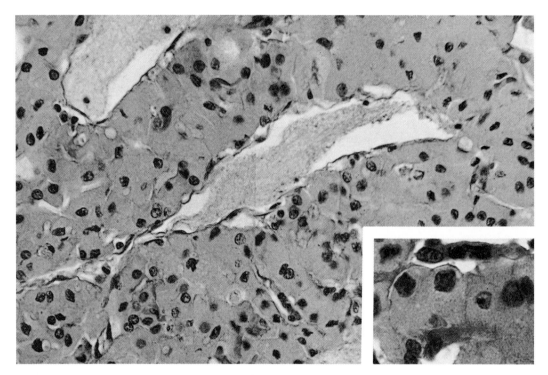

Figure 164
ONCOCYTIC CARCINOMA
Pulmonary metastasis of an oncocytic carcinoma with trabecular pattern of growth. The inset shows the abundant granular acidophilic cytoplasm and irregularly shaped hyperchromatic nuclei. (Fig. 100 from Fascicle 4, Second Series.)

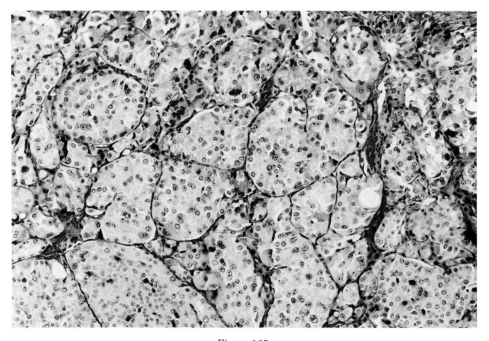

Figure 165
ONCOCYTIC CARCINOMA
This tumor shows a distinct nesting of tumor cells. The pattern is analogous to that seen in poorly differentiated (insular) carcinoma and should be regarded as a sign of probable aggressive behavior.

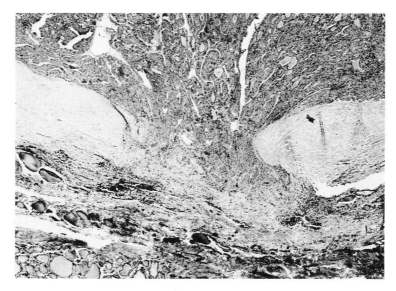

Figure 166
ONCOCYTIC CARCINOMA
Capsular invasion is present in this oncocytic carcinoma.

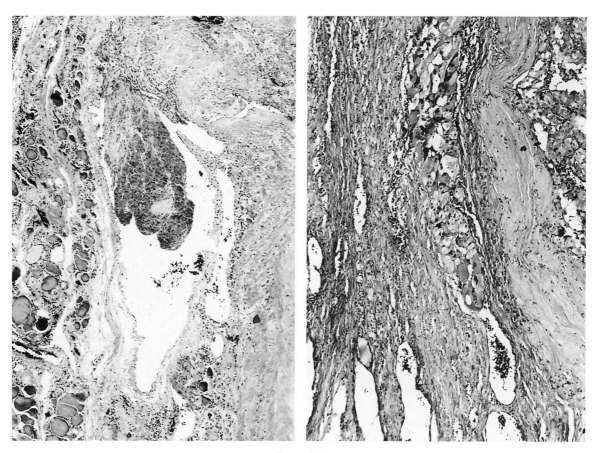

Figure 167
ONCOCYTIC CARCINOMA
Blood vessel invasion is present in this oncocytic carcinoma.

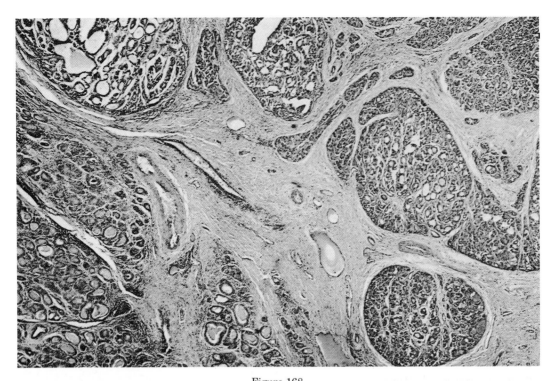

Figure 168
ONCOCYTIC CARCINOMA
This illustration shows the characteristic multinodular pattern of invasion at the periphery.

is hyperplastic or neoplastic and, if neoplastic, whether it is benign or malignant. However, two neoplasms of the region deserve mention because of their uncanny resemblance to oncocytic thyroid carcinoma at the H&E level. One, not surprisingly, is oncocytoma (benign or malignant) of parathyroid glands (37,42). The other is the oncocytic variant of thyroid medullary carcinoma (see page 233). Laboratory data, ultrastructural evaluation, and immunohistochemical stains may be necessary to rule out these possibilities.

Ultrastructural and Immunohistochemical Features. These features of oncocytic carcinomas are not significantly different from those described for the oncocytic adenomas (see page 165).

Cytological Features. These are also discussed in the section on Oncocytic Adenomas.

Other Special Techniques. Ebner and coworkers (30) found that the increase of mitochondria in these tumors was accompanied by increased enzymatic activity of respiratory complexes I, II, IV, and V.

Expression of the p21 *ras* oncogene product has been found consistently in both benign and malignant oncocytic tumors. The significance of this finding is unknown (35).

DNA analysis, by either flow-cytometric or microspectrophotometric techniques, has shown a high incidence of polyploidy and aneuploidy in these tumors. This finding is anticipated on the basis of the abnormal nuclear features as detected morphologically (30). Most studies indicate that aneuploidy in histologically malignant tumors statistically correlates with higher invasiveness and clinical malignancy (27,28,31,38). The most impressive results in this regard are those of Rainwater and coworkers (38): in a series of 37 oncocytic carcinomas, none of the patients with diploid or polyploid carcinomas died, but 11 of the 19 patients (58 percent) with aneuploid carcinoma did. However, there is no convincing evidence that the information obtained from this technique adds a great deal to the diagnostic conclusions derived from the pathologic evaluation; it certainly cannot be used currently to either document or rule out malignancy. Specifically, and despite some statements to the contrary (32), there does not appear to be any unfavorable prognostic significance for abnormal DNA content in histologically benign oncocytic neoplasms (27,28,31).

Spread and Metastasis. Direct spread into the perithyroid soft tissues is more common in oncocytic carcinoma than in the conventional follicular carcinoma. This is probably also true for distant metastases. The most common sites are lung and bone, followed by regional lymph nodes (40). The latter are more frequent than for conventional follicular carcinoma but substantially less so than for papillary carcinoma (41). Some of these metastases occur very late in the course of the disease (up to 10 years or more), emphasizing the need for long-term follow-up (34).

Treatment. It is generally agreed that widely invasive oncocytic carcinomas should be treated by total or near-total thyroidectomy (34,36). Most minimally invasive tumors are also treated in this fashion (36), but there is no available evidence that doing so produces better results than performing a more conservative operation. Adjunctive therapeutic modalities such as suppression, radioactive iodine, or external irradiation are of little or no value.

Prognosis. The overall 5-year survival rate for oncocytic carcinoma has ranged between 50 and 60 percent in most series. It is directly dependent on the degree of invasiveness and is therefore substantially better for minimally invasive than for widely invasive tumors. Obviously, blood-borne metastases impact greatly on survival (29). Interestingly, this is also true for regional nodal metastases. In contrast, this parameter has no prognostic significance in papillary carcinoma.

A difficult and currently unresolved issue is whether oncocytic carcinomas are more malignant than follicular carcinomas of nononcocytic type with a similar size and degree of invasiveness. Some series suggest that this might be the case (39).

PAPILLARY ONCOCYTIC NEOPLASMS

As already stated, most oncocytic thyroid neoplasms exhibit follicular, trabecular, and/or solid patterns of growth. For this reason, they are regarded by most as a subtype of follicular neoplasms. In some of these tumors, particularly those

with a macrofollicular pattern of growth, the septa separating the follicles are very thin, so that when cut tangentially, they may simulate papillae. This feature has no diagnostic significance (fig. 169).

There are, however, rare oncocytic neoplasms that exhibit a papillary configuration throughout, a feature that is analogous in all regards to that seen in papillary carcinoma. These papillae are lined by a single layer of oncocytic cells of either cuboidal or columnar shape (fig. 170). The nuclei, although vesicular, usually lack a well-developed ground-glass appearance. Some of these tumors are invasive and seem to behave similarly to conventional papillary carcinoma; i.e., they have a tendency for regional lymph node involvement. Their long-term behavior is said to

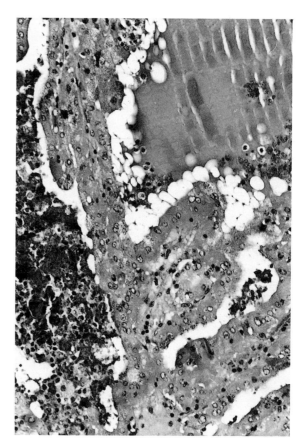

Figure 169
PSEUDOPAPILLARY FORMATIONS IN
ONCOCYTIC ADENOMA
The pseudopapillary formations in this oncocytic thyroid tumor resulted from tangential sectioning of the septa separating dilated follicles.

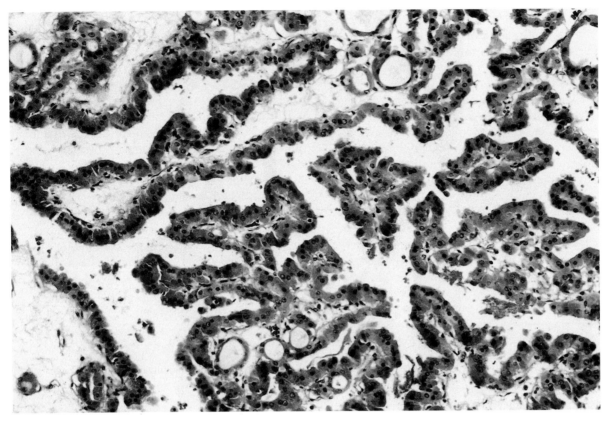

Figure 170
ONCOCYTIC PAPILLARY NEOPLASM
This oncocytic neoplasm has a well-developed papillary pattern of growth.

be comparable to that of their nononcocytic counterparts (44), but our own (limited) experience suggests that they might behave more aggressively (43). In the reported series of papillary carcinoma, the incidence of the oncocytic type has ranged from 1.1 to 11.3 percent. This probably reflects differences in diagnostic criteria (45). We suspect that the higher figures derive from the inclusion of other types of papillary carcinoma, as discussed on page 72. For these invasive papillary neoplasms exhibiting true oncocytic features, we prefer the designation *oncocytic papillary carcinoma*.

Other oncocytic papillary neoplasms are totally encapsulated and exhibit no signs of either capsular or vascular invasion (43). The position of these lesions in the classification scheme of thyroid neoplasia remains controversial. They could be regarded as encapsulated papillary carcinomas of oncocytic type, conversely, they could be viewed as oncocytic adenomas with papillary hyperplasia, by use of a similar reasoning to that applied to nononcocytic follicular adenomas (see page 38). We favor the latter interpretation because we have found no documentation of metastases in our series or in those of others (43,44). However, because we consider the issue unresolved, we recommend that these tumors be designated for now with the noncommittal term *encapsulated papillary oncocytic neoplasms*. A conservative surgical approach seems justified in view of the above findings.

REFERENCES

Tumors with Oncocytic Features
(Hürthle Cell Tumors)

1. Clark OH, Gerend PL. Thyrotropin receptor-adenylate cyclase system in Hürthle cell neoplasms. J Clin Endocrinol Metab 1985;61:773–8.
2. Flint A, Lloyd RV. Hürthle-cell neoplasms of the thyroid gland. Pathol Annu 1990;25(Pt. 1):37–52.
3. Hamperl H. Benign and malignant oncocytoma. Cancer 1962;15:1019–27.
4. Hedinger CE, Williams ED, Sobin LH. Histological typing of thyroid tumours. In: Hedinger CE, ed. International histological classification of tumours; Vol 11. 2nd ed. Berlin: Springer-Verlag, 1988.
5. Nesland JM, Sobrinho-Simões MA, Holm R, Sambade MC, Johannessen JV. Hürthle-cell lesions of the thyroid: a combined study using transmission electron microscopy, scanning electron microscopy, and immunocytochemistry. Ultrastruct Pathol 1985;8:269–90.
6. Tallini G, Carcangiu ML, Rosai J. Oncocytic neoplasms of the thyroid gland. Acta Pathol Jpn 1992;42:305–15.

Oncocytic Adenoma (Hürthle Cell Adenoma)

7. Axiotis CA, Merino MJ, Ain K, Norton JA. Papillary endothelial hyperplasia in the thyroid following fine-needle aspiration. Arch Pathol Lab Med 1991;115:240–2.
8. Bondeson L, Bondeson A-G, Ljungberg O, Tibblin S. Oxyphil tumors of the thyroid: follow-up of 42 surgical cases. Ann Surg 1981;194:677–80.
9. Bronner MP, LiVolsi VA. Oxyphilic (Askanazy/Hürthle cell) tumors of the thyroid. Microscopic features predict biologic behavior. Surg Pathol 1988;1:137–50.
10. Caplan RH, Abellera RM, Kisken WA. Hürthle cell tumors of the thyroid gland. A clinicopathologic review and long-term follow-up. JAMA 1984;251:3114–7.
11. Carcangiu ML, Bianchi S, Savino D, Voynick IM, Rosai J. Follicular Hürthle cell neoplasms of the thyroid gland. A study of 153 cases. Cancer 1991;68:1944–53.
12. Flint A, Lloyd RV. Hürthle-cell neoplasms of the thyroid gland. Pathol Annu 1990;25(Pt. 1):37–52.
13. Gerken K, Nunez C, Broughan T, Esselstyn C, Sebek B. Clinical outcome of Hürthle cell tumors of the thyroid [Abstract]. Am J Clin Pathol 1988;90:498A.
14. Gosain AK, Clark OH. Hürthle cell neoplasms. Malignant potential. Arch Surg 1984;119:515–9.
15. Hedinger CE, Williams ED, Sobin LH. Histological typing of thyroid tumours. In: Hedinger CE, ed. International histological classification of tumours; Vol 11. 2nd ed. Berlin: Springer-Verlag, 1988.
16. Heppe H, Armin A, Calandra DB, Lawrence AM, Paloyan E. Hürthle cell tumors of the thyroid gland. Surgery 1985;98:1162–5.
17. Horn RC. Hürthle cell tumors of the thyroid. Cancer 1954;7:234–44.
18. Johnson TL, Lloyd RV, Burney RE, Thompson NW. Hürthle cell thyroid tumors. An immunohistochemical study. Cancer 1987;59:107–12.
19. Kini SR, Miller JM, Abrash MP, Gaba A, Johnson T. Post fine needle aspiration biopsy infarction in thyroid nodules [Abstract]. Mod Pathol 1988;1:48A.
20. Kini SR, Miller JM, Hamburger JI. Cytopathology of Hürthle cell lesions of the thyroid gland by fine needle aspiration. Acta Cytol 1981;25:647–52.
21. Matias C, Moura Nunes JF, Sobrinho LG, Soares J. Giant mitochondria and intramitochondrial inclusions in benign thyroid lesions. Ultrastruct Pathol 1991;15:221–9.
22. McLeod MK, Thompson NW. Hürthle cell neoplasms of the thyroid. Otolaryngol Clin North Am 1990;23:441–52.
23. Nesland JM, Sobrinho-Simões MA, Holm R, Sambade MC, Johannessen JV. Hürthle-cell lesions of the thyroid: a combined study using transmission electron microscopy, scanning electron microscopy, and immunocytochemistry. Ultrastruct Pathol 1985;8:269–90.
24. Ortmann M, Vierbuchen M, Koller G, Fisher R. Renal oncocytoma. I. Cytochrome c oxidase in normal and neoplastic renal tissue as detected by immunohistochemistry: a valuable aid to distinguish oncocytomas from renal cell carcinomas. Virchows Arch [Cell Pathol] 1988;56:165–73.
25. Ruchti C, Komor J, König MP. Grosszellige Tumoren (sogenannte Hürthlezell-Tumoren) der Schilddrüse. Helv Chir Acta 1976;43:129–32.
26. Thompson NW, Dunn EL, Batsakis JG, Nishiyama RH. Hürthle cell lesions of the thyroid gland. Surg Gynecol Obstet 1974;139:555–60.

Oncocytic Carcinoma (Hürthle Cell Carcinoma)

27. Bondeson L, Azavedo E, Bondeson A-G, Caspersson T, Ljungberg O. Nuclear DNA content and behavior of oxyphil thyroid tumors. Cancer 1986;58:672–5.
28. Bronner MP, Clevenger CV, Edmonds PR, Lowell DM, McFarland MM, LiVolsi VA. Flow cytometric analysis of DNA content in Hürthle cell adenomas and carcinomas of the thyroid. Am J Clin Pathol 1988;89:764–9.
29. Carcangiu ML, Bianchi S, Savino D, Voynick IM, Rosai J. Follicular Hürthle cell neoplasms of the thyroid gland. A study of 153 cases. Cancer 1991;68:1944–53.
30. Ebner D, Rödel G, Pavenstaedt I, Haferkamp O. Functional and molecular analysis of mitochondria in thyroid oncocytoma. Virchows Arch [Cell Pathol] 1991;60:139–44.
31. el-Naggar AK, Batsakis JG, Luna MA, Hickey RC. Hürthle cell tumors of the thyroid. A flow cytometric DNA analysis. Arch Otolaryngol Head Neck Surg 1988;114:520–1.
32. Flint A, Davenport RD, Lloyd RV, Beckwith AL, Thompson NW. Cytophotometric measurements of Hürthle cell tumors of the thyroid gland. Correlation with pathologic features and clinical behavior. Cancer 1988;61:110–3.

33. González-Cámpora R, Herrero-Zapatero A, Lerma E, Sanchez F, Galera H. Hürthle cell and mitochondrion-rich cell tumors. Correlation with pathologic features and clinical behavior. Cancer 1986;57:1154–63.

34. Gundry SR, Burney RE, Thompson NW, Lloyd R. Total thyroidectomy for Hürthle cell neoplasm of the thyroid. Arch Surg 1983;118:529–32.

35. Johnson TL, Lloyd RV, Thor A. Expression of *ras* oncogene p21 antigen in normal and proliferative thyroid tissues. Am J Pathol 1987;127:60–5.

36. McLeod MK, Thompson NW. Hürthle cell neoplasms of the thyroid. Otolaryngol Clin North Am 1990; 23:441–52.

37. Obara T, Fujimoto Y, Yamaguchi K, Takanashi R, Kino I, Sasaki Y. Parathyroid carcinoma of the oxyphil cell type. A report of two cases, light and electron microscopic study. Cancer 1985;55:1482–9.

38. Rainwater LM, Farrow GM, Hay ID, Lieber MM. Oncocytic tumours of the salivary gland, kidney, and thyroid: nuclear DNA patterns studied by flow cytometry. Br J Cancer 1986;53:799–804.

39. Schröder S, Pfannschmidt N, Dralle H, Arps H, Böcker W. The encapsulated follicular carcinoma of the thyroid. Virchows Arch [A] 1984;402:259–73.

40. Tollefsen HR, Shah JP, Huvos AG. Hürthle cell carcinoma of the thyroid. Am J Surg 1975;130:390–4.

41. Watson RG, Brennan MD, Goellner JR, van Heerden JA, McConahey WM, Taylor WF. Invasive Hürthle cell carcinoma of the thyroid: natural history and management. Mayo Clin Proc 1984;59:851–5.

42. Wolpert HR, Vickery AL Jr, Wang C-A. Functioning oxyphil cell adenomas of the parathyroid gland. A study of 15 cases. Am J Surg Pathol 1989;13:500–4.

Papillary Oncocytic Neoplasms

43. Barbuto D, Carcangiu ML, Rosai J. Papillary Hürthle cell neoplasms of the thyroid gland. A study of 20 cases [Abstract]. Mod Pathol 1990;3:7A.

44. Beckner M, Oertel J. Papillary carcinomas of the oxyphil cell subtype [Abstract]. Lab Invest 1987;56:5A.

45. Sobrinho-Simões MA, Nesland JM, Holm R, Sambade MC, Johannessen JV. Hürthle cell and mitochondrion-rich papillary carcinomas of the thyroid gland: an ultrastructural and immunocytochemical study. Ultrastruct Pathol 1985;8:131–42.

TUMORS WITH CLEAR CELL FEATURES

Definition. Included in this chapter are primary thyroid neoplasms in which 75 percent or more of the tumor cells show marked cytoplasmic clearing.

General Considerations. Older classification schemes of thyroid tumors often include a category of clear cell carcinoma, implying the existence of a distinctive type of thyroid neoplasm that is always malignant. We believe that neither assumption is correct. Instead, we view cytoplasmic clear changes in follicular cells as a secondary event that can result from a variety of mechanisms and can occur in practically any of the major tumor types (2). Thus, we view this situation as not substantially different from that of other organs. In the lung, for instance, the belief in the existence of a clear cell carcinoma existed for many years; it has now been convincingly shown that clear cell changes can occur in any of the major types of lung carcinomas and that these changes, albeit morphologically spectacular, have no significant impact in the natural history of the tumor (10).

There are several mechanisms by which a follicular cell can acquire a clear cytoplasmic appearance when examined in H&E-stained sections. The most important are the following.

Cytoplasmic vesicles. At the ultrastructural level, these are membrane-bound structures of relatively uniform diameter that contain an electron-lucent material. Although the appearance of most is nondescript, the presence of distorted residual cristae in some of these structures suggests that, in most instances, these vesicles represent massively dilated mitochondria. Others may represent dilated secretory vesicles, whereas still others may have derived from the endoplasmic reticulum or Golgi apparatus (9,15).

When the cytoplasmic clearing is due to vesicle accumulation, the cells appear clear at the H&E level but still retain a fine granularity, which could be graphically depicted as having the appearance of a washed-out oncocyte. The nucleus is usually centrally located and has smooth contours. The cell membrane is sharply outlined, a feature shared by most other types of follicular clear cells.

Glycogen. This type of clear cell tends to be larger than the preceding type, and the clearing is more complete. Instead of a fine granularity, an empty cytoplasm is seen with an appearance that has been classically compared to that of a vegetable cell. The glycogen, which tends to be scattered throughout the cytoplasm, can be demonstrated by the PAS reaction, by other glycogen stains, or by ultrastructural examination. The nucleus is usually centrally located and has smooth contours, as in the preceding type.

Lipid. This type of alteration, which can present in association with glycogen particles, presents in its fully developed form as an accumulation of cytoplasmic vesicles that are small to medium sized and that typically indent the centrally located nucleus. This results in an appearance similar to either a lipoblast or a spongiocyte from the *fasciculata* layer of the adrenal cortex. The lipid present in these vacuoles can be demonstrated with oil red O or other fat stains in wet (non–paraffin-embedded) formalin-fixed tissue or by ultrastructural examination.

Thyroglobulin. Under some conditions, thyroglobulin accumulates in the cytoplasm in the form of small or large membrane-bound aggregates. Most of these formations have a homogeneous or granular acidophilic appearance, but others have a very light staining quality; i.e., they appear clear on H&E sections. When the aggregates are smaller, the nucleus retains its central position, and it may acquire indentations similar to those seen as a result of cytoplasmic lipid accumulation. When large, the aggregates displace the nucleus laterally and distort it in such a way as to create a signet-ring cell configuration.

Mucin. If the cytoplasmic clearing seen in follicular cells has a slight basophilic quality, the probability that this is due to the accumulation of mucosubstances should be considered and further investigated with mucin stains such as Alcian blue. The source of the mucin deposition, which is sometimes accompanied by a similar deposition extracellularly, is not easily apparent. However, it should be remembered that thyroglobulin is a glycoprotein and that the number of acidic groups in it can range widely. It is therefore possible that some instances of clear cell thyroid tumors of mucinous type are related to the accumulation of highly acidic forms of thyroglobulin.

Tumor Types. Clear cell changes have been described in nearly all major types of benign and malignant thyroid neoplasms. It should also be pointed out that they are not restricted to neoplastic conditions. They have also been observed in some forms of dyshormonogenetic goiter (1), in conventional nodular hyperplasia, and in Hashimoto thyroiditis. In the latter disorder, they seem to be the result of vesicular swelling of mitochondria in the oncocytic follicular cells that are an integral part of the disease. Primary thyroid tumors in which clear cell changes have been documented include the following types.

Oncocytic neoplasms. There is probably no type of thyroid follicular cell that is more prone to undergo secondary clear changes than the oncocyte, whether neoplastic or not. Thus, the change can be observed in any thyroid disorder in which oncocytes occur, such as Hashimoto thyroiditis, nodular hyperplasia, and benign and malignant oncocytic tumors. The mechanism is apparently the same in all and is related to vesicular swelling of mitochondria. In the oncocytic neoplasms, the change can be focal or extensive. The oncocytes and the clear cells may be segregated in nests or closely intermingled (figs. 171, 172). Sometimes, transitional forms between these two cell types are evident. The most spectacular of these is the tall cuboidal or columnar cell in which the basal cytoplasm is oncocytic and the apical cytoplasm is clear (fig. 173) (4). This change can also occur in oncocytic neoplasms of other sites, such as salivary glands.

The reasons for the mitochondrial swelling are unknown. Some authors have suggested that the vesicular cytoplasmic formation may be induced by thyroid-stimulating hormone overstimulation of these cells (11), but this hypothesis remains unsubstantiated.

This type of clear cell change occurs in both benign and malignant oncocytic tumors. The criteria for distinguishing them are the same as for oncocytic (or, for that matter, follicular) tumors in general; however, there is a disproportionately high number of malignant cases (80

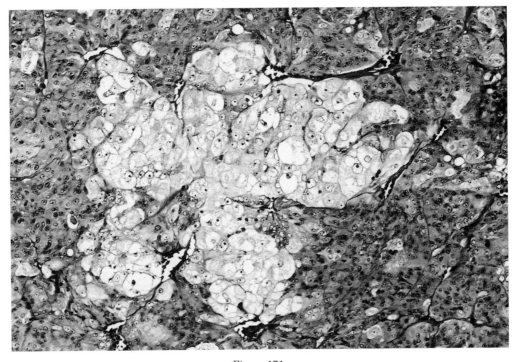

Figure 171
ONCOCYTIC TUMOR WITH FOCAL CLEAR CELL CHANGE
The two components are sharply segregated in this example. The clear cells have more abundant cytoplasm, larger nuclei, and more prominent nucleoli than the oncocytic elements that surround them.

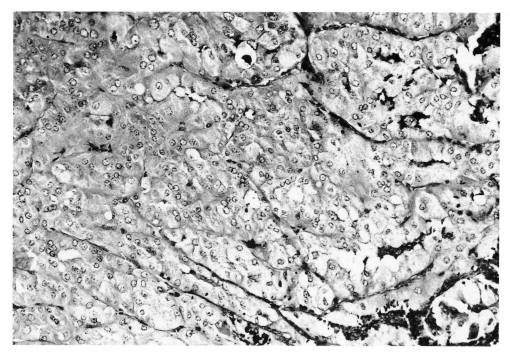

Figure 172
ONCOCYTIC TUMOR WITH CLEAR CELL CHANGE
In this tumor, the transition from one area to the other is gradual, with many cells exhibiting transitional features.

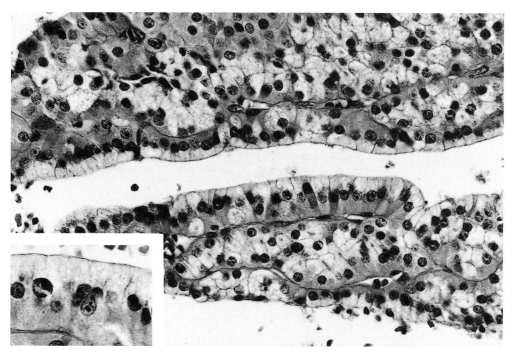

Figure 173
ONCOCYTIC TUMOR WITH CLEAR CELL CHANGE
In this illustration, the two patterns coexist in the same cell. This is particularly obvious in the columnar cell component of the tumor (inset). The nucleus is centrally located, the basilar portion of the cytoplasm is oncocytic, and the apical portion is clear.

percent in one series [2]) among the oncocytic tumors with clear cell changes compared with oncocytic neoplasms in general. The finding of clear cell changes in an oncocytic neoplasm should therefore heighten the suspicion of carcinoma and lead to a careful search for confirmatory evidence.

Follicular neoplasms. This group represents the prototypic example of clear cell thyroid tumor, and the one probably referred to in most articles dealing with thyroid as *clear cell tumor*, *clear cell carcinoma*, *hypernephroid tumor*, and *parastruma* (7,17,20). Some have been included in the category of atypical adenoma only because their cytoplasm was clear (8).

The criteria for malignancy are the same as for follicular tumors in general, i.e., capsular and/or blood vessel invasion (fig. 174). When thus defined, both benign and malignant forms will be identified, and the former will predominate (2). In some instances, scattered follicles of nondescript appearance are seen among those composed of clear cells. The pattern of growth is usually follicular, but it may be solid and/or trabecular (fig.

175). It is possible that some of the tumors that are entirely composed of clear cells represent oncocytic neoplasms in which the cytoplasmic clearing has proceeded to its ultimate expression. This is suggested by the fact that, ultrastructurally, the change is due in most cases to vesicles that appear similar to those of clear cell oncocytomas. In other instances, the change is the result of glycogen accumulation or dilatation of granular endoplasmic reticulum (fig. 176) (9). There is immunoreactivity for thyroglobulin in most cells, but it is usually mild to moderate. In general, the more clear the cell, the less prominent the thyroglobulin staining (3). Although the existence of benign clear cell follicular tumors of the thyroid with the features described above is now widely accepted, the index of suspicion for malignancy should be raised if this clear cell change is widespread and/or combined with oncocytic features.

Although a small to moderate number of glycogen granules can occasionally be detected in the cytoplasm of follicular clear cells by special

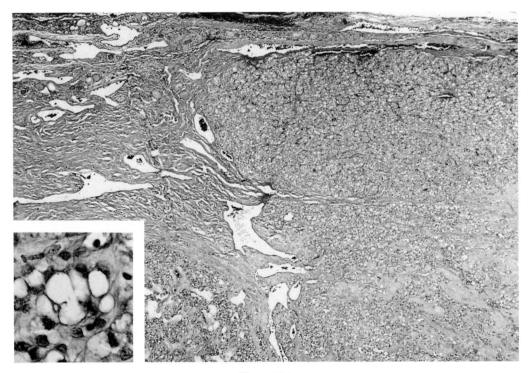

Figure 174
FOLLICULAR CARCINOMA WITH CLEAR CELL CHANGE
The tumor exhibits extensive capsular invasion. The inset shows the clear cell appearance of the cytoplasm of the tumor cells, many of which have a signet-ring appearance.

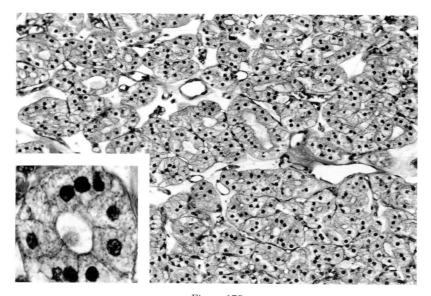

Figure 175
(Figures 175 and 176 are from the same patient)
FOLLICULAR NEOPLASM WITH PROMINENT CLEAR CELL CHANGE
As shown in the inset, the follicular cells, although clear, retain some cytoplasmic granularity. This is a useful feature in the differential diagnosis with metastatic renal cell carcinoma.

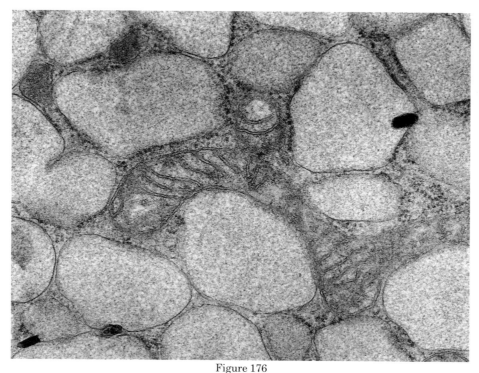

Figure 176
FOLLICULAR TUMOR WITH PROMINENT CLEAR CELL CHANGE
The clear cell change seen in this electron micrograph is due to marked dilatation of the cisternae of the granular endoplasmic reticulum. This is an unusual occurrence. X49,050. (Courtesy of Dr. Robert Erlandson, Memorial Sloan-Kettering Cancer Center, New York, NY.)

stains or electron microscopy, the existence of a glycogen-rich clear cell follicular adenoma has not been proved (20). Before such a diagnosis is considered, the more probable alternative of a metastatic clear cell carcinoma (particularly from the kidney) should be ruled out.

Signet-ring follicular adenoma and carcinoma. As the name indicates, these tumors are characterized by the fact that many of their follicular cells exhibit a large cytoplasmic vacuole that displaces the nucleus laterally, leading to a signet-ring configuration (18). The content of the cytoplasmic vacuole may appear clear, homogeneously acidophilic, or granular in H&E sections. The nucleus may retain its original round or oval shape, but more often it acquires a semilunar shape, which heightens the resemblance of the cell to a signet ring (figs. 177, 178). Usually these cells alternate with others that have a more conventional appearance. Ultrastructurally, the vacuoles represent either intracellular lumina bordered by microvilli or distended vesicles (17).

A variant is the follicular adenoma in which the intracytoplasmic vacuoles are small and the nucleus remains centrally located. This may represent an early stage of the cell destined to become of signet-ring type. In these tumors, the stroma tends to be hyaline and is occasionally peppered with fine particles of calcium salts.

Immunohistochemical studies have shown that these cytoplasmic vacuoles, whether small or large, are strongly reactive for thyroglobulin (pl. XXI-A). Interestingly, they can also be positive for mucin stains, a fact that has led to the alternative designations *signet-ring cell mucinous adenoma* (6) or *mucin-producing microfollicular adenoma* (16). It has been suggested that the mucin reactivity is due to the presence of protein-polysaccharide complexes derived from partial degradation of thyroglobulin (14). It has been further suggested that the intracellular accumulation of thyroglobulin results from an inability of the cell to excrete it, perhaps due to a deletion in one or more of the many proteins

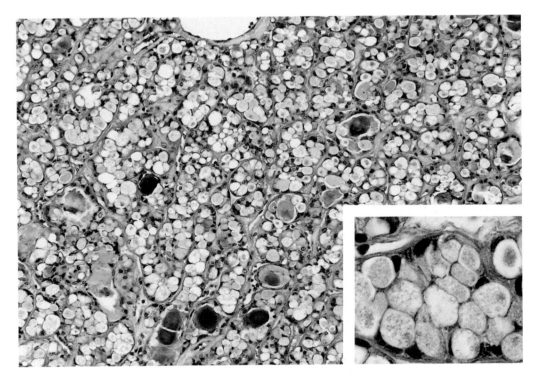

Figure 177
SIGNET-RING FOLLICULAR ADENOMA
Most of the tumor cells have a signet-ring appearance resulting from the intracellular accumulation of thyroglobulin. The inset shows the fine basophilic granularity present within the cytoplasm, and the nuclear displacement.

PLATE XXI

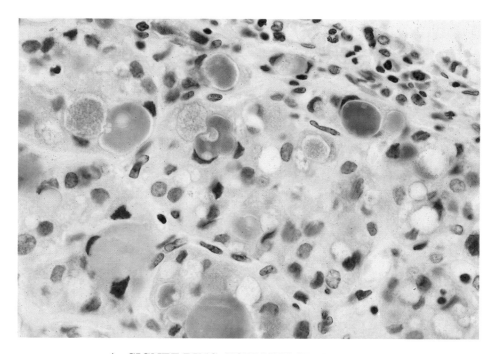

A. SIGNET-RING FOLLICULAR ADENOMA
Strong intracytoplasmic immunoreactivity for thyroglobulin is evident in this signet-ring follicular adenoma.

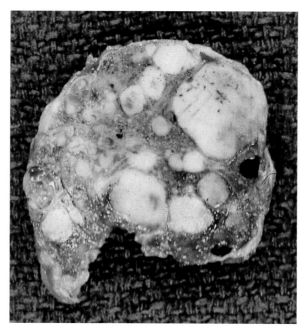

**B. NODULAR HYPERPLASIA WITH
CLEAR CELL CHANGE**
The clear cell-containing nodules are variously sized,
whitish gray, and well circumscribed.

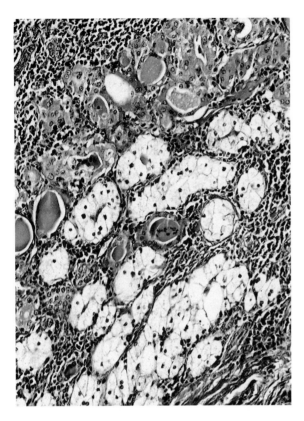

Figure 181
CLEAR CELL CHANGE IN
HASHIMOTO THYROIDITIS
An area of cytoplasmic clear cell changes in
Hashimoto thyroiditis is shown in this illustration. This
probably represents secondary clear cell transformation
in oncocytic cells.

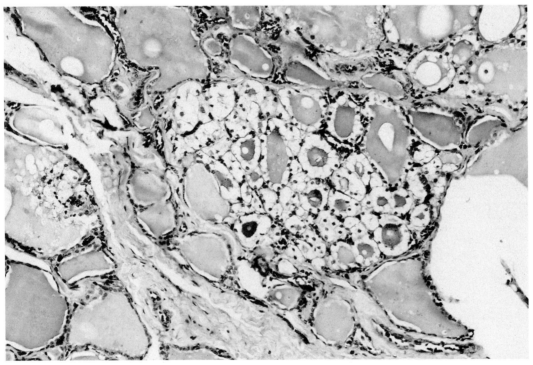

Figure 182
CLEAR CELL CHANGE IN NODULAR HYPERPLASIA
This figure illustrates focal cytoplasmic clear cell change in nodular hyperplasia.

REFERENCES

1. Batsakis JG, Nishiyama RH, Schmidt RW. "Sporadic goiter syndrome": a clinicopathologic analysis. Am J Clin Pathol 1963;39:241–51.

2. Carcangiu ML, Sibley RK, Rosai J. Clear cell change in primary thyroid tumors. A study of 38 cases. Am J Surg Pathol 1985;9:705–22.

3. Civantos F, Albores-Saavedra J, Nadji M, Morales AR. Clear cell variant of thyroid carcinoma. Am J Surg Pathol 1984;8:187–92.

4. Dickersin GR, Vickery AL Jr, Smith SB. Papillary carcinoma of the thyroid oxyphil cell type, "clear cell" variant. Am J Surg Pathol 1980;4:501–9.

5. Fisher ER, Kim WS. Primary clear cell thyroid carcinoma with squamous features. Cancer 1977;39:2497–502.

6. Gherardi G. Signet ring cell 'mucinous' thyroid adenoma: a follicle cell tumour with abnormal accumulation of thyroglobulin and a peculiar histochemical profile. Histopathology 1987;11:317–26.

7. Harach HR, Virgili E, Soler G, Zusman SB, Saravia-Day E. Cytopathology of follicular tumours of the thyroid with clear cell change. Cytopath 1991;2:125–35.

8. Hazard JB, Kenyon R. Atypical adenoma of the thyroid. Arch Pathol 1954;58:554–63.

9. Ishimaru Y, Fukuda S, Kurano R, Miura K, Tajiri J, Maeda K. Follicular thyroid carcinoma with clear cell change showing unusual ultrastructural features. Am J Surg Pathol 1988;12:240–6.

10. Katzenstein A-L, Prioleau PG, Askin FB. The histologic spectrum and significance of clear-cell change in lung carcinoma. Cancer 1980;45:943–7.

11. Kniseley RM, Andrews GA. Transformation of thyroidal carcinoma to clear-cell type. Am J Clin Pathol 1956;26:1427–38.

12. Landon G, Ordoñez NG. Clear cell variant of medullary carcinoma of the thyroid. Hum Pathol 1985;16:844–7.

13. Meissner WA, Adler A. Papillary carcinoma of the thyroid. A study of the pathology of two hundred twenty-six cases. Arch Pathol 1958;66:518–25.

14. Mendelsohn G. Signet-ring-simulating microfollicular adenoma of the thyroid. Am J Surg Pathol 1984;8:705–8.

15. Mochizuki M, Saito K, Kanazawa K. Benign follicular thyroid nodule composed of signet-ring-like cells with PAS-negative thyroglobulin accumulation in dilated rough endoplasmic reticulums. Acta Pathol Jpn 1992;42:111–4.

16. Rigaud C, Peltier F, Bogomoletz WV. Mucin producing microfollicular adenoma of the thyroid. J Clin Pathol 1985;38:277–80.

17. Schröder S, Böcker W. Clear-cell carcinomas of thyroid gland: a clinicopathological study of 13 cases. Histopathology 1986;10:75–89.

18. _____, Böcker W. Signet-ring-cell thyroid tumors. Follicle cell tumors with arrest of folliculogenesis. Am J Surg Pathol 1985;9:619–29.

19. _____, Hüsselmann H, Böcher W. Lipid-rich cell adenoma of the thyroid gland. Report of a peculiar thyroid tumour. Virchows Arch [A] 1984; 404:105–8.

20. Stoll W, Lietz H. Zur Kenntnis und Problematik des hellzelligen Adenomes in der Schilddrüse. Virchows Arch [A] 1973;361:163–73.

21. Variakojis D, Getz ML, Paloyan E, Straus FH. Papillary clear cell carcinoma of the thyroid gland. Hum Pathol 1975;6:384–90.

22. Wassef M, Monteil JP, Bourgeon F, Le Charpentier Y. Carcinome indifférencié à cellules claires de la thyroide. Intérêt diagnostique de l'étude ultrastructurale. Ann Pathol 1981;1:95–8.

23. Woolner LB, Beahrs OH, Black BM, McConahey WM, Keating FR Jr. Classification and prognosis of thyroid carcinoma. A study of 885 cases observed in a thirty year period. Am J Surg 1961;102:354–87.

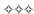

TUMORS WITH SQUAMOUS FEATURES

There is a large variety of thyroid neoplasms that exhibit focal or extensive squamous differentiation. Most of them have been discussed elsewhere in this Fascicle, but they are listed here in a single section for comparative and differential-diagnostic purposes.

- **Papillary Carcinoma**

    Squamous metaplasia is a common event in this tumor, having been reported in 20 to 40 percent of the cases. The squamous component has an appearance that is very well differentiated, analogous to that seen in adenoacanthomas of the endometrium and other organs (see page 72).

- **Mucoepidermoid Carcinoma**

    Mucoepidermoid carcinoma is a term that has been proposed for a rare malignant thyroid neoplasm exhibiting a combination of squamous and mucin-secreting features. The age of presentation in the reported cases has ranged from 10 to 56 years (4,9,12,14). Microscopically, the squamous areas are arranged in solid sheets with horny pearl formation, whereas the mucinous cells are often seen lining duct-like formations. A close intermingling of the two components is the rule (fig. 183). The stroma is markedly fibrotic, and psammoma bodies have been detected in several of the cases (fig. 184). The mucinous material is positive with Mayer's mucicarmine and Alcian blue stains. Immunohistochemically, the tumor cells are positive for keratin and CEA, the latter predominating in the duct-like elements. Although thyroglobulin was reported to be negative in the original series, more recent studies have shown that it is often expressed (16). Neuroendocrine markers, including calcitonin, are generally absent. Lymph node metastases to the neck are common, but no distant metastases or deaths from this tumor have been reported.

    The origin of mucoepidermoid carcinoma of the thyroid remains controversial. It has been suggested that the tumor might be related to the intrathyroidal solid cell nests thought to represent vestiges of the ultimobranchial body (see page 12) (4,7,8). The other possibility,

which we favor, is that this tumor is of metaplastic follicular cell derivation. Actually, some features suggest that mucoepidermoid carcinoma is histogenetically related to papillary carcinoma, a tumor well known for its tendency to undergo squamous metaplastic changes. It shares with that entity the presence of prominent fibrosis and psammoma bodies and the tendency for regional nodal metastases. Furthermore, it has been reported in association with conventional papillary carcinoma (4), and we have seen a case in which a typical thyroglobulin-positive papillary carcinoma merged imperceptibly with a thyroglobulin-negative mucoepidermoid carcinoma, the latter component having metastasized to a regional lymph node. A similar case

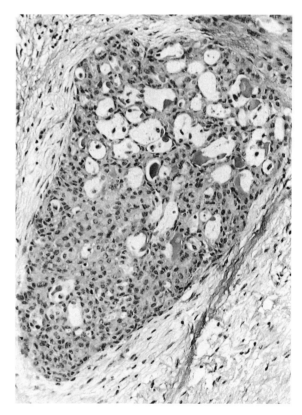

Figure 183

MUCOEPIDERMOID CARCINOMA

This tumor shows a combination of squamous and mucin-producing features accompanied by microcystic formation. The nest of tumor cells is surrounded by cellular stroma.

has been reported by Bondeson and coworkers (2). It is also interesting that one of the reported cases of mucoepidermoid carcinoma exhibited undifferentiated (anaplastic) areas and that another contained areas with an insular pattern (4).

- **Sclerosing Mucoepidermoid Carcinoma with Eosinophilia**

The descriptive term *sclerosing mucoepidermoid carcinoma with eosinophilia* has been proposed for a morphologically distinctive low-grade malignant neoplasm arising in thyroid glands affected by Hashimoto thyroiditis, often of the fibrous type (3). At the gross level, the tumor is white, homogeneous, firm, and either poorly or well circumscribed (pl. XXII-A). Microscopically, strands and small nests of squamoid tumor cells that exhibit mild-to-moderate nuclear pleomorphism, distinct nucleoli, and pale cytoplasm are seen infiltrat-

ing an abundant, dense, fibrohyaline stroma (fig. 185). Foci of definite squamous differentiation and pools of mucin are often present (fig. 186). The tumor cells are immunoreactive for keratin but not for thyroglobulin or calcitonin. Stains for mucin are focally positive in the squamoid islands. A striking feature of the tumor is the heavy infiltration of the stroma and many of the tumor islands by mature eosinophils (fig. 187). Extrathyroidal extension can occur, together with perineurial and vascular permeation. Only two of the cases we have seen (one included in the original report) have resulted in regional lymph node metastases. There have been no distant metastases and no tumor deaths.

The exact position of this tumor type in the scheme of thyroid malignancies remains to be

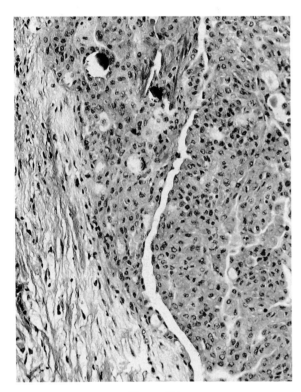

Figure 184
MUCOEPIDERMOID CARCINOMA
A solid nest of squamous cells is combined with foci exhibiting mucin production. The dense fibrosis and the formation of psammoma bodies suggest a link with papillary carcinoma.

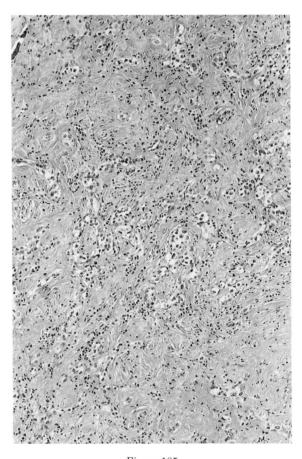

Figure 185
SCLEROSING MUCOEPIDERMOID
CARCINOMA WITH EOSINOPHILIA
Small irregular strands of tumor cells are seen growing in a dense fibrous stroma infiltrated by inflammatory elements.

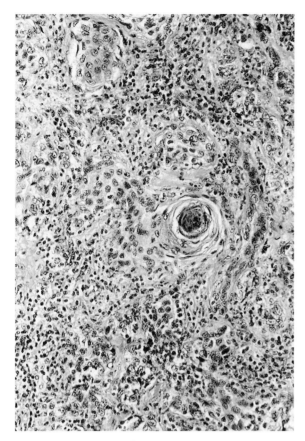

Figure 186
SCLEROSING MUCOEPIDERMOID CARCINOMA
WITH EOSINOPHILIA

In this area, the neoplastic nests show foci of obvious squamous change. (Fig. 5 from Chan JK, Albores-Saavedra J, Battifora H, Carcangiu ML, Rosai J. Sclerosing mucoepidermoid thyroid carcinoma with eosinophilia. A distinctive low-grade malignancy arising from the metaplastic follicles of Hashimoto's thyroiditis. Am J Surg Pathol 1991;15:438–48.)

determined. It shares many features with the reported cases of mucoepidermoid carcinoma, of which it may simply represent a variant; however, other features of this tumor and its constant association with Hashimoto thyroiditis deserve a separate description.

In regard to histogenesis, an origin from the benign squamous nests that are often found in Hashimoto thyroiditis (particularly its fibrous variant) is suggested by the close intermingling and occasional merging with these structures. The marked tissue eosinophilia is analogous to that described in carcinomas of other sites, such as oral cavity, vulva, and cervix and

ascribed to the secretion of eosinophil chemotactic factors by the tumor cells. Interestingly, most of those tumors have shown features of squamous differentiation (11).

- **Squamous Cell and Undifferentiated Carcinoma**

The name *squamous cell carcinoma* has been applied in the literature to primary malignant thyroid neoplasms with obvious squamous differentiation and marked cytologic atypia. It is rare in its pure form. When associated with mucin production, it has been designated *adenosquamous carcinoma* (13). In most cases, the squamous component merges with undifferentiated areas, so that the tendency has been to place the tumor into the undifferentiated (anaplastic) category. A residual component of papillary carcinoma is sometimes found in these neoplasms (fig. 188).

- **Carcinoma with Thymus-Like Differentiation ("CASTLE")**

This unusual intra- or perithyroidal carcinoma is characterized by a lobular pattern of growth, lymphocytic infiltration, and occasional perivascular space formation. It is thought to arise from thymic or related branchial pouch derivatives (see page 284).

- **Follicular Neoplasms**

In contrast to papillary carcinoma, the occurrence of squamous metaplasia in follicular neoplasms of either benign or malignant type is extremely rare (fig. 189). One such case, developing in a follicular carcinoma, has been reported as *adenoacanthoma* (15) (see page 195).

- **Medullary Carcinoma**

A squamous variety of this tumor has been recently described (see page 233).

- **Secondary Carcinoma**

The thyroid can be invaded by direct extension of squamous cell carcinoma of pharynx, larynx, trachea, esophagus, or adjacent metastatic lymph nodes, and it can be colonized through blood-borne metastases by squamous cell carcinoma of distant sites, particularly lung (see page 289).

- **Non-Neoplastic Conditions**

Epithelial nests of squamoid or squamous appearance can be seen in a variety of non-neoplastic conditions, of which Hashimoto thyroiditis is the most important (fig. 190). They can also appear in other types of thyroiditis, in

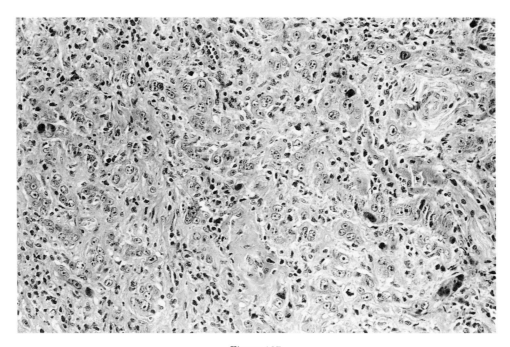

Figure 187
SCLEROSING MUCOEPIDERMOID CARCINOMA WITH EOSINOPHILIA
The tumor cells grow as small cords and individual elements in a fibrous stroma densely infiltrated by eosinophils. The nuclei are large and vesicular, and the nucleoli are prominent. (Fig. 8 from Chan JK, Albores-Saavedra J, Battifora H, Carcangiu ML, Rosai J. Sclerosing mucoepidermoid thyroid carcinoma with eosinophilia. A distinctive low-grade malignancy arising from the metaplastic follicles of Hashimoto's disease. Am J Surg Pathol 1991;15:438–48.)

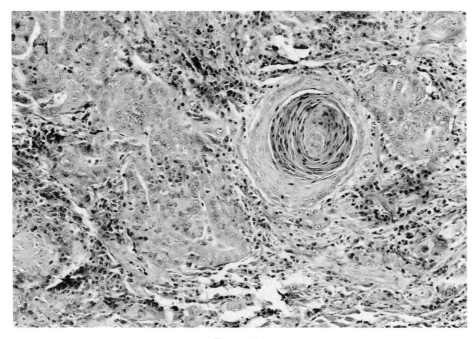

Figure 188
PAPILLARY CARCINOMA WITH SQUAMOUS METAPLASIA
This papillary carcinoma has a keratin pearl indicative of squamous metaplasia.

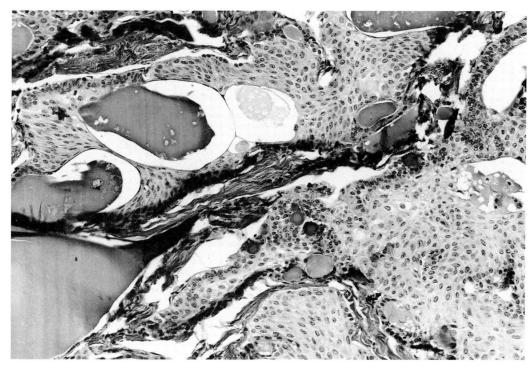

Figure 189
FOLLICULAR ADENOMA WITH SQUAMOUS METAPLASIA
The cytologic and architectural features of this tumor were benign throughout.

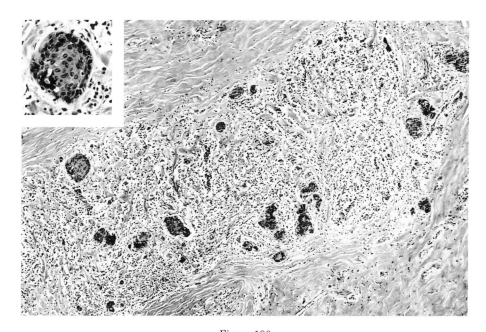

Figure 190
HASHIMOTO THYROIDITIS WITH SQUAMOUS METAPLASIA
The small and irregular metaplastic squamous follicles are typical of the fibrous type of
Hashimoto thyroiditis. The inset shows the well-developed squamous nature of the follicle and
the absence of a lumen.

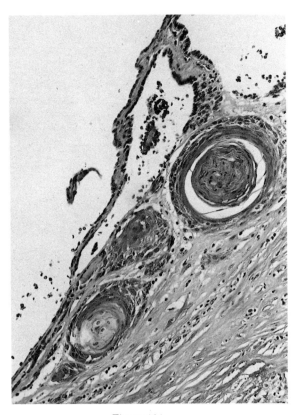

Figure 191

NODULAR HYPERPLASIA WITH
FOCAL SQUAMOUS METAPLASIA

The situation illustrated here is probably the result
of degenerative and necrotic changes. Two well-formed
squamous pearls are seen.

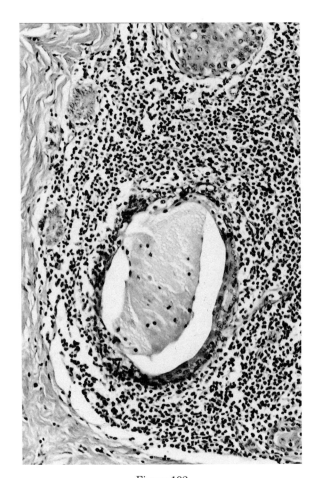

Figure 192

HASHIMOTO THYROIDITIS

This metaplastic follicle from a case of fibrous variant of
Hashimoto thyroiditis shows a dilated lumen filled with
mucinous material.

the atrophic and fibrotic gland accompanying myxedema, and in nodular hyperplasia (adenomatoid goiter) (fig. 191). The nests can be solid or cystic and are sometimes accompanied by mucin deposition (pl. XXII-B; fig. 192). They are invariably positive immunohistochemically for keratin and often for CEA (pl. XXII-B) (17). Some have also been found to be reactive for thyroglobulin, whereas others may contain or be surrounded by clusters of C cells (5,6). The source of these structures is probably multifactorial. Some (perhaps most) represent metaplastic folli-

cles. Others may be remnants from branchial pouches, whether the third or fourth (in which case they may have the appearance of thymic nests) or the fifth, which corresponds to the ultimobranchial body (in which case they may contain C cells) (see page 12). The solid and cystic formations that have been described with great frequency in the neonatal thyroid are probably of branchial pouch derivation (1), and are also probably the source for the gross cystic formations occasionally seen accompanying Hashimoto thyroiditis (10).

PLATE XXII

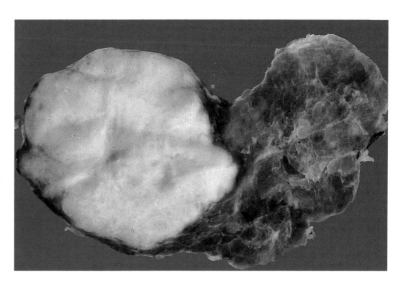

A. SCLEROSING MUCOEPIDERMOID CARCINOMA WITH EOSINOPHILIA ARISING IN HASHIMOTO THYROIDITIS

In this case, the tumor has an unusually well-circumscribed appearance. The dense fibrosis that is characteristic of this tumor is well appreciated.

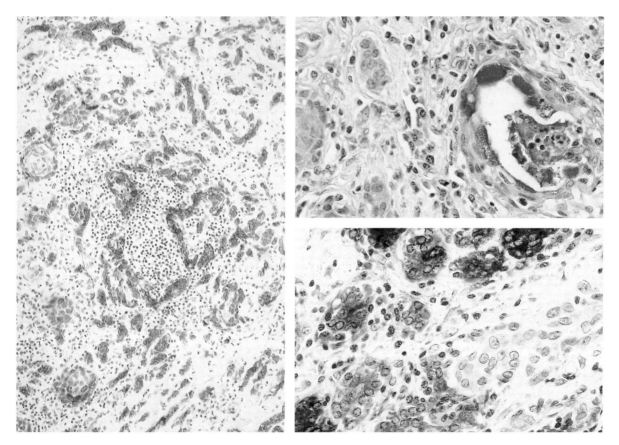

B. METAPLASTIC THYROID FOLLICLES IN FIBROUS HASHIMOTO THYROIDITIS

Strong immunoreactivity for keratin is evident in the field on the left. Some of the metaplastic follicles have intraluminal and intracytoplasmic mucin, as evidenced by the Mayer's mucicarmine stain (top right). The metaplastic squamous follicles are negative for thyroglobulin, in contrast to the adjacent follicles (bottom right).

REFERENCES

1. Beckner ME, Shultz JJ, Richardson T. Solid and cystic ultimobranchial body remnants in the thyroid. Arch Pathol Lab Med 1990;114:1049–52.
2. Bondeson L, Bondeson A-G, Thompson NW. Papillary carcinoma of the thyroid with mucoepidermoid features. Am J Clin Pathol 1991;95:175–9.
3. Chan JK, Albores-Saavedra J, Battifora H, Carcangiu ML, Rosai J. Sclerosing mucoepidermoid carcinoma of the thyroid with eosinophilia. A distinctive low-grade malignancy arising from the metaplastic follicles of Hashimoto's thyroiditis. Am J Surg Pathol 1991;15: 438–48.
4. Franssila KO, Harach HR, Wasenius V-M. Mucoepidermoid carcinoma of the thyroid. Histopathology 1984;8:847–60.
5. Harach HR. Histological markers of solid nests of the thyroid, with some emphasis on their expression in thyroid ultimobranchial-related tumors. Acta Anat (Basel) 1985;124:111–6.
6. ————. Solid cell nests of the thyroid. J Pathol 1988;155:191–200.
7. ————. Thyroid follicles with acid mucins in man: a second kind of follicles? Cell Tissue Res 1985; 242:211–5.
8. ————, Day ES, de Strizic NA. Mucoepidermoid carcinoma of the thyroid. Report of a case with immunohistochemical studies. Medicina (Buenos Aires) 1986;46:213–6.
9. Katoh R, Sugai T, Ono S, et al. Mucoepidermoid carcinoma of the thyroid gland. Cancer 1990;65:2020–7.
10. Louis DN, Vickery AL Jr, Rosai J, Wang CA. Multiple branchial cleft-like cysts in Hashimoto's thyroiditis. Am J Surg Pathol 1989;13:45–9.
11. Lowe D, Jorizzo J, Hutt MS. Tumor-associated eosinophilia: a review. J Clin Pathol 1981;34:1343–8.
12. Mizukami Y, Matsubara F, Hashimoto T, et al. Primary mucoepidermoid carcinoma in the thyroid gland. Cancer 1984;53:1741–5.
13. Nicolaides AR, Rhys Evans P, Fisher C. Adenosquamous carcinoma of the thyroid gland. J Laryngol Otol 1989;103:978–9.
14. Rhatigan RM, Roque JL, Bucher RL. Mucoepidermoid carcinoma of the thyroid gland. Cancer 1977;39:210–4.
15. Mahoney JP, Saffos RO, Rhatigan RM. Follicular adenoacanthoma of the thyroid gland. Histopathology 1980;4:547–57.
16. Sambade C, Franssila K, Basìlio-de-Oliveira CA, Sobrinho-Simões M. Mucoepidermoid carcinoma of the thyroid revisited. Surg Pathol 1990;3:271–80.
17. Vollenweider I, Hedinger C. Solid cell nests (SCN) in Hashimoto's thyroiditis. Virchows Arch [A] 1988; 412:357–63.

✧✧✧

TUMORS WITH MUCINOUS FEATURES

It is sometimes assumed that, if a thyroid neoplasm is positive for mucin stains, it must be of metastatic nature and that mucin positivity in a tumor at another site (e.g., lymph node or lung) rules out a thyroid origin. These assumptions are incorrect. The number of primary thyroid neoplasms in which mucosubstances have been detected is substantial (11). We are referring not only to the presence of extracellular hyaluronic acid and/or related polysaccharides (a rather nonspecific phenomenon) but also to the occurrence of acid glycoproteins detectable by Mayer's mucicarmine or Alcian blue in the cytoplasm of the tumor cells or in the lumina of the follicles. In the case of the follicular cells, it has been pointed out that thyroglobulin is a sialic acid–containing glycoprotein and that the mucin that is detected in some tumors may therefore be an abnormal form of this substance (7). The following thyroid neoplasms have been found to contain mucin.

- **Signet-Ring Follicular Adenoma**
  The intracellular thyroglobulin that accumulates in this rare variant of follicular adenoma is often mucin-positive, although usually weakly (see page 188) (pl. XXIII-A) (7,10). This is also true for the even rarer malignant counterpart of this tumor, follicular carcinoma with signet-ring features.
- **Mucoepidermoid Carcinoma and Sclerosing Mucoepidermoid Carcinoma with Eosinophilia**
  In these tumors, the mucin deposition is accompanied by squamous metaplasia. They are discussed on pages 195–197.
- **Mucinous Carcinoma**
  A few cases of mucinous or mucin-producing (adeno)carcinoma of the thyroid are on record (3,4,5,9,12). Postulated sources for this tumor include metaplastic follicles and ultimobranchial body remnants. Some are probably closely related to mucoepidermoid carcinoma, but their exact place in the scheme of thyroid neoplasia is still uncertain. Actually, the impression derived from the individual case reports is not that of a definite entity but rather of a heterogeneous group of tumors sharing the feature of mucin secretion (pl. XXIII-B; fig. 193).

- **Papillary Carcinoma**
  It has been shown that papillary thyroid carcinoma metastatic to cervical lymph nodes exhibits intracytoplasmic mucin positivity in 17 percent of cases (2). An even higher percentage was recorded by Mlynek and coworkers (11) in their study of primary tumors of this microscopic type.
- **Undifferentiated Carcinoma**
  Some otherwise undifferentiated carcinomas show focal mucin positivity, almost always in intimate admixture with squamoid or squamous foci (see page 136) (1).

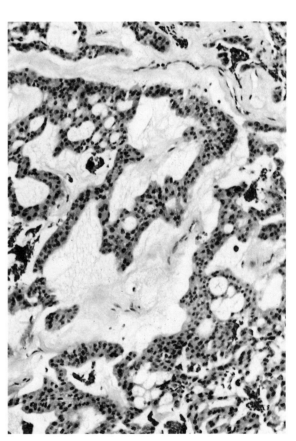

Figure 193
FOLLICULAR CARCINOMA
WITH MUCIN PRODUCTION

In this follicular neoplasm with a trabecular pattern of growth, there is extensive mucinous deposition in the extracellular space. Tumors with this appearance are sometimes designated *mucinous carcinomas*.

PLATE XXIII

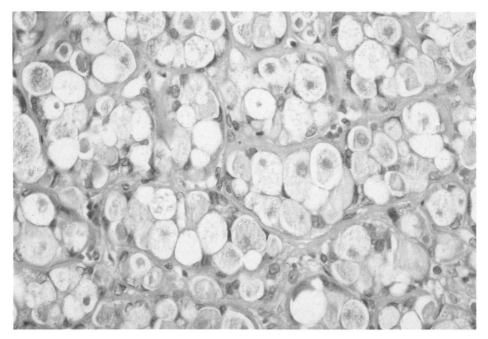

A. SIGNET-RING FOLLICULAR ADENOMA
The presence of acidic mucin is indicated in this signet-ring adenoma by the strong intracytoplasmic positivity for Alcian blue.

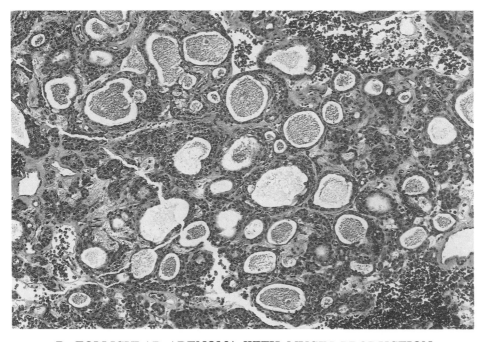

B. FOLLICULAR ADENOMA WITH MUCIN PRODUCTION
The intraluminal content of this follicular adenoma is granular and basophilic, indicative of the presence of acidic mucosubstances. Mucin stains were strongly positive.

- **Medullary Carcinoma**

In about 10 percent of all cases of medullary carcinoma, positivity for mucin is found in the cytoplasm of the tumor cells (see page 213) (6,13). A mixed medullary-mucinous (amphicrine) carcinoma of the thyroid has been reported (8).

- **Secondary Carcinoma**

A variety of mucin-producing adenocarcinomas can metastasize to the thyroid. Those from the gastrointestinal tract and breast are the most common (see page 289).

REFERENCES

1. Carcangiu ML, Steeper T, Zampi G, Rosai J. Anaplastic thyroid carcinoma. A study of 70 cases. Am J Clin Pathol 1985;83:135–58.

2. Chan JK, Tse CC. Mucin production in metastatic papillary carcinoma of the thyroid. Hum Pathol 1988;19:195–200.

3. Cruz MC, Marques LP, Sambade CC, Sobrinho-Simões MA. Primary mucinous carcinoma of the thyroid. Surg Pathol 1991;4:266–73.

4. Deligdisch L, Subhani Z, Gordon RE. Primary mucinous carcinoma of the thyroid gland: report of a case and ultrastructural study. Cancer 1980;45:2564–7.

5. Diaz-Perez R, Quiroz H, Nishiyama RH. Primary mucinous adenocarcinoma of thyroid gland. Cancer 1976;38:1323–5.

6. Fernandes BJ, Bedard YC, Rosen I. Mucus-producing medullary cell carcinoma of the thyroid gland. Am J Clin Pathol 1982;78:536–40.

7. Gherardi G. Signet ring cell 'mucinous' thyroid adenoma: a follicle cell tumour with abnormal accumulation of thyroglobulin and a peculiar histochemical profile. Histopathology 1987;11:317–26.

8. Golouh R, Us-Krasovecf M, Auersperg M, Jancar J, Bondi A, Eusebi V. Amphicrine-composite calcitonin and mucin-producing carcinoma of the thyroid. Ultrastruct Pathol 1985;8:197–206.

9. Harada T, Shimaoka K, Hiratsuka M, Hirokawa M, Tsukayama C. Mucin-producing carcinoma of the thyroid gland—a case report and review of the literature. Jpn J Clin Oncol 1984;14:417–24.

10. Mendelsohn G. Signet cell simulating microfollicular adenoma of the thyroid. Am J Surg Pathol 1984;8:705–8.

11. Mlynek ML, Richter HJ, Leder LD. Mucin in carcinomas of the thyroid. Cancer 1985;56:2647–50.

12. Sobrinho-Simões MA, Nesland JM, Johannessen JV. A mucin-producing tumor in the thyroid gland. Ultrastruct Pathol 1985;9:277–81.

13. Zaatari GS, Saigo PE, Huvos AG. Mucin production in medullary carcinoma of the thyroid. Arch Pathol Lab Med 1983;107:70–4.

MEDULLARY CARCINOMA

Definition. Medullary carcinoma is a malignant tumor of the thyroid composed of cells showing evidence of C cell differentiation and usually containing calcitonin (42). These tumors have also been referred to as *solid amyloidotic carcinomas* and as *C cell carcinomas* (1).

General Features. Horn (46) first described a distinctive morphologic variant of thyroid carcinoma characterized by sharply defined rounded or ovoid compact cell groups in 1951. Hazard and coworkers (41) subsequently defined the major histologic features of this tumor type, including the presence of stromal amyloid, and suggested the name medullary carcinoma for it. Williams (108) later proposed that these tumors originated from the parafollicular or C cells of the thyroid.

Medullary carcinomas account for up to 10 percent of all thyroid malignancies (76,89). These tumors can occur sporadically or in familial forms, with an autosomal dominant pattern of inheritance. In most large series, the sporadic tumors account for up to 70 percent of all cases.

Sporadic (nonfamilial) forms of medullary carcinoma occur with equal frequency in different parts of the world, and little is known about their etiology and pathogenesis (58). In rare instances, these tumors may arise in the setting of Hashimoto disease, but this association is probably coincidental (102). There are some data to support the view that chronic hypercalcemia may be associated with an increased incidence of these tumors (59). In contrast to their relative rarity in humans, medullary carcinomas occur commonly in many strains of rats, and their incidence increases progressively with the age of the population (10). The chronic administration of vitamin D3 has been reported to increase the frequency of medullary carcinomas in rats, whereas animals on a vitamin D–deficient diet had a lower incidence of C cell tumors than did control animals maintained on a normal diet (98,99). C cell neoplasms also occur commonly in bulls, where they are known as *ultimobranchial neoplasms* (8).

The incidence of medullary thyroid carcinoma is apparently not increased in human subjects treated by irradiation to the head and neck area.

However, data in experimental animals suggest that rats treated with low doses of ^{131}I have an increased incidence of C cell tumors (98,99). Interestingly, high calcium levels in drinking water did not seem to potentiate the carcinogenic effects of irradiation on C cells in these experiments (98,99).

Medullary carcinomas of the familial type may occur in association with adrenal medullary and parathyroid proliferative abnormalities (type IIA or II multiple endocrine neoplasia [MEN]) or together with proliferation of mucosal and ocular nerves, adrenal medullary proliferative lesions, and marfanoid habitus (type IIB or III MEN) (pl. XXIV-A) (3,19,37,65,78,88,89). In rare instances, familial forms of medullary carcinoma may occur without other associated endocrine abnormalities (Table 2) (91).

Cytogenetic studies have mapped the gene for the MEN IIA syndrome to a locus near the centromere of chromosome 10 (87). The availability of polymorphic DNA probes for this region of chromosome 10 has permitted the use of restriction-fragment–length polymorphisms to identify carriers of the gene for this disorder (90). If further studies confirm linkage to the same locus

Table 2

FAMILIAL MEDULLARY THYROID CARCINOMA SYNDROMES

Medullary Carcinoma Alone

MEN IIA (II)

C Cell Hyperplasia – Medullary Carcinoma

Adrenal Medullary Hyperplasia –
Pheochromocytoma

Parathyroid Hyperplasia – Adenoma

MEN IIB (III)

C Cell Hyperplasia – Medullary Carcinoma

Adrenal Medullary Hyperplasia –
Pheochromocytoma

Gastrointestinal and Ocular Ganglioneuromas

Skeletal Abnormalities

---

on chromosome 10 in families with medullary thyroid carcinoma alone and in families with MEN IIB, the prospects for recognizing those individuals at risk for the development of this form of hereditary thyroid cancer will improve greatly (49,62,71,91).

Boultwood and coworkers (11) have examined medullary carcinomas for the expression of the N- and c-*myc* oncogenes. Elevated levels of N-*myc* were noted in 6 of 21 cases, whereas the levels of c-*myc* were increased in 1 of 21 cases. Neither N- nor c-*myc* could be demonstrated in normal C cells with in situ hybridization techniques. There was no consistent correlation of N-*myc* positivity and tumor grade in this series. Elevated levels of H-*ras* have also been noted in medullary carcinoma.

Clinical Features. The sporadic form of medullary thyroid carcinoma is primarily a tumor of middle-aged adults with a slightly higher incidence in women (ratio of women to men, 1.3:1). Chong and coworkers (21) reported a mean age at diagnosis of 51 years, whereas Lips and coworkers (58) reported a mean age of 36 years, based on several large series. Generally, patients with the sporadic form of the disease present with unilateral involvement of the gland with or without associated cervical nodal metastases. In rare cases, they may present with evidence of metastatic disease (2). The tumor generally pursues an indolent course, with 5-year survival rates in the range of 60 to 70 percent after thyroidectomy.

In patients with medullary thyroid carcinoma associated with MEN IIA, the mean age at diagnosis for the thyroid tumors is 20 years, and there is a slightly higher incidence in women (ratio of women to men 1.3:1)(33,52,58). Patients often present with evidence of multicentric tumors involving both lobes of the thyroid gland. The tumors are generally slow growing, and the prognosis is similar to that observed in patients with the sporadic form of the disease. With the routine use of prospective screening studies in high-risk patients, the mean age at diagnosis has become progressively younger.

Medullary thyroid carcinomas associated with the type IIB (III) syndrome occur at a mean age of 15 years (11,19,20). In the series reported by Carney and coworkers (19), one affected individual was found to have elevated plasma calcitonin at 8 months of age, and evidence of bilateral medullary thyroid carcinoma was documented at surgery at the age of 15 months. As is the case in sporadic and MEN IIA–associated medullary thyroid carcinomas, the incidence is slightly higher in women (ratio of women to men, 1.3:1). The medullary carcinomas in this syndrome are aggressive neoplasms that tend to metastasize early and have a poor prognosis (17,19,20,69).

Patients with sporadic and familial medullary thyroid carcinomas may present with evidence of a variety of signs and symptoms in addition to the presence of a thyroid mass (7). For example, they may present with severe watery diarrhea similar to that seen in patients with the Verner-Morrison syndrome. Numerous factors, including prostaglandins, biogenic amines, vasoactive intestinal peptide, kinins, and calcitonin itself, have been implicated in the pathogenesis of the diarrhea (110). Both the carcinoid and Cushing syndromes have been reported in patients with these tumors, presumably due to the synthesis and secretion of serotonin or related amines and ACTH by the tumors, respectively (101,111).

In patients with MEN IIA, the signs and symptoms of the thyroid tumors may be masked by symptomatology related to adrenal medullary or parathyroid disease (26). The pheochromocytomas in patients with MEN IIA and IIB are most commonly bilateral and multicentric and are often preceded in their development by adrenal medullary hyperplasia (20,27). The latter condition is often accompanied by increased synthesis and secretion of catecholamines, particularly epinephrine (27). Patients with adrenal medullary hyperplasia may present with episodic hypertension or cardiac arrhythmias. It is important, therefore, that patients undergoing surgery for medullary thyroid carcinomas be tested preoperatively for catecholamine abnormalities. Hyperparathyroidism may mask the symptoms and signs of thyroid neoplasms in patients with MEN IIA (78). However, hyperparathyroidism is generally an uncommon presentation for MEN IIA and does not occur in association with the MEN IIB syndrome (79).

Laboratory Diagnosis. In 1962, Copp and coworkers (22) reported the discovery of a novel calcium-lowering hormone that was called thyrocalcitonin. Subsequent immunofluorescence studies showed that calcitonin was present in the clear cells or parafollicular cells of the thyroid, which were subsequently named C cells. Williams' (108) studies established that the cells of medullary carcinomas resembled parafollicular cells, and subsequent morphological, immunohistochemical, and ultrastructural studies confirmed the parafollicular or C cell origin of these tumors (108).

The laboratory diagnosis of medullary thyroid carcinoma of both sporadic and familial types depends on the demonstration of increased levels of calcitonin in the serum (3,31,65,104). Because most patients with the sporadic form of the disease present with nodular thyroid glands, with or without nodal involvement, the initial diagnostic work-up most commonly includes a thyroid scan with or without a fine-needle aspiration biopsy. A diagnosis of medullary carcinoma in a needle-biopsy specimen may be confirmed by the demonstration of calcitonin in the tumor cells by immunohistochemistry. Analysis of plasma levels of calcitonin both basally and after the administration of calcium and pentagastrin can be used to confirm the diagnosis. Measurements of calcitonin can be used to monitor the presence of residual, recurrent, or metastatic disease in the postoperative period (103). In general, the extent of elevation of plasma calcitonin has correlated with the tumor burden, but in some cases of metastatic disease, calcitonin levels have fallen (100).

The observation that calcitonin secretion could be stimulated by the administration of secretagogues such as calcium or pentagastrin has formed the basis for large-scale screening studies aimed at the early detection of familial C cell neoplasms (33,36,97,105). In the series reported by Gagel and coworkers (33), 12 individuals (mean age, 38.5 years) from a large MEN IIA kindred had thyroidectomies on the basis of abnormal calcitonin levels discovered between 1969 and 1971. All of these patients had bilateral medullary carcinomas with associated C cell hyperplasia, and 7 of these patients also had lymph node metastases. In the same series, 23 patients (mean age 11.8 years) had thyroidectomies as a result of calcitonin abnormalities that were discovered after 1971. From this group, 13 patients had C cell hyperplasia without evidence of an associated carcinoma, 9 patients had C cell hyperplasia with associated microscopic medullary carcinomas, and 1 patient had no apparent C cell abnormality. In general, the extent of elevation

of calcitonin in the serum could not be used to distinguish those patients with C cell hyperplasia alone from those who had microscopic carcinomas together with C cell hyperplasia.

The levels of katacalcin parallel those of calcitonin in individuals with medullary thyroid carcinoma (51). Plasma levels of calcitonin gene–related peptide, on the other hand, are increased in only about 50 percent of patients with medullary carcinoma. Both histaminase (4) and CEA (13) are elevated in the plasma of most patients with medullary thyroid carcinomas.

Gross Features. Medullary carcinomas vary in size from those that are just barely visible at the gross level to those that replace the entire thyroid (pl. XXIV-B; pl.XXV-A and B; pl. XXVI-A) (41,109). The larger tumors are generally sharply circumscribed but nonencapsulated lesions. However, in rare instances, they may be surrounded by a fibrous connective capsule. On cross section, the tumors are typically tan to pink, with a soft-to-firm consistency. Others are quite firm and fibrotic, with areas of granular yellow discoloration that represent focal calcifications. The smaller tumors typically occur at the junction of the upper and middle thirds of the thyroid lobes, corresponding to an area in which the C cells normally predominate. Such tumors are typically firm and yellow to white, with indistinct borders that appear to infiltrate the adjacent thyroid parenchyma (6). When the tumors become very large, they may replace the entire lobe and extend directly into the perithyroidal soft tissue and trachea. Whereas the sporadic tumors most commonly present as unilateral lesions, familial tumors characteristically involve both lobes of the gland.

Microscopic Features. Most sporadic and familial medullary carcinomas are nonencapsulated tumors that show a solid pattern of growth. They exhibit a wide spectrum of histologic patterns that may mimic other types of primary thyroid malignancies, including follicular, papillary, and undifferentiated carcinomas (40,64,109).

The prototypic medullary carcinoma shows a lobular, trabecular, insular, or sheet-like growth pattern (figs. 194–199). Although most of the tumors appear sharply circumscribed at the gross level, microscopic examination most often reveals extension of the tumor into the adjacent normal thyroid tissue. Individual tumor cells

PLATE XXIV

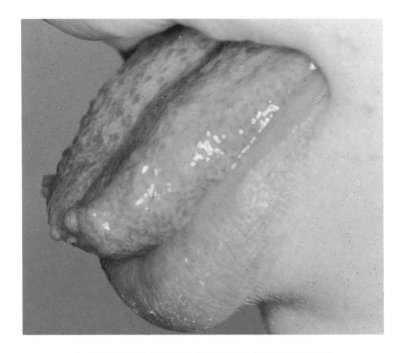

**A. MULTIPLE ENDOCRINE NEOPLASIA
TYPE IIB (MEN IIB)**
The surface of the patient's tongue shows multiple neuromas.

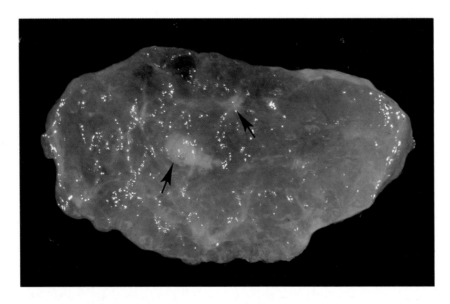

**B. FAMILIAL MEDULLARY THYROID CARCINOMA
ASSOCIATED WITH MEN IIA**
Multiple foci of tumor (arrows) are present within this lobe of the thyroid.

PLATE XXV

FAMILIAL MEDULLARY CARCINOMA ASSOCIATED WITH MEN IIA

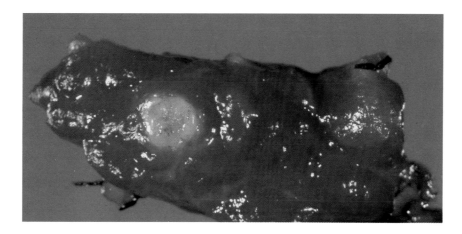

A. A single nodule of tumor is present in this lobe of the thyroid.

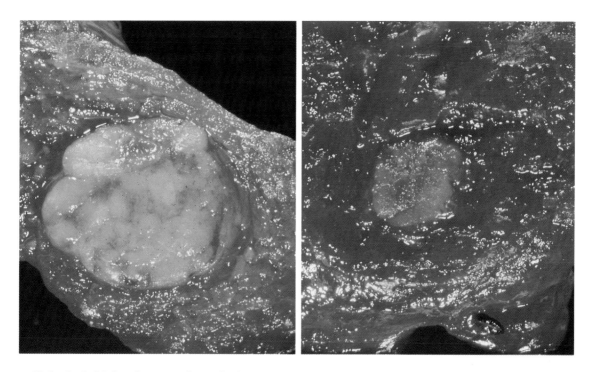

B. In the left lobe, the tumor has a fleshy appearance and appears well circumscribed (left). In the right lobe, the tumor nodule appears finely granular on cross section (right).

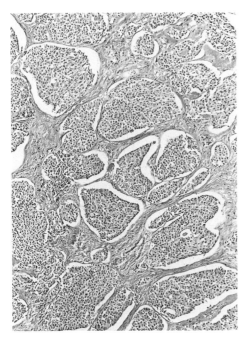

Figure 194
MEDULLARY THYROID CARCINOMA,
LOBULAR PATTERN

The lobular pattern of growth of this tumor is
accentuated by some degree of shrinkage artifact.

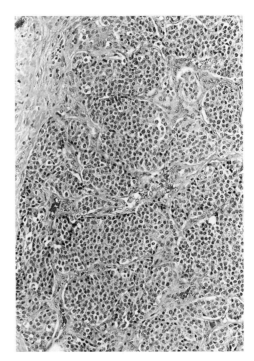

Figure 195
(Figures 195 and 196 are from the same patient)
MEDULLARY THYROID CARCINOMA
This tumor is composed of round cells.

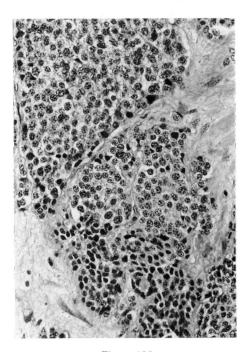

Figure 196
MEDULLARY THYROID CARCINOMA

This tumor is composed of round cells. The
nuclei have a plasmacytoid appearance.

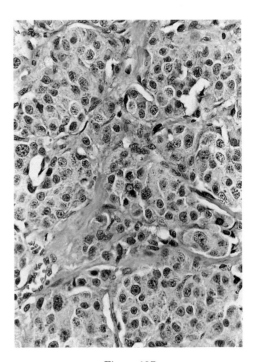

Figure 197
MEDULLARY THYROID CARCINOMA

This tumor is composed of polygonal cells with
abundant cytoplasm.

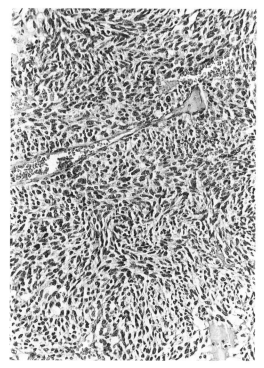

Figure 198
MEDULLARY THYROID CARCINOMA, SOLID
PATTERN
This tumor is composed of small spindle cells.

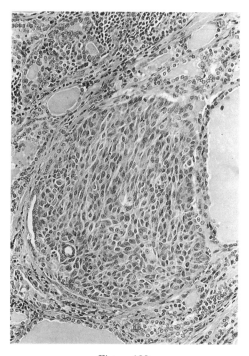

Figure 199
MEDULLARY THYROID CARCINOMA
This tumor is composed of spindle cells.

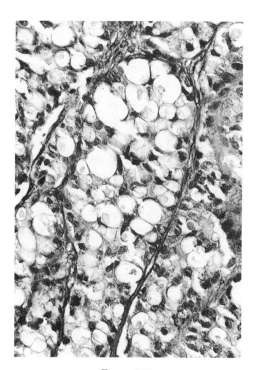

Figure 200
MEDULLARY THYROID CARCINOMA,
MUCINOUS TYPE

Most of the cells of this tumor have large
mucin-filled vacuoles.

may be round (figs. 195, 196), polygonal (fig. 197), or spindle shaped (figs. 198, 199), with frequent admixtures of these cell types. Occasional small cell variants may resemble oat cell carcinomas. In the round- and polygonal-type cells, the nuclei are round to oval, with coarsely clumped or speckled chromatin and inconspicuous nucleoli (figs. 195–197). Binucleated cells are commonly present, and giant cells with multiple nuclei may be evident (53). Occasional nuclei may contain cytoplasmic pseudoinclusions similar to those seen in papillary carcinomas (fig. 197). In those tumors with a spindle cell morphology, the nuclei are elongated (fig. 199). The nuclei commonly exhibit a moderate degree of variation in size. In most cases, overall mitotic activity is low (55).

The cytoplasm of the tumor cells is generally eosinophilic or amphophilc and finely granular. However, in some cases, the cytoplasm appears clear. Occasional mucin-positive cytoplasmic vacuoles may be apparent in some cases (fig. 200) (30). Zaatari and coworkers (116) have found mucicarmine-positive deposits in 42 percent of medullary thyroid carcinomas. In 17 percent of their cases, the mucosubstances were exclusively extracellular, in 8 percent they were only intracellular, and in 17 percent they were both intra- and extracellular. Receptors for *U. europaeus*-I lectin, concanavalin A, *Ricinus communis*, succinylated wheat-germ agglutinin, and glycine MAX(SBA) have been identified in many cases (61); however, there are considerable differences in lectin affinity among individual examples.

Foci of necrosis, hemorrhage, and mitotic activity are uncommon in small medullary carcinomas. In the series of MEN IIA–associated medullary carcinomas reported by Bigner and coworkers (6), mitotic activity, areas of necrosis, and anaplastic foci were rarely seen in tumors that measured less than 1.5 cm. In larger tumors, mitotic activity and necrosis were more frequent. Lymphatic and vascular invasion may be seen at the advancing front of the tumor (fig. 201). In advanced cases, foci of lymphatic invasion may be seen in the contralateral lobe. In rare cases, patients with occult primaries may present with metastatic disease (2,107).

Stromal amyloid deposits have been identified in up to 80 percent of cases (pl. XXVI-B; fig. 202) (14,106). The amyloid deposits are Congo red–positive and show typical green birefringence in polarized light (pl. XXVI-C). In sections stained with crystal violet, the amyloid deposits are typically metachromatic. Ultrastructurally, the amyloid deposits have a fibrillar structure that is identical to that seen in other forms of amyloidosis (fig. 203). Immunohistochemical studies with antibodies to calcitonin generally show positive staining in the amyloid deposits. These observations have suggested that the amyloid is derived from calcitonin or one of its precursors (106).

In addition to amyloid, the stroma also contains variable amounts of collagen (fig. 203). Occasional medullary carcinomas may consist predominantly of stromal elements and amyloid. Such cases may be difficult to distinguish from amyloid goiters (fig. 204) (50). In some instances, the amyloid deposits may induce a foreign-body reaction, and amyloid may be seen within the cytoplasm of the accompanying giant cells.

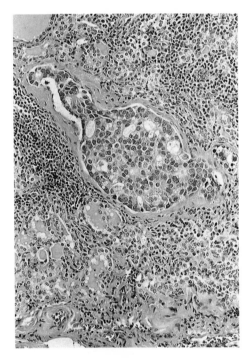

Figure 201
MEDULLARY THYROID CARCINOMA
This tumor has an area of vascular invasion.

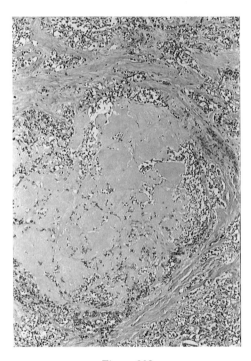

Figure 202
MEDULLARY THYROID CARCINOMA
Prominent amyloid deposits can be seen in this tumor.

PLATE XXVI

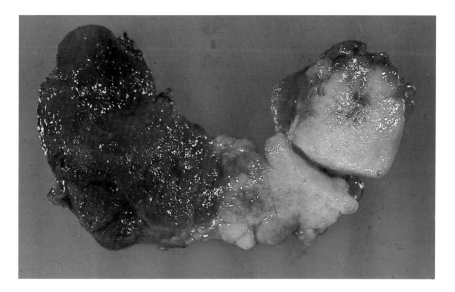

A. NONFAMILIAL MEDULLARY THYROID CARCINOMA
The entire left lobe and isthmus are involved by tumor.

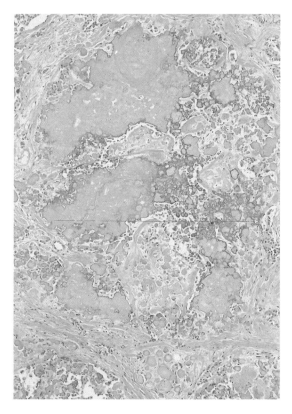

B. MEDULLARY THYROID CARCINOMA
The tumor is replaced almost entirely by amyloid deposits that are focally calcified at their peripheries.

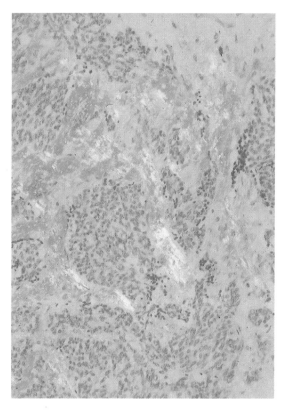

C. MEDULLARY THYROID CARCINOMA
This example is stained with Congo red and photographed in partially polarized light. The amyloid deposits exhibit green birefringence.

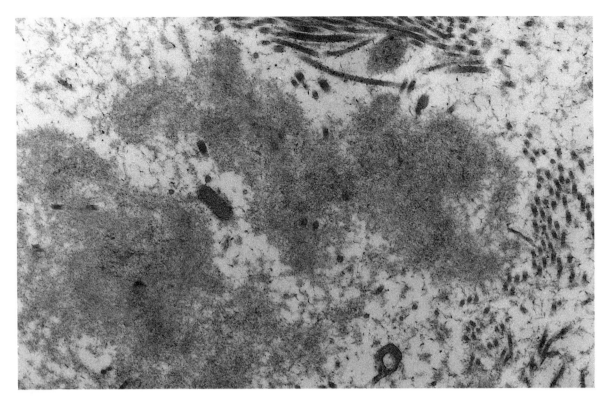

Figure 203

MEDULLARY THYROID CARCINOMA

Amyloid deposits are visible in this electron micrograph. In many areas, the amyloid deposits have an amorphous appearance. In other areas, there is a finely fibrillary structure. Collagen fibrils are evident at the periphery of the amyloid. X29,700.

The stromal element of medullary carcinomas shows frequent areas of calcification (pl. XXVI-B), and occasional tumors may contain true psammoma bodies.

Sporadic medullary carcinomas show the same wide spectrum of histopathologic features as the familial neoplasms; however, a number of other characteristics may serve to distinguish these two tumor groups (9,31,77). As noted earlier, familial tumors occur at a younger age and may be associated with adrenal medullary, parathyroid, and neural abnormalities. The familial medullary carcinomas are typically bilateral (pl. XXV-B) (19,20,26). In the series reported by Block and coworkers (9), bilateral tumors were found in 40 of 41 familial cases. The single exception occurred in an individual with agenesis of the left thyroid lobe. In contrast, 24 patients with sporadic disease had unilateral tumor nodules (pl. XXVI-A). However, it should be noted that patients with large sporadic medullary carcinomas may have metastases to the contralateral lobe that may occasionally be confused with bilateral primary tumors.

An important feature that distinguishes familial from sporadic medullary carcinoma is the presence of C cell hyperplasia in the former group (fig. 205) (9,112). In individuals with familial disease, foci of C cell hyperplasia are typically seen adjacent to the tumors. Moreover, foci of hyperplasia and early carcinoma are apparent in sections away from the main neoplasm. Briefly, early (microscopic) carcinomas are characterized by the extension of C cells through the follicular basement membrane into the thyroid interstitium (26,84). Early medullary carcinoma, as seen in the setting of familial disease, is discussed in detail in the section on C Cell Hyperplasia. The finding of C cell hyperplasia in an individual with apparent sporadic disease should alert both the

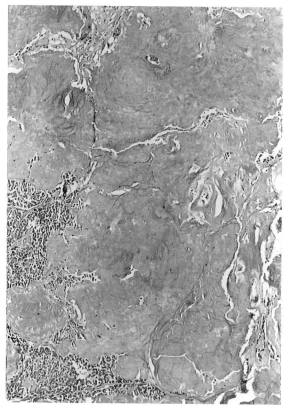

Figure 204
MEDULLARY THYROID CARCINOMA
Extensive amyloid deposits are present in this tumor.

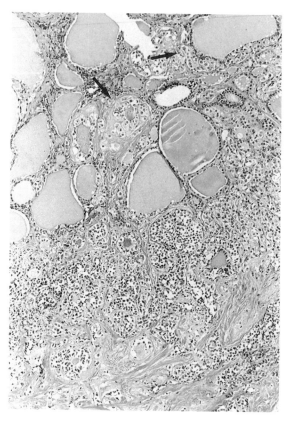

Figure 205
FAMILIAL MEDULLARY THYROID CARCINOMA
The invasive tumor is present at the bottom of the figure.
C cell hyperplasia is present adjacent to the tumor (arrows).

pathologist and clinician to the possibility of familial disease, and appropriate clinical testing should be performed in family members.

In some instances, it may be extremely difficult to distinguish intrathyroidal metastases from foci of C cell hyperplasia or early carcinomas. In cases of metastatic disease, tumor emboli are found within the vascular and/or lymphatic channels. In contrast to foci of C cell hyperplasia or early carcinoma, the tumor cells in intrathyroidal metastases are generally more pleomorphic and typically exhibit strong positive staining for CEA (26,28). When tumor has extended beyond the confines of the vascular and/or lymphatic wall, it may infiltrate the thyroid in a manner similar to that observed in small primary or microscopic carcinomas. The presence of C cell hyperplasia adjacent to such lesions may indicate a primary rather than metastatic tumor. Occasional medullary carcinomas may show a prominent inflammatory infil-

trate, suggesting the possibility of a cellular immune response to a tumor-associated antigen (fig. 206) (35,73).

Histochemical Features. Argyrophilia, as demonstrated by the Grimelius stain, has been reported in more than 90 percent of medullary thyroid carcinomas (fig. 207). In most cases, individual tumor cells show reactivity that is weak to moderate, with occasional strongly stained cells dispersed throughout (26,86). The most intensely positive cells often have a dendritic morphology. Although the Masson-Fontana argentaffin stain is usually negative, occasional tumors may contain rare scattered argentaffin cells.

The tumor cells may show focal PAS and Alcian blue positivity. However, the PAS positivity does not appear to be related to glycogen even in those tumors with a clear cytoplasm. The tumor stroma typically shows evidence of Alcian blue and PAS positivity. Both extra- and intracellular

217

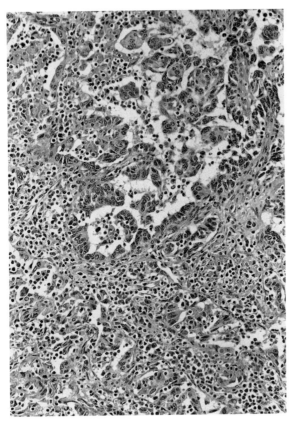

Figure 206
MEDULLARY THYROID CARCINOMA
This tumor shows an extensive inflammatory cell infiltrate. In some areas, the tumor cells are arranged in a papillary pattern.

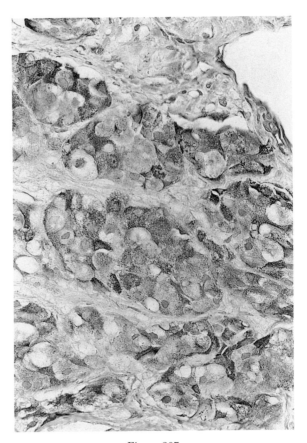

Figure 207
MEDULLARY THYROID CARCINOMA
Most of the tumor cells in this example contain fine argyrophilic granules. Grimelius stain.

mucin positivity are evident with mucicarmine stains in a high proportion of cases. Mucicarmine positivity in the tumor cells is present in the form of a large droplet, which may compress the nucleus to produce a signet-ring–type appearance. Signet-ring cells may indicate the possibility of a mucinous tumor of gastrointestinal origin when they are present in metastatic sites (30).

Immunohistochemical Features. Medullary thyroid carcinoma cells are typically positive for low–molecular-weight keratin proteins (24,93). However, in different areas of the same tumor, there may be considerable variation in staining intensity (pl. XXVII-A). High–molecular-weight keratins are rarely expressed. Vimentin immunoreactivity is variably present within the tumor cells, and some tumors have been reported to contain subpopulations of neurofilament-positive cells.

Medullary thyroid carcinomas demonstrate positive staining with antibodies directed at a variety of nonhormonal constituents of neuroendocrine cells. Thus, these tumors are typically positive for neuron-specific enolase, histaminase, synaptophysin, and chromogranins (24,38,44, 66,101). Neuron-specific enolase, however, is also expressed in a variety of non–C cell neoplasms and should not be used as the only marker to distinguish medullary carcinomas from other thyroid malignancies (pl. XXVII-B). Chromogranin, on the other hand, is a more specific marker for medullary thyroid carcinoma and may be more sensitive than calcitonin as a marker for this tumor type (pl. XXVII-C) (80). Synaptophysin is also commonly expressed in medullary carcinomas (38). Histaminase is typically expressed in carcinomas but not in hyperplastic foci (66).

Calcitonin is present in approximately 80 percent of medullary thyroid carcinomas (pl. XXVIII-A and B). Although many cases show extensive calcitonin immunoreactivity, occasional cases may show small and focal areas of positivity (75). The calcitonin gene–related peptide has also been localized in a high proportion of cases (51,94). In situ hybridization analyses with probes for calcitonin and calcitonin gene–related peptide mRNAs typically give positive signals within these tumors (60).

A variety of other peptides have been localized by immunohistochemistry within the tumors, and their presence has been confirmed by radioimmunoassays of tissue extracts (44). Both somatostatin (85,86,96,114) and bombesin (gastrin-releasing peptide) (63,95,115) are present in subpopulations of normal C cells. Both of these peptides are also commonly found in medullary thyroid carcinomas (32). In general, somatostatin immunoreactivity is present in single cells or in small cell groups, which most often represent less than 5 percent of the entire tumor cell population (85). The somatostatin cells often have a dendritic configuration with branching processes extending between adjacent tumor cells. Reubi and coworkers (72) detected somatostatin receptors in 4 of 19 tumors.

Other peptides that have been reported in cases of medullary thyroid carcinoma include ACTH (111) and other pro-opiomelanocortin–related peptides (β-endorphin) (70,74), Leu-enkephalin, neurotensin, substance P, vasoactive intestinal peptide, chorionic gonadotropin, and prolactin-stimulating factors may also be present (7). In rare instances, these tumors may contain subpopulations of cells immunoreactive for glucagon, gastrin, and insulin (86,101).

Both serotonin and catecholamines have also been demonstrated in medullary thyroid carcinomas (87,101). In the study reported by Uribe and coworkers (101), serotonin immunoreactivity was identified by immunohistochemistry in 14 of 20 cases. One of the serotonin-positive cases reported by this group was negative for calcitonin but was strongly positive by the Grimelius argyrophil stain. Similar to the distribution of peptide hormones in these tumors, serotonin immunoreactivity is most often present in cells with a dendritic morphology.

CEA levels are typically increased in the plasma of patients with medullary thyroid carci-noma compared with patients with papillary, follicular, or anaplastic carcinomas (13,25,48, 67, 82). Correlative immunohistochemical studies have revealed that almost 100 percent of medullary carcinomas are positive for this marker (pl. XXVIII-C). Several groups have demonstrated that some medullary carcinomas may lose their capacity to synthesize and secrete calcitonin while maintaining their capacity for CEA production. Immunohistochemical analyses have further shown that calcitonin-negative areas in such tumors frequently exhibit CEA positivity. In patients with medullary carcinoma, the finding of persistently elevated CEA levels in the face of decreasing calcitonin levels predicts aggressive disease (67). High levels of histaminase have been detected in the plasma and tissue extracts of patients with medullary carcinoma (66). No consistent lectin-binding pattern has been detected in medullary thyroid carcinoma (92).

Ultrastructural Features. A characteristic feature of medullary carcinoma cells at the ultrastructural level is the presence of membrane-bound secretory granules that represent the storage sites of calcitonin and other hormonal products (figs. 208, 209) (12,23,47). At least two different types of secretory granules have been identified in hyperplastic and neoplastic C cells. The larger granules (type I) have an average diameter of 280 nm with moderately electron-dense, finely granular contents that are closely applied to the limiting membranes of the granules. Smaller granules (type II) have an average diameter of 130 nm with more electron-dense contents that are separated from the limiting membranes by a narrow electron-lucent space (23). Capella and coworkers (16) described cells with the ultrastructural features of somatostatin-, serotonin-, and ACTH-containing cells in cases of medullary carcinoma.

Generally, neoplastic C cells have smaller numbers of secretory granules than do normal or hyperplastic C cells (26). Although both type I and type II granules are present in neoplastic C cells, they tend to have a higher proportion of type II granules. Moreover, neoplastic C cells more commonly show morphologic evidence of active protein synthesis, including the presence of prominent Golgi regions, abundant stacks of granular endoplasmic reticulum, and frequent cytoplasmic polyribosomes.

PLATE XXVII

MEDULLARY THYROID CARCINOMA

These photographs illustrate the appearance of various immunostains in medullary thyroid carcinoma.

A. The field shown in Plate XXVII–A is stained for low–molecular-weight keratins with the immunoperoxidase technique. Many of the cells show strong cytokeratin positivity.

B. The field shown in Plate XXVII–B is stained for neuron-specific enolase with the immunoperoxidase technique. Tumor cells within a vascular channel show strong staining.

C. The field shown in Plate XXVII–C is stained for chromogranin A with the immunoperoxidase technique. Most of the cells show intense granular cytoplasmic staining.

PLATE XXVII

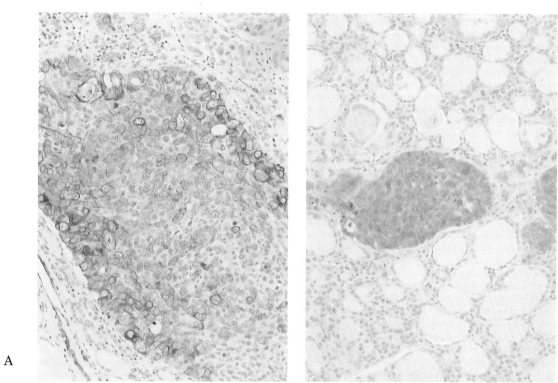

A

B

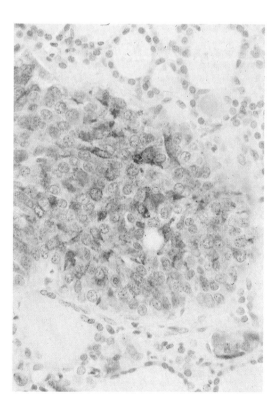

C

PLATE XXVIII

MEDULLARY THYROID CARCINOMA

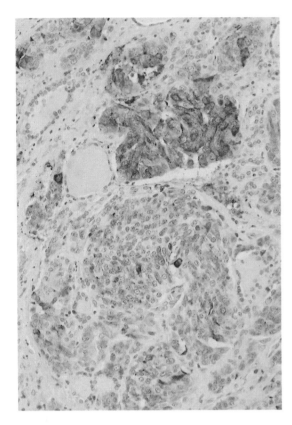

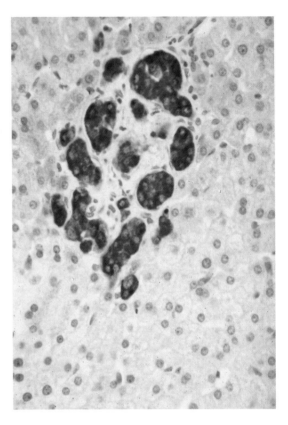

A. This example is stained for calcitonin with the immunoperoxidase technique. Some areas are intensely stained while others show relatively weak immunoreactivity.

B. This example, which was metastatic to liver, is stained for calcitonin with the immunoperoxidase technique. Tumor cells show intense cytoplasmic staining.

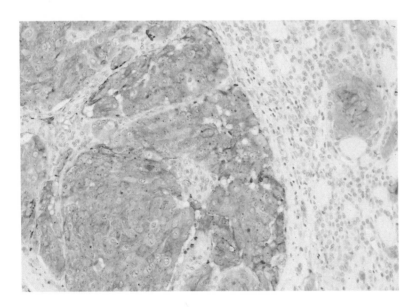

C. This example is stained for CEA with the immunoperoxidase technique. Intense staining is present in all of the tumor cells.

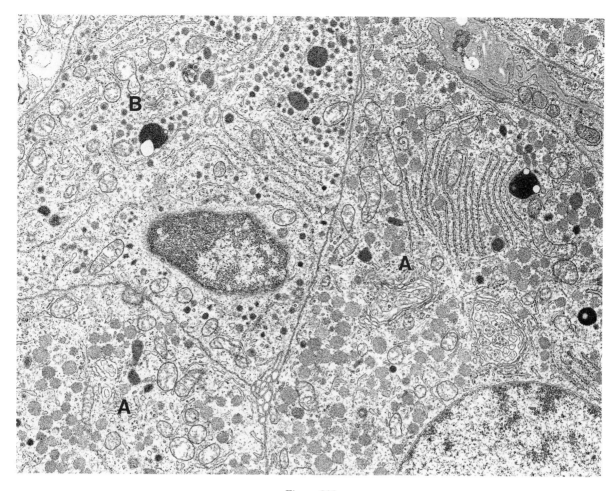

Figure 208

MEDULLARY THYROID CARCINOMA

As seen in this electron micrograph, some cells contain a predominance of large type I granules (A), whereas others contain a predominance of smaller type II granules (B). X10,701.

Cytologic Features. In fine-needle aspiration biopsy specimens, medullary carcinomas are variably cellular, depending on the amount of stromal fibrosis and amyloid deposition within any individual tumor (figs. 210, 211) (34,54). Typically, the tumor cells are present singly or in loosely cohesive groups with poorly defined cell borders. Syncytial groupings of tumor cells are rarely present. Medullary carcinomas in cytologic preparations are characteristically pleomorphic (figs. 210, 211). Whereas some cells are small and round, others may be cuboidal, polyhedral, or spindle shaped. Occasional tumors may be dominated by one cell type.

As described by Kini and coworkers (54), the tumor cell nuclei tend to be located eccentrically within the cytoplasm. This feature imparts a plasmacytoid appearance to the cells. Individual nuclei may be round, ovoid, or elongated, and bi- or multinucleated forms are common. Considerable nuclear pleomorphism may be evident in some cases. The chromatin is generally coarsely granular, and nucleoli are usually inconspicuous. Intranuclear cytoplasmic inclusions similar to those found in papillary carcinomas may be seen in some cases; however, medullary carcinoma cells lack the nuclear grooves that are usually present in papillary neoplasms.

The cytoplasm of the tumor cells is generally pale and vaguely fibrillary in Papanicolaou-stained preparations. The cells may exhibit fine cytoplasmic processes that are similar to those

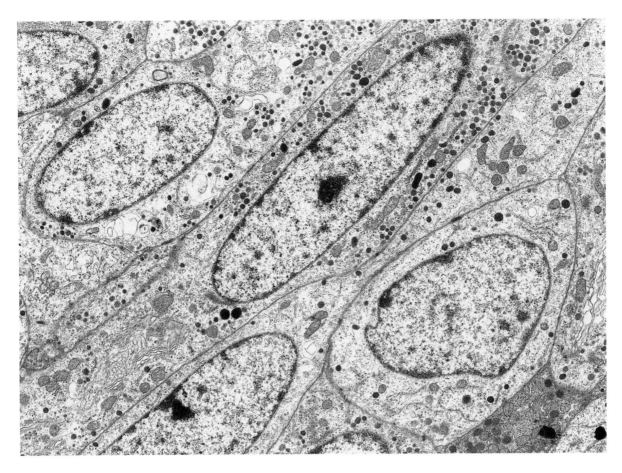

Figure 209
MEDULLARY THYROID CARCINOMA, SPINDLE CELL TYPE
The cells of this tumor are sparsely granulated. X6006.

seen in histologic preparations. In air-dried Wright-Giemsa–stained slides, some of the cells may contain fine cytoplasmic granules that are positively stained for calcitonin by immunofluorescence or immunoperoxidase procedures. Amyloid deposits may be impossible to distinguish from colloid in Papanicolaou stains (fig. 212). However, Congo red stains may be performed to confirm the presence of amyloid in suspected cases of medullary carcinoma.

Generally, medullary carcinoma tends to be overdiagnosed in cytologic preparations (54). These tumors may bear a striking resemblance to oncocytic neoplasms, which often also have an eccentrically placed nucleus; however, oncocytes typically have a more granular or dense cytoplasm, nuclei with finely granular chromatin and prominent nucleoli. Medullary carcinomas

may also be difficult to distinguish from some cases of anaplastic carcinoma of follicular origin. The cytologic diagnosis of medullary carcinoma should therefore be confirmed by immunohistochemical staining of the smears for calcitonin or measurements of serum calcitonin levels.

Differential Diagnosis. Medullary carcinomas may mimic a wide variety of benign and malignant primary thyroid neoplasms (68). True papillary variants of medullary carcinoma are rare, as discussed on page 230. The pseudopapillary variants, which result from artifactual separation of groups of tumor cells, are considerably more common. Papillary carcinomas of follicular cell origin are characterized by alignment of tumor cells on fibrovascular cores. The nuclei are generally irregular and overlapping and often have a ground-glass appearance with

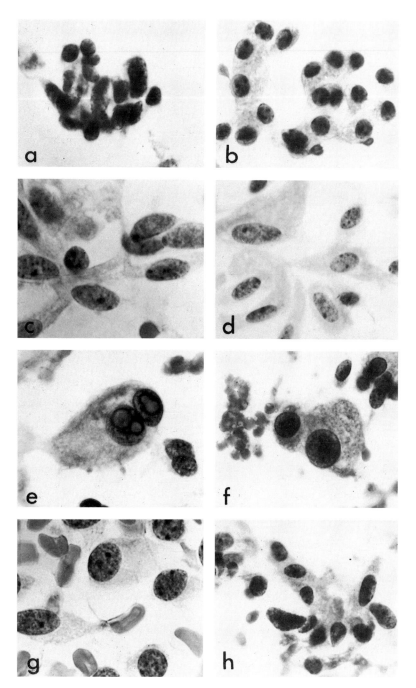

Figure 210
MEDULLARY CARCINOMA, VARIOUS CELL TYPES

Some of the cell types in medullary carcinoma include small cells with dense chromatin and scanty cytoplasm (A), small cuboidal cells (B), short, spindle-shaped cells with plump nuclei (C), delicate, spindle-shaped cells with cytoplasmic projections (D), large, oval cells with binucleation and intranuclear cytoplasmic inclusions (E), triangular cells and small round carcinoid-like cells (F), plasmacytoid cells with rudimentary cytoplasmic processes (G), and medium-sized cuboidal and oval cells with eccentric nuclei and cytoplasmic processes (H). Papanicolaou stains. (Fig. 10.9 from Kini SR. Thyroid. In: Kline TS, ed. Guides to Clinical Aspiration Biopsy; Vol 3.New York: Igaku-Shoin, 1987.)

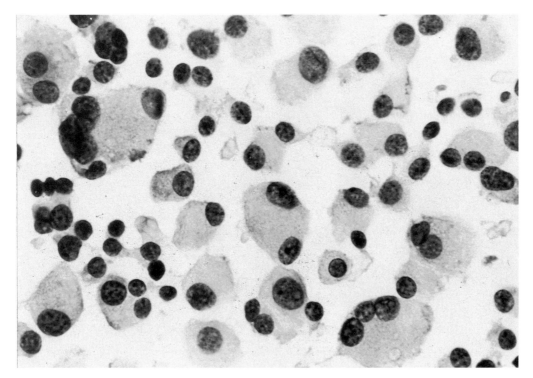

Figure 211
MEDULLARY CARCINOMA CELLS WITH MARKED PLEOMORPHISM
This illustration shows an admixture of carcinoid-type cells, plasmacytoid cells, polyhedral cells, and triangular cells with eccentric nuclei and multinucleation. Papanicolaou stain. (Fig. 10.10 from Kini SR. Thyroid. In: Kline TS, ed. Guides to Clinical Aspiration Biopsy; Vol 3. New York: Igaku-Shoin, 1987.)

or without pseudoinclusions and nuclear grooves. Nuclei of medullary carcinoma cells, on the other hand, often have coarsely punctate chromatin, and nuclear pseudoinclusions are considerably less prominent than in papillary carcinomas.

Occasional papillary carcinomas may contain abundant stromal collagen with foci of hyalinization that may mimic amyloid deposits. The often solid growth pattern of sclerosing variants of papillary carcinoma together with the prominent stroma may be confused histologically with medullary carcinoma; however, the sclerosing variants of papillary carcinoma are negative for amyloid, lack calcitonin immunoreactivity, and are positive for thyroglobulin. Foci of calcification are relatively common in the stromal regions of medullary carcinoma; however, true psammoma bodies are uncommon.

Medullary carcinomas often contain follicular structures and must therefore be distinguished from follicular carcinomas. Entrapped residual normal thyroid follicles are encountered fre-quently in medullary carcinomas. Both the colloid and follicular cells are typically thyroglobulin positive and calcitonin negative. The surrounding medullary carcinoma cells are typically calcitonin positive. Occasional medullary carcinomas may exhibit a follicular pattern of growth. Other areas of such tumors may show typical features of medullary carcinoma, including the presence of amyloid. In the exceptional cases of pure follicular variants of medullary carcinoma, immunoperoxidase studies for both calcitonin and thyroglobulin may be essential to resolve the diagnostic dilemma. Follicular variants of medullary carcinoma are calcitonin positive but are thyroglobulin negative. Mixed follicular and C cell tumors, which may show extensive follicular areas, are positive for both thyroglobulins and calcitonin, as discussed on page 238 (45). Some of these mixed tumors may be responsive to radioactive iodine treatment, as discussed on page 238 (43,45).

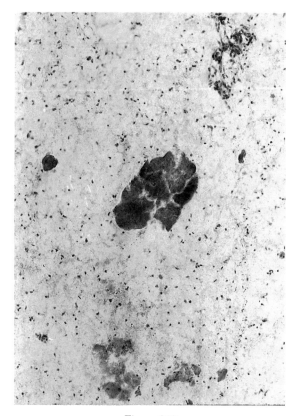

Figure 212
MEDULLARY THYROID CARCINOMA
A large amyloid deposit is present in this field. Fine-needle aspiration biopsy specimen. Congo red stain.

Occasional medullary carcinomas may be difficult to distinguish from amyloid-containing plasmacytomas. However, the tumor cells in plasmacytomas are typically positive for immunoglobulins.

The hyalinizing trabecular adenoma, which is discussed on page 31, is typically encapsulated, as are occasional variants of medullary thyroid carcinoma (18). A trabecular pattern of growth may be seen both in the hyalinizing adenomas and in medullary carcinomas, although it is less common in medullary carcinoma. Both lesions may show hyalinization and focal calcification, but the presence of amyloid is typical of medullary carcinoma. Follicle formation may be apparent in both tumors, but the formation of papillary structures is more typical of trabecular adenomas. Medullary carcinomas are calcitonin positive and thyroglobulin negative, whereas the reverse is true of hyalinizing trabecular adenomas.

Medullary carcinomas must be distinguished from poorly differentiated or insular thyroid carcinomas, as discussed on page 123. The insular carcinomas are characterized by the presence of solid islands of tumor cells containing occasional small follicles. The stroma of insular carcinomas is typically negative for amyloid, whereas the tumor cells are thyroglobulin positive but calcitonin negative.

Because medullary carcinomas often exhibit a solid pattern of growth without formation of follicles or papillae, they have in the past been classified as undifferentiated (anaplastic) carcinomas. Medullary carcinomas of spindle and giant cell types may be distinguished from undifferentiated carcinomas and sarcomas on the basis of calcitonin immunoreactivity in the former group. Moreover, spindle and giant cell forms of medullary carcinoma may show foci of more typical medullary carcinoma on extensive sectioning.

Studies reported by Nieuwenhuizjen-Kruseman and coworkers (138) have suggested that certain anaplastic thyroid carcinomas may, in fact, represent medullary carcinomas. In a series of 14 anaplastic carcinomas, including giant cell, spindle cell, and small cell variants, 9 cases exhibited both argyrophilia and calcitonin immunoreactivity. Martinelli and coworkers (135) described a case of anaplastic medullary carcinoma that, in addition to argyrophilia and calcitonin immunoreactivity, also displayed mucinous and squamous differentiation. Anaplastic transformation of medullary carcinoma has also been reported by Zeman and coworkers (140). However, other authors have not been able to confirm the presence of calcitonin in anaplastic thyroid carcinomas. In a study of 70 anaplastic carcinomas, including giant cell, spindle cell, and squamoid variants, Carcangiu and coworkers (122) did not find any cases that showed calcitonin immunoreactivity.

The small cell malignant tumors of the thyroid are discussed on pages 230 and 231. Most small cell tumors in this site represent malignant lymphomas, as demonstrated by positivity for leukocyte-common antigen and other markers of lymphoid cells. The small cell variants of medullary carcinoma are typically positive for calcitonin by immunohistochemistry or give positive signals for calcitonin mRNA when in situ hybridization techniques are used. The "primary oat cell carcinomas" of the thyroid are negative for calcitonin and calcitonin mRNA (29).

Medullary carcinomas may show oncocytic or clear cell features. These tumors are typically positive for calcitonin. Clear cell and oncocytic variants of follicular tumors are typically calcitonin negative but give positive reactions for thyroglobulin.

In rare instances, parathyroid adenomas may present as intrathyroidal masses. Such tumors are typically encapsulated and are composed of cords and nests of chief cells that have small, centrally placed nuclei and relatively clear or vacuolated cytoplasm. The chief cells are negative for calcitonin but may exhibit weak reactivity for chromogranin.

A variety of tumors may metastasize to the thyroid gland, as discussed on page 289. Metastases from renal cell carcinoma may mimic clear cell variants of medullary carcinoma, particularly because some renal tumors may contain amyloid deposits. However, metastatic renal cell carcinomas are negative for calcitonin. Metastatic bronchogenic oat cell carcinomas may be difficult to differentiate from small cell variants of medullary carcinoma because both tumors may be positive for calcitonin and bombesin. Similarly, thyroid metastases from carcinoids of bronchopulmonary or gastrointestinal origin may be positive for both calcitonin and bombesin.

Spread and Metastasis. The probability of nodal metastasis generally increases with the size of the primary tumor. Initial sites of metastasis include the central lymph nodes and the lateral cervical nodes (pl. XXIX-A; fig. 213). The tumor may also metastasize to a variety of distant sites, including lung, liver, and bone. The adrenals are also common sites of metastasis, and in patients with MEN IIA and IIB, metastases to pheochromocytomas may also be evident.

Treatment. The definitive treatment for sporadic and familial medullary carcinoma is total thyroidectomy. In addition, the lymph nodes of the central compartment of the neck are removed during the primary surgical procedure, both for tumor staging and for the prevention of subsequent appearance of metastases at these sites. If there is no evidence of central nodal metastasis, a surgical cure is likely and further neck dissection is probably unnecessary (75).

In patients with palpable primary tumors, cervical lymph node metastases are likely to be found. However, the value of neck dissections

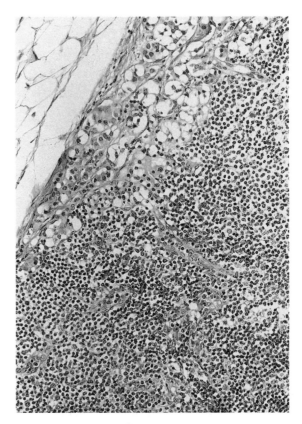

Figure 213
MEDULLARY THYROID CARCINOMA
METASTATIC TO A CERVICAL LYMPH NODE
Groups of tumor cells have focally replaced the peripheral sinus in this lymph node.

in these instances has been questioned. Recent studies have demonstrated normalization of serum calcitonin values in up to one third of such patients with evidence of elevated serum calcitonin levels and no radiologically detectable disease who were treated by neck dissection (39).

Prognosis. Patients with medullary thyroid carcinoma show considerable variation in overall survival (113). In most large series, the 5-year survival rates are 60 to 70 percent, whereas 10-year survivals have ranged from 40 to 50 percent (76,81). Survival is correlated significantly with age and sex of the patient and stage of the disease. Patients less than 40 years old at the time of diagnosis have a significantly better prognosis than older patients, even when individuals with the familial form of the disease are excluded from analysis. In addition, women have a better prognosis than men.

The probability of nodal metastasis is positively correlated with the size of the primary neoplasm. The studies of Bigner and coworkers (6) on familial medullary carcinomas demonstrated that approximately 20 percent of patients with tumors measuring less than 0.7 cm had nodal metastases. In contrast, nodal metastases were found in 80 percent of patients whose tumors were greater than 1.5 cm in diameter, whereas 30 percent of patients whose tumors measured between 0.7 and 1.5 cm had nodal metastases. In general, the levels of calcitonin parallel the extent of disease (103).

The prognosis for patients with early stages of disease is considerably better than that for patients with more advanced stages (81). Significant survival differences are noted when comparing patients with or without perithyroidal soft tissue involvement (pT4 vs. pT1–3). Regional nodal metastases (N0 vs. N1) and distant metastases (M0 vs. M1) are both correlated with decreased survival probability.

Schröder and coworkers (81) reported no differences in survival when they compared different histologic patterns of the primary tumors (spindle cell vs. polygonal cell type or other morphologies). However, other authors reported that a small cell anaplastic morphology is associated with a poor prognosis. In a study of 249 medullary carcinomas, Bergholm and coworkers (5) noted that tumors with less than 10 percent calcitonin-immunoreactive cells were more aggressive than calcitonin-rich tumors containing more than 50 percent calcitonin-immunoreactive cells. These findings essentially support the earlier studies of Lippman and coworkers (57), who also noted a more aggressive clinical course in patients with calcitonin-poor tumors. However, other authors have not confirmed these observations (5).

The presence of peptides including bombesin, somatostatin, and neurotensin did not appear to affect prognosis in the series of cases reported by Schröder and coworkers or in other series (81). Similarly, the numbers of S-100–positive dendritic cells do not appear to affect prognosis significantly. Leu-M1 is a myelomonocytic marker that has been detected in a variety of epithelial tumors, including papillary carcinomas of the thyroid (83). Medullary thyroid carcinomas also frequently express Leu-M1, and the degree of staining has been found to correlate with prognosis. In a series of 39 medullary carcinomas (T1-3 M0), local recurrences occurred three times and death from tumor occurred four times more commonly in medullary carcinomas, with more than 15 percent staining of tumor cells than in tumors with only slight or absent staining for Leu-M1 (83).

Prominent mitotic activity has been associated with poor prognosis. In the series of MEN IIA patients reported by Bigner and coworkers (6), mitotic figures were more common in tumors of patients who died of metastatic disease. More recent studies with flow cytometry revealed a worse prognosis for tumors that have a higher proportion of cells in S phase, G1 phase, and M phase. In reported series, a benign course of disease was twice as frequent among patients with diploid tumors as compared to those with aneuploid tumors.

The impact of amyloid content on prognosis has been controversial. Schröder and coworkers (81) concluded that amyloid-free tumors did not differ significantly from those neoplasms that contained amyloid . Bergholm and coworkers (5), on the other hand, concluded that the presence of amyloid confers a significantly better prognosis.

MEDULLARY CARCINOMA VARIANTS

Tubular (Follicular) Variant

Medullary carcinomas may be composed in part of tubular or follicular structures and may resemble follicular carcinomas (fig. 214) (121, 128,133,139). The tumors should also be distinguished from mixed medullary and follicular carcinomas (see page 238) and from medullary carcinomas with entrapped normal follicles (pl. XXIX-B). The tumor cells in the tubular variant form follicular structures that are lined by cells that resemble those in the more typical or solid areas of the tumor. The lumina of the follicular structures may appear empty or may contain an eosinophilic material resembling colloid.

Lertprasertsuke and coworkers (133) studied the immunohistochemical and ultrastructural characteristics of one case of the follicular variant of medullary carcinoma. The tumor cells, both in the follicular and solid areas, stained positively for calcitonin, calcitonin gene–related peptide, somatostatin, and serotonin. The cells

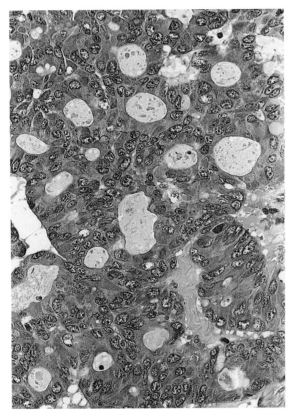

Figure 214
MEDULLARY THYROID CARCINOMA
TUBULAR (FOLLICULAR) VARIANT
This figure illustrates the tubular (follicular) variant of medullary thyroid carcinoma.

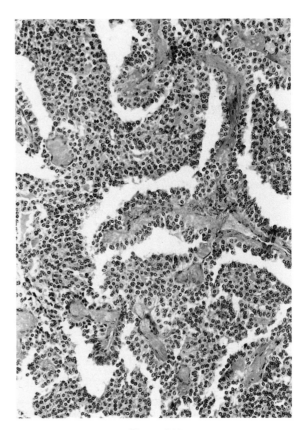

Figure 215
MEDULLARY THYROID CARCINOMA
This tumor shows a pseudopapillary pattern of growth.

and luminal contents were completely unreactive for thyroglobulin. Ultrastructurally, the cells contained variable numbers of secretory granules, apical microvilli, and well-developed desmosomes near the luminal poles. Similar foci of follicular differentiation have been noted in serial passages of a transplantable rat medullary thyroid carcinoma, suggesting that neoplasms derived from C cells retain their capacity for glandular differentiation.

Although the origin of the intraluminal eosinophilic material is unknown, our studies suggest that it may represent secreted calcitonin and other proteins. Immunoperoxidase studies of the follicular contents have revealed variable degrees of immunoreactivity for calcitonin. In contrast, the luminal contents seen in entrapped follicles stain positively for thyroglobulin, as do the surrounding compressed follicular cells.

Papillary Variant

In rare instances, medullary carcinomas may exhibit true papillary patterns of growth in which the constituent tumor cells are aligned along fibrovascular stalks. In the cases described by Kakudo and coworkers (130), the tumors also contained solid foci characteristic of typical medullary carcinomas. The presence of calcitonin-immunoreactivity serves to distinguish the papillary variant of medullary carcinoma from papillary carcinomas of follicular cell origin.

More common than the true papillary variant of medullary carcinoma is the "pseudopapillary" variant (fig. 215). Its appearance in medullary carcinomas results from artifactual separation of groups of tumor cells. As a result, groups of tumor cells may appear to be attached to the stromal components of the neoplasm with intervening empty-appearing spaces.

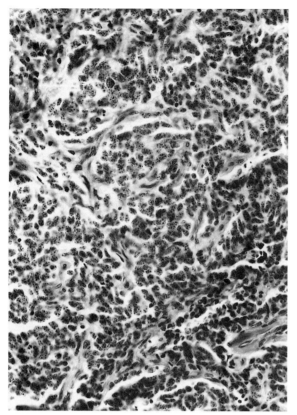

Figure 216
MEDULLARY THYROID CARCINOMA,
SMALL CELL VARIANT
This figure illustrates the small cell variant of medullary thyroid carcinoma.

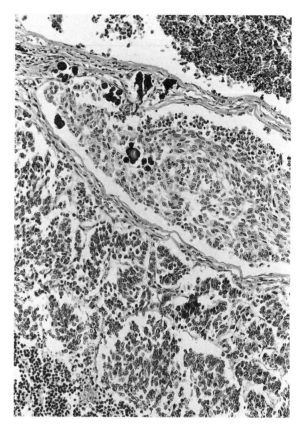

Figure 217
MEDULLARY THYROID CARCINOMA,
SMALL CELL VARIANT
Foci of calcification are evident in this tumor.

Small Cell Variant

The small cell variant of medullary thyroid carcinoma is characterized by the presence of cells with hyperchromatic nuclei that are round to ovoid and small amounts of cytoplasm (figs. 216–218) (117,136). These tumors most closely resemble the intermediate variant of small cell bronchogenic carcinomas. The small cell variant of medullary carcinoma may be difficult to distinguish on morphologic grounds from malignant lymphomas of the thyroid. The presence of leukocyte-common antigen or immunoglobulin heavy and light chains (see page 269) is diagnostic of malignant lymphoma. The presence of calcitonin, calcitonin gene–related peptide, or other peptides (bombesin, somatostatin) is characteristic of C cell differentiation in such neoplasms (pl. XXIX-C).

The small cell variant of medullary carcinoma may exhibit a compact, trabecular, or diffuse pattern of growth (figs. 216–218). Overall mitotic activity is high, and the tumors often show foci of necrosis. This variant may occur in a pure form or may be admixed with more typical areas of medullary carcinoma. Stromal amyloid deposits may be absent from this type of tumor. The tumor cells may be negative for calcitonin but frequently exhibit immunoreactivity for CEA, as do other types of medullary carcinoma. The prognosis of the small cell variant is less favorable than that for typical medullary carcinomas.

Eusebi and coworkers (125) have reported two cases of small cell carcinoma of the thyroid that were classified as apparent primary oat cell carcinomas. Both tumors were positive for chromogranin A and synaptophysin but negative for thyroglobulin and calcitonin by immunohistochemistry. Both tumors were negative for calcitonin mRNA when in situ

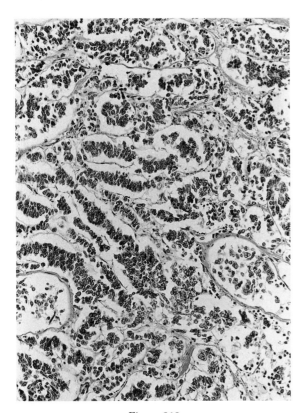

Figure 218
MEDULLARY THYROID CARCINOMA,
SMALL CELL VARIANT
This tumor shows a trabecular growth pattern.

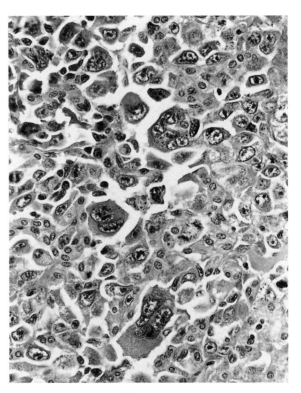

Figure 219
MEDULLARY THYROID CARCINOMA
This tumor contains clusters of giant cells.

hybridization procedures were used. On the basis of these studies, Eusebi and coworkers concluded that such cases should be separated from the small cell anaplastic variants of medullary carcinoma and should be classified as oat cell or small cell carcinomas.

Giant Cell Variant

Isolated tumor giant cells characterized by multiple nuclei and abundant eosinophilic cytoplasm may be found in occasional medullary thyroid carcinomas of both familial and sporadic types (fig. 219). However, some medullary carcinomas may contain a predominance of giant cells that resemble the syncytial trophoblastic cells of choriocarcinoma. Typically, the giant cell areas are admixed with foci of more typical medullary carcinoma. The tumor giant cells are variably positive for calcitonin, and the stroma may contain amyloid deposits. The prognosis for medul-

lary carcinomas of giant cell type is considerably better than that for anaplastic giant cell carcinomas of follicular origin.

Clear Cell Variant

Medullary carcinomas may be composed wholly or partly of cells with optically clear cytoplasm (fig. 220). Landon and Ordòñez (132) described a medullary carcinoma composed predominantly of large polygonal cells with clear cytoplasm. In other areas, the tumor was composed of spindle-shaped cells with faintly eosinophilic cytoplasm. The tumor cells in this case were negative for mucins and did not contain appreciable amounts of glycogen. The tumor cells stained positively for calcitonin and contained secretory granules ultrastructurally. The patient developed widespread bone metastases 6 years after thyroidectomy. Clear cell medullary carcinomas can be distinguished from clear cell variants of follicular neoplasms with thyroglobulin immunohistochemistry.

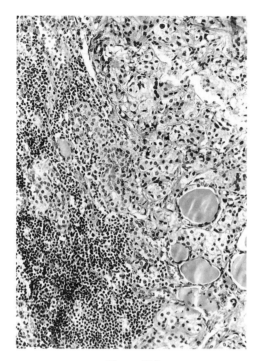

Figure 220
MEDULLARY THYROID CARCINOMA
This tumor is composed in part of cells with clear cytoplasm.

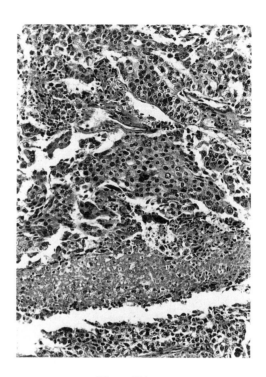

Figure 221
MEDULLARY THYROID CARCINOMA
This tumor shows foci of necrosis and is composed in part

Melanotic (Pigmented) Variant

Melanin pigment has been described in a variety of peptide and amine-producing endocrine tumors, including thymic carcinoids and medullary thyroid carcinomas. Marcus and coworkers (134) described a case of nonfamilial medullary thyroid carcinoma that contained collections of dendritic argentaffin-positive cells (pl. XXIX-D). The dendritic cells were negative for calcitonin by immunohistochemistry, whereas the remaining cells within the tumor were positive. Ultrastructurally, the argentaffin-positive cells contained typical melanosomes. Beerman and coworkers (118) demonstrated both melanosomes and calcitonin-containing secretory granules within the same cells.

Oncocytic (Oxyphilic) Variant

Rare examples of medullary carcinoma composed predominantly of oncocytic cells have been reported (pl. XXX) (124,127). In the case reported by Dominguez-Malagon and coworkers (124), 60 to 70 percent of the tumor cells were of the oncocytic type, whereas the remainder of the

tumor had the features of a conventional medullary carcinoma. The tumor cells showed a trabecular pattern of growth and were separated by an amyloid-free fibrous stroma. Ultrastructurally, the tumor cells contained numerous mitochondria with few dispersed membrane-bound secretory granules. The oncocytic tumor cells exhibited strong positivity for chromogranin, calcitonin, and CEA but were negative for thyroglobulin.

Squamous Variant

Dominguez-Malagon and coworkers (124) reported a single case of medullary thyroid carcinoma that showed extensive foci of squamous carcinoma that were well to moderately differentiated (fig. 221). The authors noted transitional areas between the squamous and endocrine areas of the tumor. This case was calcitonin negative but showed diffuse positivity for neuron-specific enolase and chromogranin and focal positivity for CEA. The stroma showed focal amyloid deposition. Schröder and coworkers (81) noted areas of squamous differentiation in metastatic medullary carcinoma.

PLATE XXIX

A. METASTATIC MEDULLARY THYROID CARCINOMA
This illustration shows a lymph node with metastatic medullary thyroid carcinoma.

B. MEDULLARY THYROID CARCINOMA
This example is stained for thyroglobulin with the immunoperoxidase technique. The tumor cells are negative, but there is reactivity in the entrapped follicular cells.

C. MEDULLARY THYROID CARCINOMA, SMALL CELL VARIANT
This example is stained for calcitonin with the immunoperoxidase technique. Most of the tumor cells are stained positively.

D. MEDULLARY THYROID CARCINOMA, MELANOTIC VARIANT
Scattered tumor cells are filled with melanin pigment.

PLATE XXIX

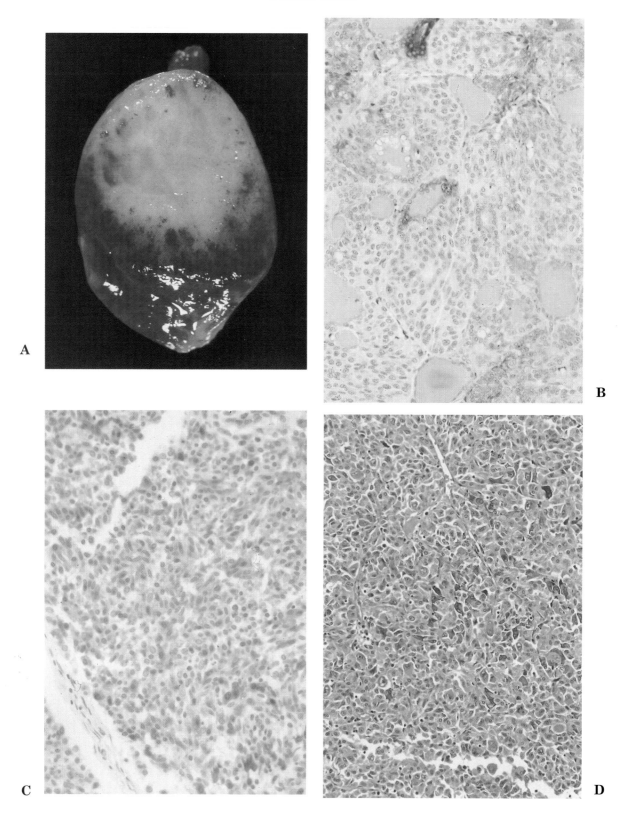

PLATE XXX

MEDULLARY THYROID CARCINOMA, ONCOCYTIC VARIANT

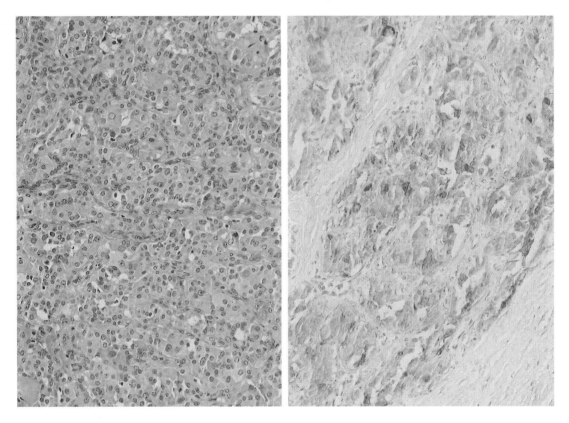

A. The tumor on the left is stained with H&E. The cells have granular eosinophilic cytoplasm. The tumor on the right is stained for calcitonin with the immunoperoxidase technique. Many of the cells are strongly stained.

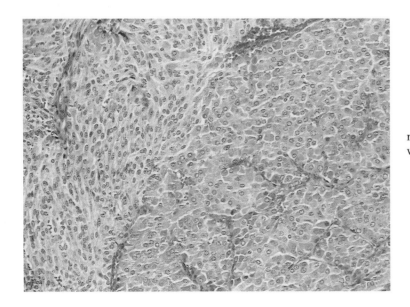

B. This illustration shows medullary thyroid carcinoma with oncocytic foci.

Amphicrine (Composite Calcitonin and Mucin-Producing) Variant

Mucicarmine-positive cells have been reported in up to 25 percent of medullary thyroid carcinomas. Golough and coworkers (126) reported a case of medullary carcinoma in which approximately 30 percent of the tumor cells resembled signet-ring cells (pl. XXXI-A). Combined Alcian blue and Grimelius stains revealed that approximately 5 percent of the tumor cells were both alcianophilic and argyrophilic or calcitonin positive. Ultrastructurally, these cells contained both membrane-bound secretory granules and finely reticulated mucin deposits.

Paraganglioma-Like Variant

Occasional medullary carcinomas may be encapsulated and may be arranged in a broad trabecular pattern with an amyloid-negative hyalinized stroma (fig. 222) (123). Huss and Mendelsohn (129) reported two such cases that presented as encapsulated neoplasms resembling hyalinizing trabecular adenoma. In con-trast to the latter (129), those cases were calcitonin positive (123). Rare examples of true paragangliomas have been reported to involve the thyroid gland.

Encapsulated Medullary Carcinoma

Most neoplastic proliferations of C cells have been considered to represent carcinomas, but occasional examples of lesions classified as adenomas have been reported (119). In 1988, Kodama and coworkers (131) reported two cases of C cell adenoma, each measuring 4 cm in diameter (fig. 223). One of the tumors was almost completely encapsulated, whereas the other lacked a connective tissue capsule. Each tumor was composed of cells that were fusiform to cuboidal, with small elliptical nuclei. Neither tumor contained calcification or amyloid deposits. In contrast to most medullary thyroid carcinomas, plasma levels of CEA were within normal limits, and there was no immunoreactive CEA within the tumor cells. On the other hand, serum calcitonin levels were markedly elevated, and the tumors stained

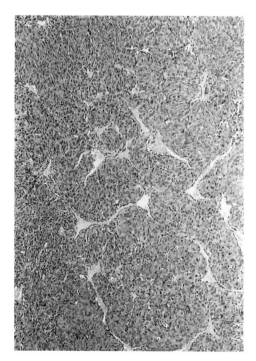

Figure 222
MEDULLARY THYROID CARCINOMA

This tumor shows a paraganglioma-like pattern in many areas.

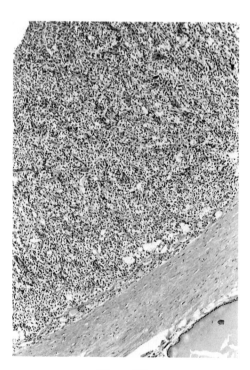

Figure 223
MEDULLARY THYROID CARCINOMA

This field shows the encapsulated type of medullary thyroid carcinoma.

strongly for this peptide. Whether the C cell adenoma exists as a valid entity is a debatable issue. Some authors have considered encapsulated C cell neoplasms to represent encapsulated medullary carcinomas (137). Until more data are accrued, it seems prudent to regard all C cell neoplasms as carcinomas.

MIXED MEDULLARY-FOLLICULAR CARCINOMA

Mixed medullary and follicular carcinomas are composed of cells that show evidence of C cell and follicular differentiation histologically and contain calcitonin or other neuropeptides and thyroglobulin (42,143). These rare neoplasms, which have also been referred to as intermediate carcinomas (147), must be distinguished from medullary carcinomas with entrapped normal follicles and from the follicular variant of medullary carcinoma (141–143,146–150). The existence of such mixed tumors may explain the rare cases of medullary carcinoma that have the ability to incorporate radioactive iodine (144).

The cellular origin of these neoplasms is unknown, but several studies have noted their similarities to the ultimobranchial neoplasms of bulls (147). It has been suggested that such mixed tumors could arise from uncommitted stem cells of the ultimobranchial body that would have the potential to differentiate into either C cells or follicular cells (147). Alternatively, this phenomenon could result from activation of neuropeptide genes in follicular tumors. It is also possible, although unlikely, that these neoplasms represent collision tumors (146,150).

At the gross level, mixed medullary and follicular carcinomas may be partially encapsulated or nonencapsulated and invade the surrounding thyroid parenchyma or soft tissues of the neck. Microscopically, these tumors have been described as solid and follicular, with or without cribriform areas (figs. 224–227). The solid areas resemble typical medullary carcinomas and are characterized by polyhedral cells arranged in compact lobules and trabeculae (figs. 224, 225). The intervening stroma is generally devoid of amyloid deposits. The follicular regions generally have a microfollicular pattern, although large follicles may be evident in some cases. In contrast to med-

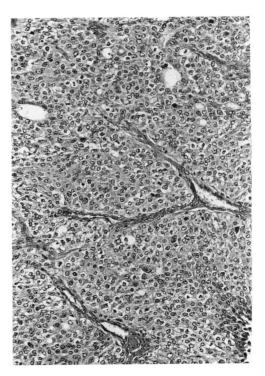

Figure 224
MIXED MEDULLARY-FOLLICULAR CARCINOMA
The tumor cells in this area show a lobular growth pattern. (Courtesy of Dr. O. Ljungberg, Malmo, Sweden.)

ullary carcinoma with entrapped normal follicles, the nuclei of the follicular areas of mixed tumors have features similar to those seen in the solid areas (figs. 226, 227). In rare instances, some of the tumors have a component of indifferent cells with tubules and cystic structures reminiscent of ultimobranchial elements.

Immunohistochemical analyses have revealed that the mixed medullary and follicular carcinomas invariably contain thyroglobulin (pl. XXXI-B). In the series of 14 cases reported by Ljungberg and coworkers (147), 4 also contained calcitonin, 8 contained somatostatin, and 10 had neurotensin-immunoreactive cells. Holm and coworkers (145) successfully colocalized thyroglobulin and calcitonin or calcitonin gene–related peptide in 8 cases of mixed medullary-follicular carcinoma. Tumor cells in regional node metastases also coexpressed thyroglobulin and one of the neuropeptides. Ultrastructural studies have revealed that some of the tumor cells contain secretory granules of the C cell type, whereas others exhibit dilated cisternae of endoplasmic reticulum similar to those observed in follicular cells (145).

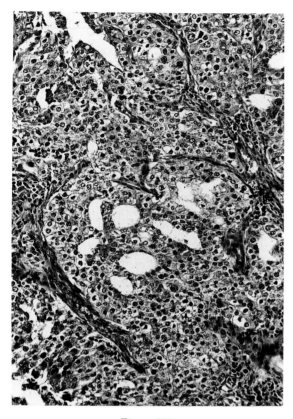

Figure 225
MIXED MEDULLARY-FOLLICULAR CARCINOMA
The tumor shows scattered, early follicle-like areas.
(Courtesy of Dr. O. Ljungberg, Malmo, Sweden.)

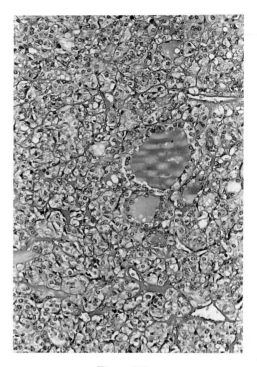

Figure 226
MIXED MEDULLARY-FOLLICULAR CARCINOMA
These tumor cells form colloid-containing follicles.
(Courtesy of Dr. O. Ljungberg, Malmo, Sweden.)

MIXED MEDULLARY-PAPILLARY CARCINOMA

Albores-Saavedra and coworkers (151) described a rare variant of medullary carcinoma
that contained intimately admixed populations
of cells with the characteristic clear nuclei of
papillary carcinoma. Cells with the phenotype of
papillary carcinoma were thyroglobulin positive
and calcitonin and CEA negative. The cells of the
medullary component, on the other hand, were
thyroglobulin negative but CEA and calcitonin
positive. Admixtures of the papillary and medullary elements were identified both in the primary tumors and in the nodal metastases.
Whether these rare tumors arise from a stem cell
capable of dual differentiation into follicular and
C cell elements or they arise as a result of separate neoplastic transformation of C cells and
follicular cells is unknown at present.

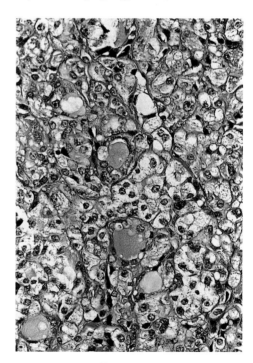

Figure 227
MIXED MEDULLARY-FOLLICULAR CARCINOMA
Many of the cells in this tumor have a clear cytoplasm.
(Courtesy of Dr. O. Ljungberg, Malmo, Sweden.)

239

PLATE XXXI

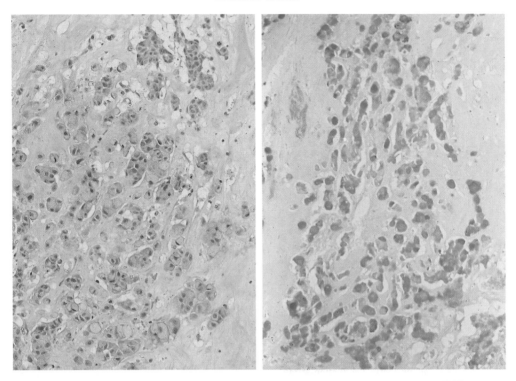

A. MEDULLARY THYROID CARCINOMA, AMPHICRINE TYPE

In the field on the left, H&E stain shows cells with vacuolated cytoplasm. In the field on the right, Alcian blue and immunoperoxidase stain for calcitonin is demonstrated. Some tumor cells contain both calcitonin and mucin. (Courtesy of Dr. Vincenzo Eusebi, Bologna, Italy.)

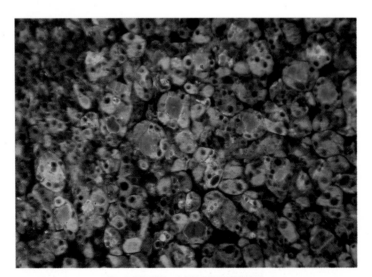

B. MIXED MEDULLARY-FOLLICULAR CARCINOMA

An immunofluorescence preparation is shown. Thyroglobulin is stained with a fluorescein-labeled antibody (green), and calcitonin is stained with a rhodamine-labeled antibody (orange). (Courtesy of Dr. O. Ljungberg, Malmo, Sweden.)

REFERENCES

Medullary Carcinoma

1. Albores-Saavedra J, LiVolsi VA, Williams ED. Medullary carcinoma. Semin Diagn Pathol 1985;2:137–46.

2. Aldabagh SM, Trujillo YP, Taxy JB. Occult medullary thyroid carcinoma. Unusual histologic variant presenting with metastatic disease. Am J Clin Pathol 1986;85:247–50.

3. Al Saadi AA. Management and prevention of familial medullary carcinoma of the thyroid. Prog Clin Biol Res 1979;34:343–50.

4. Baylin SB, Beaven MA, Engelman K, Sjoerdsma A. Elevated histaminase activity in medullary carcinoma of the thyroid gland. N Engl J Med 1972;283:1239–44.

5. Bergholm V, Adami H-O, Auer G, et al. Histopathologic characteristics and nuclear DNA content as prognostic factors in medullary thyroid carcinoma. A nationwide study in Sweden. The Swedish MTC study group. Cancer 1989;64:135–42.

6. Bigner SH, Cox EB, Mendelsohn G, Baylin SB, Wells SA Jr, Eggleston JC. Medullary carcinoma of the thyroid in the multiple endocrine neoplasia IIA syndrome. Am J Surg Pathol 1981;5:459–72.

7. Birkenhäger JC, Upton GV, Seldenrath HJ, Krieger DT, Tashjian AH Jr. Medullary thyroid carcinoma: ectopic production of peptides with ACTH-like, corticotrophin-releasing factor-like and prolactin production-stimulating activities. Acta Endocrinol (Copenh) 1976;83:280–92.

8. Black HE, Capen CC, Young DM. Ultimobranchial thyroid neoplasms in bulls. A syndrome resembling medullary thyroid carcinoma in man. Cancer 1973;32:865–78.

9. Block MA, Jackson CE, Greenwald KA, Yott JB, Tashjian AH Jr. Clinical characteristics distinguishing hereditary from sporadic medullary thyroid carcinoma. Treatment implications. Arch Surg 1980;115:142–8.

10. Boorman GA, Hollander CF. Animal models of human disease. Medullary carcinoma of the thyroid. Am J Pathol 1976;83:237–40.

11. Boultwood J, Wyllie FS, Williams ED, Winford-Thomas D. N-*myc* expression in neoplasia of human thyroid C-cells. Cancer Res 1988;48:4073–7.

12. Braunstein H, Stephens CL, Gibson RL. Secretory granules in medullary carcinoma of the thyroid. Electron microscopic demonstration. Arch Pathol 1968;85:306–13.

13. Burtin P, Calmettes C, Fondaneche MC. CEA and non-specific cross-reacting antigen (NCA) in medullary carcinomas of the thyroid. Int J Cancer 1979;23:741–5.

14. Bussolati G, Monga G. Medullary carcinoma of the thyroid with atypical patterns. Cancer 1979;44:1769–77.

15. _____, Pearse AG. Immunofluorescent localization of calcitonin in the C cells of the pig and dog thyroid. J Clin Endocrinol 1967;37:205–9.

16. Capella C, Bordi C, Monga G, et al. Multiple endocrine cell types in thyroid medullary carcinoma. Evidence for calcitonin, somatostatin, ACTH, 5HT and small granule cells. Virchows Arch [A] 1978;377:111–28.

17. Carney JA, Hayles AB. Alimentary tract manifestations of multiple endocrine neoplasia, type 2b. Mayo Clin Proc 1977;52:543–8.

18. _____, Ryan J, Goellner JR. Hyalinizing trabecular adenoma of the thyroid gland. Am J Surg Pathol 1986;10:672–9.

19. _____, Sizemore GW, Hayles AB. Multiple endocrine neoplasia, type 2b. Pathobiol Annu 1978;8:105–53.

20. _____, Sizemore GW, Tyce GM. Bilateral adrenal medullary hyperplasia in multiple endocrine neoplasia, type 2: the precursor of bilateral pheochromocytoma. Mayo Clin Proc 1975;50:3–10.

21. Chong GC, Beahrs OH, Sizemore GW, Woolner LH. Medullary carcinoma of the thyroid. Cancer 1973;35:695–704.

22. Copp DH, Cameron EC, Cheney BA, Davidson AG, Henze KG. Evidence for calcitonin—a new hormone from the parathyroid that lowers serum calcium. Endocrinology 1962;70:638–49.

23. Dämmrich J, Ormanns W, Schäffer R. Electron microscopic demonstration of calcitonin in human medullary carcinoma of the thyroid by the immuno gold staining method. Histochemistry 1984;81:369–72.

24. DeLellis RA. Endocrine tumors. In: Colvin RB, Bhan AK, McCluskey RT, eds. Diagnostic immunopathology. New York: Raven Press, 1988:301–38.

25. _____, Rule AH, Spiler I, Nathanson L, Tashjian AH Jr, Wolfe HJ. Calcitonin and carcinoembryonic antigen as tumor markers in medullary thyroid carcinoma. Am J Clin Pathol 1978;70:587–94.

26. _____, Wolfe HJ. The pathobiology of the human calcitonin (C)-cell: a review. Pathol Annu 1981;16:25–52.

27. _____, Wolfe HJ, Gagel RF, et al. Adrenal medullary hyperplasia. A morphometric analysis in patients with familial medullary thyroid carcinoma. Am J Pathol 1976;83:177–96.

28. _____, Wolfe HJ, Rule AH. Carcinoembryonic antigen as a tissue marker in medullary thyroid carcinoma [Letter]. N Engl J Med 1979;299:1082.

29. Eusebi V, Damiani S, Riva C, Lloyd RV, Capella C. Calcitonin free oat cell carcinoma of the thyroid gland. Virchows Arch [A] 1990;417:267–71.

30. Fernandes BJ, Bedard YC, Rosen I. Mucus-producing medullary cell carcinoma of the thyroid gland. Am J Clin Pathol 1982;78:536–40.

31. Franc B, Caillou B, Carrier AM, et al. Immunohistochemistry in medullary thyroid carcinoma: prognosis and distinction between hereditary and sporadic tumors. Henry Ford Hosp Med J 1987;35:139–42.

32. Franc B, Chayvialle JA, Modigliani E, et al. Plasma and tumor levels of somatostatin (SRIF) and somatostatin immunohistochemistry in medullary thyroid carcinoma: apparently discrepant results. Henry Ford Hosp Med J 1987;35:147–8.

33. Gagel RF, Tashjian AH Jr, Cummings T, et al. The clinical outcome of prospective screening for multiple endocrine neoplasia type 2a. N Engl J Med 1988;318:478–84.

34. Geddie WR, Bedard YC, Strawbridge HT. Medullary carcinoma of the thyroid in fine-needle aspiration biopsies. Am J Clin Pathol 1984;82:552–8.

35. George JM, Williams MA, Almoney R, Sizemore G. Medullary carcinoma of the thyroid. Cellular immune response to tumor antigen in a heritable human cancer. Cancer 1975;36:1658–61.

36. Goltzman D, Potts JT Jr, Ridgway RC, Maloof F. Calcitonin as a tumor marker. Use of the radioimmunoassay for calcitonin in the postoperative evaluation of patients with medullary thyroid carcinoma. N Engl J Med 1974;290:1035–9.

37. Gorlin RJ, Sedano HO, Vickers RA, Cervenka J. Multiple mucosal neuromas, pheochromocytoma and medullary carcinoma of the thyroid—a syndrome. Cancer 1968;22:293–9.

38. Gould VE, Wiedenmann B, Lee I, et al. Synaptophysin expression in neuroendocrine neoplasms as determined by immunocytochemistry. Am J Pathol 1987;126:243–57.

39. Grauer A, Raue F, Gagel RF. Changing concepts in the management of hereditary and sporadic medullary thyroid carcinoma. Endocrinol Metab Clin North Am 1990; 19:613–35.

40. Hazard JB. The C cells (parafollicular cells) of the thyroid gland and medullary thyroid carcinoma. A review. Am J Pathol 1977;88:213–50.

41. _____, Hawk WA, Crile G Jr. Medullary (solid) carcinoma of the thyroid; a clinicopathologic entity. J Clin Endocrinol Metab 1959;19:152–61.

42. Hedinger CHR, Williams ED, Sobin LH, et al. Histological typing of thyroid tumors. WHO international classification of tumors. 2nd ed. Springer-verlag. Berlin 1988.

43. Hellman DE, Kartchner M, Van Antwerp JD, Salmon SE, Patton DD, O'Mara R. Radioiodine in the treatment of medullary carcinoma of the thyroid. J Clin Endocrinol Metab 1979;48:451–8.

44. Holm R, Sobrinho-Simões M, Nesland JM, Gould VE, Johannessen JV. Medullary thyroid carcinoma of the thyroid gland: an immunocytochemical study. Ultrastruct Pathol 1985;8:25–41.

45. _____, Sobrinho-Simões M, Nesland JM, Sambade C, Johannessen JV. Medullary carcinoma of the thyroid gland with thyroglobulin immunoreactivity. A special entity? Lab Invest 1987;57:258–68.

46. Horn RC. Carcinoma of the thyroid. Description of a distinctive morphological variant and report of 7 cases. Cancer 1951;4:697–707.

47. Huang SN, Goltzman D. Electron and immunoelectron microscopic study of thyroidal medullary carcinoma. Cancer 1978;41:2226–35.

48. Ishikawa N, Hamada S. Association of medullary carcinoma of the thyroid with carcinoembryonic antigen. Br J Cancer 1976;34:111–5.

49. Jackson CE, Block MA, Greenawald KA, Tashjian AH Jr. The two-mutational-event theory in medullary thyroid cancer. Am J Hum Genet 1979;31:704–10.

50. James PD. Amyloid goitre. J Clin Pathol 1972;25:683–6.

51. Johannsen L, Daa Schroder H, Schifter S. Calcitonin gene-related peptide and calcitonin in MEN-2 and sporadic pheochromocytomas: an immunohistochemical study. Henry Ford Hosp Med J 1987;35:115–7.

52. Kakudo K, Carney JA, Sizemore GW. Medullary carcinoma of the thyroid. Biologic behavior of the sporadic and familial neoplasm. Cancer 1985;55:2818–21.

53. _____, Miyauchi A, Ogihara T, et al. Medullary carcinoma of the thyroid. Giant cell type. Arch Pathol Lab Med 1978;102:445–7.

54. Kini SR. Thyroid. In: Kline TS, ed. Guides to clinical aspiration biopsy; Vol. 3. New York: Igaku-shoin, 1987;156–9.

55. Lee TK, Myers RT, Marshall RB, Bond MG, Kardon B. The significance of mitotic rate: a retrospective study of 127 thyroid carcinomas. Hum Pathol 1985;16:1042–6.

56. Lertprasertsuke N, Kakudo K, Nakamura A, et al. C cell carcinoma of the thyroid. Follicular variant. Acta Pathol Jpn 1989;39:393–9.

57. Lippman SM, Mendelsohn G, Trump DL, Wells SA Jr, Baylin SB. The prognostic and biological significance of cellular heterogeneity in medullary thyroid carcinoma: a study of calcitonin, L-dopa decarboxylase, and histaminase. J Clin Endocrinol Metab 1982;54:233–40.

58. Lips CJ, Vasen HF, Lamers CB. Multiple endocrine neoplasia syndromes. CRC Crit Rev Oncol Hematol 1988;2:117–84.

59. LiVolsi VA, Feind CR. Incidental medullary thyroid carcinoma in sporadic hyperparathyroidism. An expansion of the concept of C-cell hyperplasia. Am J Clin Pathol 1979;71:595–9.

60. Lloyd RV. Use of molecular probes in the study of endocrine diseases. Hum Pathol 1987;18:1199–211.

61. Martin-Lacave I, Gonzalez-Campora R, Moreno Fernandez A, Sanchez Gallego F, Montero C, Galera-Davidson H. Mucosubstances in medullary carcinoma of the thyroid. Histopathology 1988;13:55–66.

62. Mathew CG, Chin KS, Easton DF, et al. A linked genetic marker for multiple endocrine neoplasia type 2A on chromosome 10. Nature 1987;328:527–8.

63. Matsubayashi S, Yanaihara C, Ohkubo M, et al. Gastrin-releasing peptide immunoreactivity in medullary thyroid carcinoma. Cancer 1984;53:2472–7.

64. Meissner WA, Warren S. Tumors of the thyroid gland. In: The atlas of tumor pathology, Series 2, Fascicle 4. Washington D.C.: Armed Forces Institute of Pathology, 1969.

65. Melvin KE, Miller HH, Tashjian AH Jr. Early diagnosis of medullary carcinoma of the thyroid by means of calcitonin assay. N Engl J Med 1971;285:1115–20.

66. Mendelsohn G, Eggleston JC, Weisburger WR, Gann DS, Baylin SB. Calcitonin and histaminase in C-cell hyperplasia and medullary thyroid carcinoma. A light microscopic and immunohistochemical study. Am J Pathol 1978;92:35–52.

67. _____, Wells SA, Baylin SB. Relationship of tissue carcinoembryonic antigen and calcitonin to tumor virulence in medullary thyroid carcinoma. An immunohistochemical study in early, localized and virulent disseminated stages of disease. Cancer 1984;54:657–62.

68. Normann T, Johannessen JV, Gautvik KM, Olsen BR, Brennhovd IO. Medullary carcinoma of the thyroid. Diagnostic problems. Cancer 1976;38:366–77.

69. Norton JA, Froome LC, Farrell RE, Wells SA Jr. Multiple endocrine neoplasia type IIb: the most aggressive form of medullary thyroid carcinoma. Surg Clin North Am 1979;59:109–18.

70. Ohashi M, Yanase T, Fujio N, Ibayashi H, Kinjo M, Matsuo H. Alpha neoendorphin-like immunoreactivity in medullary carcinoma of the thyroid. Cancer 1987; 59:277–80.

71. Ponder BA, Ponder MA, Coffey R, et al. Risk estimation and screening in families of patients with medullary thyroid carcinoma. Lancet 1988;1:397–401.

72. Reubi JC, Chayvialle JA, Franc B, Cohen R, Calmettes C, Modigliani E. Somatostatin receptors and somatostatin content in medullary thyroid carcinomas. Lab Invest 1991;64:567–73.

73. Rocklin RE, Gagel R, Feldman Z, Tashjian AH Jr. Cellular immune responses in familial medullary thyroid carcinoma. N Engl J Med 1977;296:835–8.

74. Roth KA, Bensch KG, Hoffman AR. Characterization of opioid peptides in human thyroid medullary carcinoma. Cancer 1987;59:1594–8.

75. Saad MF, Ordòñez NG, Guido JJ, Samaan NA. The prognostic value of calcitonin immunostaining in medullary carcinoma of the thyroid. J Clin Endocrinol Metab 1984;59:850–6.

76. _____, Ordòñez NG, Rashid RK, et al. Medullary carcinoma of the thyroid. A study of the clinical features and prognostic factors in 161 patients. Medicine (Baltimore) 1984;63:319–42.

77. Samaan NA, Schultz PN, Hickey RC. Medullary thyroid carcinoma: prognosis of familial versus sporadic disease and the role of radiotherapy. J Clin Endocrinol Metab 1988;67:801–5.

78. Schimke RN, Hartman WH. Familial amyloid producing medullary thyroid carcinoma and pheochromocytoma: a distinct genetic entity. Ann Intern Med 1965;63:1027–39.

79. _____, Hartman WH, Prout TE, Rimoin DL. Syndrome of bilateral pheochromocytoma, medullary thyroid carcinoma and multiple neuromas. A possible regulatory defect in the differentiation of chromaffin tissue. N Engl J Med 1968;279:1–17.

80. Schmid KW, Fischer-Colbrie R, Hagn C, Jasani B, Williams ED, Winkler H. Chromogranin A and B and secretogranin II in medullary carcinomas of the thyroid. Am J Surg Pathol 1987;11:551–6.

81. Schröder S, Böcker W, Baisch H, et al. Prognostic factors in medullary thyroid carcinoma. Survival in relation to age, sex, stage, histology, immunocytochemistry, and DNA content. Cancer 1988;61:806–16.

82. _____, Kloppel G. Carcinoembryonic antigen and nonspecific cross-reacting antigen in thyroid cancer. An immunocytochemical study using polyclonal and monoclonal antibodies. Am J Surg Pathol 1987;11:100–8.

83. _____, Schwarz W, Rehpenning W, Dralle H, Bay V, Böcker W. Leu-M1 immunoreactivity and prognosis in medullary carcinomas of the thyroid gland. J Cancer Res Clin Oncol 1988;114:291–6.

84. Schürch W, Babäi F, Boivin Y, Verdy M. Light-electron microscopic and cytochemical studies on the morphogenesis of familial medullary thyroid carcinoma. Virchows Arch [A] 1977;376:29–46.

85. Scopsi L, Ferrari C, Pilotti S, et al. Immunocytochemical localization and identification of prosomatostatin gene products in medullary carcinoma of human thyroid gland. Hum Pathol 1990;21:820–30.

86. Sikri KL, Varndell IM, Hamid QA, et al. Medullary carcinoma of the thyroid. An immunocytochemical and histochemical study of 25 cases using eight separate markers. Cancer 1985;56:2481–91.

87. Simpson NE, Kidd KK, Goodfellow PJ, et al. Assignment of multiple endocrine neoplasia type 2A to chromosome 10 by linkage. Nature 1987;328:528–9.

88. Sipple JH. The association of pheochromocytoma with carcinoma of the thyroid gland. Am J Med 1961;31:163–6.

89. Sizemore GW. Medullary carcinoma of the thyroid gland. Semin Oncol 1987;14:306–14.

90. Sobol G, Narod SA, Nakamura Y, et al. Screening for multiple endocrine neoplasia type 2a with DNA-polymorphism analysis. N Engl J Med 1989;321:996–1001.

91. _____, Narod SA, Schuffenecher I, et al. Hereditary medullary thyroid carcinoma: genetic analysis of three related syndromes. Henry Ford Hosp Med J 1989; 37:109–11.

92. Sobrinho-Simões M, Sambade C, Nesland JM, Holm R, Damjanov I. Lectin histochemistry and ultrastructure of medullary carcinoma of the thyroid gland. Arch Pathol Lab Med 1990;114:369–75.

93. Stanta G, Carcangiu ML, Rosai J. The biochemical and immunohistochemical profile of thyroid neoplasia. Pathol Annu 1988;23:129–57.

94. Steenbergh PH, Höppener JW, Zandberg J, van de Ven WJ, Jansz HS, Lips CJ. Calcitonin gene related peptide coding sequence is conserved in the human genome and is expressed in medullary thyroid carcinoma. J Clin Endocrinol Metab 1984;59:358–60.

95. Sunday ME, Wolfe HJ, Roos BA, Chin WW, Spindel ER. Gastrin-releasing peptide gene expression in developing hyperplastic and neoplastic human thyroid C-cells. Endocrinology 1988;122:1551–8.

96. Sundler F, Alumets J, Håkanson R, Björklund L, Ljungberg O. Somatostatin-immunoreactive cells in medullary carcinoma of the thyroid. Am J Pathol 1977; 88:381–6.

97. Tashjian AH Jr, Melvin KE. Medullary carcinoma of the thyroid gland. N Engl J Med 1968;279:279–83.

98. Thurston V, Williams ED. Experimental induction of C cell tumours in thyroid by increased dietary content of vitamin D3. Acta Endocrinol 1982;100:41–5.

99. Triggs SM, Williams ED. Experimental carcinogenesis in the rat thyroid follicular and C-cells. A comparison of the effect of variation in dietary calcium and of radiation. Acta Pathol 1977;85:84–92.

100. Trump DL, Mendelsohn G, Baylin SB. Discordance between plasma calcitonin and tumor-cell mass in medullary thyroid carcinoma. N Engl J Med 1979;301:253–5.

101. Uribe M, Fenoglio-Preiser CM, Grimes M, Feind C. Medullary carcinoma of the thyroid gland. Clinical, pathological, and immunohistochemical features with review of the literature. Am J Surg Pathol 1985;9:577–94.

102. Weiss LM, Weinberg DS, Warhol MJ. Medullary carcinoma arising in a thyroid with Hashimoto's disease. Am J Clin Pathol 1983;80:534–8.

103. Wells SA Jr, Baylin SB, Gann DS, et al. Medullary thyroid carcinoma: relationship of method of diagnosis to pathologic staging. Ann Surg 1978;188:377–83.

104. _____, Baylin SB, Leight GS, Dale JK, Dilley WG, Farndon JR. The importance of early diagnosis in patients with hereditary medullary thyroid carcinoma. Ann Surg 1982;195:595–9.

105. _____, Ontjes DA, Cooper CW, et al. The early diagnosis of medullary carcinoma of the thyroid gland in patients with multiple endocrine neoplasia type II. Ann Surg 1975;182:362–70.

106. Westermark P, Johnson KH. The polypeptide hormone-derived amyloid forms: nonspecific alterations or signs of abnormal peptide processing? Acta Pathol Microbiol Scand 1988;96:475–83.

107. White IL, Vimadalal SD, Catz B, van de Veld R, LaGanga T. Occult medullary carcinoma of thyroid: an unusual clinical and pathologic presentation. Cancer 1981;47:1364–8.

108. Williams ED. Histogenesis of medullary carcinoma of the thyroid. J Clin Pathol 1966;19:114–8.

109. _____, Brown CL, Doniach I. Pathological and clinical findings in a series of 67 cases of medullary carcinoma of the thyroid. J Clin Pathol 1966;19:103–13.

110. _____, Karim SM, Sandler M. Prostaglandin secretion by medullary carcinoma of the thyroid. A possible cause of the associated diarrhoea. Lancet 1968; 1:22–3.

111. _____, Morales AM, Horn RC. Thyroid carcinoma and Cushing's syndrome. A report of two cases with a review of the common features of the non-endocrine tumours associated with Cushing's syndrome. J Clin Pathol 1968;21:129–35.

112. Wolfe HJ, Melvin KE, Cervi-Skinner SJ, et al. C-cell hyperplasia preceding medullary thyroid carcinoma. N Engl J Med 1973;289:437–41.

113. Woolner LB, Beahrs OH, Black M, McConahey WM, Keating FR Jr. Classification and prognosis of thyroid carcinoma. A study of 885 cases observed in a 30 year period. Am J Surg 1961;102:354–87.

114. Yamada Y, Ito S, Matsubara Y, Kobayashi S. Immunohistochemical demonstration of somatostatin-containing cells in the human, dog, and rat thyroids. Tohoku J Exp Med 1977;122:87–92.

115. Yamaguchi K, Abe K, Adachi I, et al. Concomitant production of immunoreactive gastrin-releasing peptide and calcitonin in medullary carcinoma of the thyroid. Metabolism 1984;33:724–7.

116. Zaatari GS, Saigo PE, Huvos AG. Mucin production in medullary carcinoma of the thyroid. Arch Pathol Lab Med 1983;107:70–4.

Medullary Carcinoma Variants

117. Albores-Saavedra J, LiVolsi VA, Williams ED. Medullary carcinoma. Semin Diagn Pathol 1985;2:137–46.

118. Beerman H, Rigaud C, Bogomeletz WV, Hollander H, Veldhuizen H. Melanin production in black medullary thyroid carcinoma (MTC). Histopathology 1990;16:227–34.

119. Beskid M. Lorenc R, Rôsciszewska A. C-cell thyroid adenoma in man. J Pathol 1971;103:343–6.

120. Bronner M, LiVolsi VA, Jennings T. Paraganglioma-like adenomas of the thyroid. Surg Pathol 1988;1:383–9.

121. Bussolati G, Monga G. Medullary carcinoma of the thyroid with atypical patterns. Cancer 1979;44:1769–77.

122. Carcangiu ML, Steeper T, Zampi G, Rosai J. Anaplastic thyroid carcinoma. A study of 70 cases. Am J Clin Pathol 1985;83:135–58.

123. Carney JA, Ryan J, Goellner JR. Hyalinizing trabecular adenoma of the thyroid gland. Am J Surg Pathol 1987;10:583–91.

124. Dominguez-Malagon H, Delgado-Chavez R, Torres-Najera M, Gould E, Albores-Saavedra J. Oxyphil and squamous variants of medullary thyroid carcinoma. Cancer 1989;63:1183–8.

125. Eusebi V, Damiani S, Riva C, Lloyd RV, Capella C. Calcitonin free oat cell carcinoma of the thyroid gland. Virchows Arch [A] 1990;417:267–71.

126. Golough R, Us-Krasovec M, Auersperg M, Jancar J, Bondi A, Eusebi V. Amphicrine-composite calcitonin and mucin producing carcinoma of the thyroid. Ultrastruct Pathol 1985;8:197–206.

127. Harach HR, Bergholm U. Medullary (C-cell) carcinoma of the thyroid with features of follicular oxyphilic cell tumors. Histopathology 1988;13:645–56.

128. _____, Williams ED. Glandular (tubular and follicular) variants of medullary carcinoma of the thyroid. Histopathology 1983;7:83–97.

129. Huss LJ, Mendelsohn G. Medullary carcinoma of the thyroid gland: an encapsulated variant resembling the hyalinizing trabecular (paraganglioma-like) adenoma of thyroid. Mod Pathol 1990;3:581–5.

130. Kakudo K, Miyauchi A, Yakai SI, et al. C-cell carcinoma of the thyroid, papillary type. Acta Pathol Jpn 1979; 29:633–59.

131. Kodama T, Okamoto T, Fujimoto Y, et al. C-cell adenoma of the thyroid: a rare but distinct clinical entity. Surgery 1988;104:997–1003.

132. Landon G, Ordòñez NG. Clear cell variant of medullary carcinoma of the thyroid. Hum Pathol 1985;16:844–7.

133. Lertprasertsuke N, Kakudo K, Nakamura A, et al. C cell carcinoma of the thyroid. Follicular variant. Acta Pathol Jpn 1989;39:393–9.

134. Marcus JN, Dise CA, LiVolsi VA. Melanin production in a medullary thyroid carcinoma. Cancer 1982;49: 2518–26.

135. Martinelli G, Bazzocchi F, Govoni E, Santini D. Anaplastic type of medullary thyroid carcinoma. An ultrastructural and immunohistochemical study. Virchows Arch [A] 1983;400:61–7.

136. Mendelsohn G, Baylin SB, Bigner SH, Wells SA, Eggleston JC. Anaplastic variants of medullary thyroid carcinoma. A light microscopic and immunohistochemical study. Am J Surg Pathol 1980;4:333–41.

137. _____, Oertel JE. Encapsulated medullary thyroid carcinoma [Abstract]. Lab Invest 1981;44:43A.

138. Nieuwenhuizjen-Kruseman AC, Bosman FT, van Bergen Henegouw JC, Cramier-Knijnenburg G, Brutel de la Riviere G. Medullary differentiation of anaplastic thyroid carcinoma. Am J Clin Pathol 1982;77:541–7.

139. Valenta LJ, Michel-Bechet M, Mattson JC, Singer FR. Microfollicular thyroid carcinoma with amyloid rich stroma, resembling the medullary carcinoma of the thyroid (MCT). Cancer 1977;39:1573–86.

140. Zeman V, Nĕmec J, Platil A, et al. Anaplastic transformation of medullary thyroid cancer. Neoplasma 1978; 25:249–55.

Mixed Medullary-Follicular Carcinoma

141. Hales M, Rosenau W, Okerlund MD, Galante M. Carcinoma of the thyroid with a mixed medullary and follicular pattern: morphological, immunohistochemical, and clinical laboratory studies. Cancer 1982;50:1352–9.

142. Harach HR, Williams ED. Glandular (tubular and follicular) variants of medullary carcinoma of the thyroid. Histopathology 1983;7:83–97.

143. Hedinger C, Williams ED, Sobin LH. The WHO classification of thyroid tumors: a commentary on the second edition. Cancer 1989;63:908–11.

144. Hellman DE, Kartchner M, Van Antwerp JD, Salmon SE, Patton DD, O'Mara R. Radioiodine in the treatment of medullary carcinoma of the thyroid. J Clin Endocrinol Metab 1979;48:451–8.

145. Holm R, Sobrinho-Simões M, Nesland JM, Johannessen JV. Concurrent production of calcitonin and thyroglobulin by the same neoplastic cells. Ultrastruct Pathol 1986;10:241–51.

146. LiVolsi VA. Mixed thyroid carcinoma: a real entity? Lab Invest 1987;57:237–9.

147. Ljungberg O, Bondeson L, Bondeson AG. Differentiated thyroid carcinoma, intermediate type: a new tumor entity with features of follicular and parafollicular carcinoma. Hum Pathol 1984;15:218–28.

148. , Ericsson UB, Bondesson L, Thorell J. A compound follicular-parafollicular cell carcinoma of the thyroid: a new tumor entity? Cancer 1983;52:1053–61.

149. Pfaltz M, Hedinger CE, Mühlethaler JP. Mixed medullary and follicular carcinoma of the thyroid. Virchows Arch [A] 1983;400:53–9.

150. Sobrinho-Simões M, Nesland J, Johannessen JV. Farewell to the dual histogenesis of thyroid tumors. Ultrastruct Pathol 1985;8:iii–v.

Mixed Medullary-Papillary Carcinoma

151. Albores-Saavedra J, Gorraez de la Mora T, de la Torre-Rendon F, Gould E. Mixed medullary-papillary carcinoma of the thyroid: a previously unrecognized variant of thyroid carcinoma. Hum Pathol 1990;21:1151–5.

❖❖❖

C CELL HYPERPLASIA

Definition. C cell hyperplasia is a multifocal proliferative condition characterized by an increased mass of C cells within the follicles of the thyroid gland.

General Features. C cell hyperplasia is an uncommon entity that can be seen in association with a variety of conditions (Table 3). It had been noted initially in patients with a history of familial medullary thyroid carcinoma and abnormal calcitonin secretory reserves, as determined by calcium gluconate- and pentagastrin-provocative testing (15,23). C cell hyperplasia has been recognized as a preneoplastic condition that precedes the development of the multifocal medullary carcinomas that characterize the IIA and IIB MEN syndromes (3,10,17,21,23). The presence of C cell hyperplasia has been used as a histologic marker to distinguish sporadic and familial forms of this tumor (see page 216). C cell hyperplasia has also been reported in residual thyroid tissue after resection of an apparently sporadic medullary carcinoma.

In many rat strains, C cell hyperplasia occurs in an age-dependent manner and is frequently associated with multifocal medullary thyroid carcinomas, particularly after the age of 2 years (5). Many of the affected animals also have evidence of pheochromocytoma, pituitary adenomas, and pancreatic endocrine neoplasms.

Experimental studies have suggested that the chronic administration of calcitonin secretagogues may lead to the development of C cell hyperplasia (6). The administration of vitamin D_3 has been reported to accelerate the development of C cell hyperplasia in the rat (see page 207). C cell hyperplasia has been reported in human thyroid glands from occasional patients with hyperparathyroidism, other hypercalcemic states, and hypergastrinemia (14,22).

C cell hyperplasia has also been recognized in some patients with Hashimoto thyroiditis (4). In the case of Hashimoto thyroiditis described by Libbey and coworkers (12), both basal hypercalcitoninemia and an abnormal response to provocative testing were observed. Albores-Saavedra (1) suggested that C cell hyperplasia in patients with goitrous hypothyroidism and Hashimoto disease could result from chronic thyroid-stimulating hormone stimulation (1). In this regard, several experimental studies have suggested that both follicular and C cells might be under thyroid-stimulating hormone control.

Albores-Saavedra and coworkers (2) also observed C cell hyperplasia adjacent to approximately one third of follicular and papillary thyroid neoplasms (fig. 228). In most of the cases, C cells were diffusely hyperplastic, whereas only two cases showed evidence of nodular hyperplasia. In one patient with C cell hyperplasia adjacent to a papillary neoplasm, both basal and stimulated calcitonin levels were increased. In cases in which both thyroid lobes were examined, C cell hyperplasia was present only in the lobe containing the papillary or follicular neoplasm. Similar findings were reported by Scopsi and coworkers (18). These authors also documented the presence of C cell hyperplasia adjacent to metastases in the thyroid.

The mechanism for the development of C cell hyperplasia adjacent to follicular and papillary neoplasms is unknown. It has been suggested that the C cell hyperplasia might represent a compensatory event due to replacement of some of the C cells by follicular tumor formation (2). This view is strengthened by the observation that C cell hyperplasia has been unilateral in cases where both lobes have been available for study. It is also possible that C cell hyperplasia could result from chronic thyroid-stimulating hormone stimulation resulting from destruction of the thyroid parenchyma by tumor (2).

Table 3

SPECTRUM OF C CELL HYPERPLASIA

Type IIA (II) multiple endocrine neoplasia
Type IIB (III) multiple endocrine neoplasia
Hypercalcemia (e.g., hyperparathyroidism)
Hypergastrinemia (e.g., Zollinger-Ellison syndrome)
Hashimoto disease
Goitrous hypothyroidism and Hashimoto disease
Peritumoral (adjacent to follicular and
papillary neoplasms)

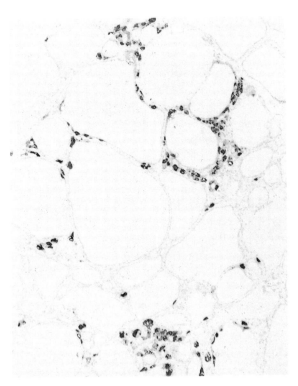

Figure 228
C CELL HYPERPLASIA

These C cells were found adjacent to follicular carcinoma. Immunoperoxidase stain for calcitonin. (Courtesy of Dr. J. Albores-Saavedra, Dallas, TX.)

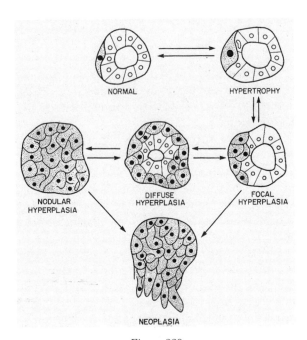

Figure 229
HISTOGENESIS OF C CELL HYPERPLASIA AND
MEDULLARY THYROID CARCINOMA

In this illustration, follicular cells have clear cytoplasm with open nuclei, whereas C cells have stippled cytoplasm with closed nuclei. C cell hyperplasia is characterized by a progressive obliteration of the follicles by C cells. Carcinoma is diagnosed when C cells penetrate the follicular basal lamina and extend into the interstitium. (Fig. 9 from DeLellis RA, Nunnemacher G, Wolfe HJ. C-cell hyperplasia: an ultrastructural analysis. Lab Invest 1977;36:237–48.)

Gross Features. The thyroid glands from patients with C cell hyperplasia associated with the MEN II syndromes most commonly show no gross abnormalities (8,9). In those patients suspected of having C cell hyperplasia, each lobe of the thyroid should be blocked in its entirety. If C cell hyperplasia is present, it will probably be found in sections corresponding to the middle thirds of the lobes.

Microscopic Features. In patients with a family history of type II MEN and abnormal calcitonin responses to calcium and pentagastrin testing, the earliest phase of C cell proliferative disease is mild diffuse C cell hyperplasia (8,9,17). This entity is characterized by increased numbers of C cells in both thyroid lobes compared with age- and sex-matched controls (fig. 229). In view of the recent studies that have shown considerable variation in C cell densities in normal glands, a diagnosis of diffuse (non-nodular) C cell hyperplasia should be made with caution (13). The process should involve both lobes, with at least 50 C cells per single low-power field. Occasional C cells in cases of diffuse hyperplasia may be enlarged and hyperchromatic. As in normal thyroid glands, C cells occupy an exclusively intrafollicular position and are separated from the interstitium by the follicular basal lamina and from the colloid by extensions of the follicular cell cytoplasm (pl. XXXII-A; figs. 230, 231) (8). In some instances, C cells may appear to be within the interstitium, but electron microscopy invariably reveals continuity of the C cells within the follicular basal lamina. The C cells in diffuse hyperplasia most commonly exhibit intense immunoreactivity for calcitonin and are well granulated ultrastructurally (8).

The proliferation of C cells within the follicle may completely surround the more centrally located follicular cells to produce a circumferential collar of C cells (figs. 229, 232–234) (3,8,17).

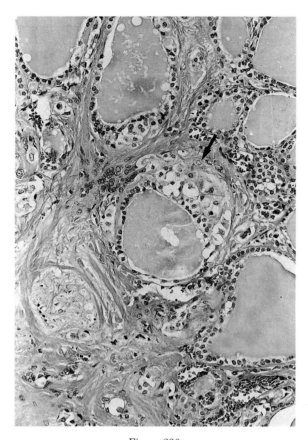

Figure 230

C CELL HYPERPLASIA ASSOCIATED WITH MEN IIA

The follicle in the center of the field shows a focal proliferation of C cells (arrow).

Nodular hyperplasia of C cells is characterized by complete obliteration of the follicular space by C cells (fig. 229; pl. XXXII-B). Because C cell nodules may be found in occasional normal glands, a definite diagnosis of nodular C cell hyperplasia should be made only when this change is extensive, bilateral, and multifocal (11,16). Immunohistochemical stains for thyroglobulin often reveal occasional thyroglobulin-positive follicular cells and deposits of colloid within the C cell–filled nodules. Similar to the C cells in diffuse C cell hyperplasia, foci of nodular C cell hyperplasia show intense reactivity for calcitonin and may show focal positivity for somatostatin and bombesin. The C cells in these foci are typically filled with type I secretory granules, and the basal lamina surrounding the C cell–filled follicles may be focally reduplicated.

Early microscopic medullary thyroid carcinoma is diagnosed when C cells extend through defects in the follicular basal lamina and infiltrate the thyroid interstitium (figs. 235, 236). Invasion in this setting is characterized by the presence of fibrosis around the infiltrating tumor cell nests. The basal lamina surrounding C-cell filled follicles may show a variety of changes, including gaps, splitting and foci of reduplication (figs. 237, 238). At the ultrastructural level, occasional tumor cells in early invasive carcinomas are devoid of basal lamina. However, most invasive tumor cells are surrounded by basal lamina that may be focally defective (8).

Differential Diagnosis. Although early studies suggested that normal adult thyroids contained fewer than 10 C cells per single low-power microscopic field, more recent studies indicate that occasional normal glands may contain up to 50 C cells per single low-power field (2,11,16). Moreover, occasional nodules composed of C cells have been identified in some normal thyroids from older individuals. The observed variations in C cell density in normal glands have important implications with respect to the diagnosis of mild C cell hyperplasia in patients from MEN II kindreds (13).

In a study of a large MEN IIA kindred, Lips and coworkers (13) identified five subjects who had thyroidectomies because of slightly increased calcitonin levels after provocative testing. Although the resected glands showed evidence of mild C cell hyperplasia, Lips and coworkers concluded that these individuals did not have MEN IIA because none of them subsequently developed pheochromocytoma or hyperparathyroidism. Moreover, all of the children of these individuals have had repeatedly normal calcitonin levels on provocative testing. These findings suggest that it may be difficult to distinguish mild forms of C cell hyperplasia in MEN IIA kindreds from occasional normal glands that may show considerable variation in C cell density. In such equivocal cases, restriction-fragment length–polymorphism analysis may be required to confirm that the patient is a carrier of the abnormal gene (20).

Foci of nodular C cell hyperplasia occasionally may be difficult to distinguish from a variety of other changes, including squamous metaplasia, solid cell nests, intrathyroidal thymic or parathyroid nests, palpation thyroiditis (multifocal granulomatous folliculitis), and tangential cuts

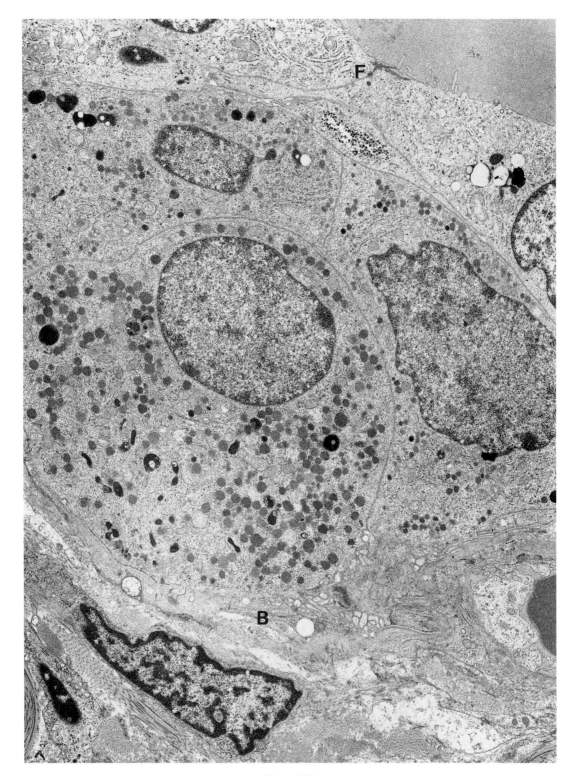

Figure 231
C CELL HYPERPLASIA ASSOCIATED WITH MEN IIA
The area shown is similar to that illustrated in figure 230. This electron micrograph shows a focal proliferation of C cells between follicular cells (F) and the follicular basal lamina (B). X8500.

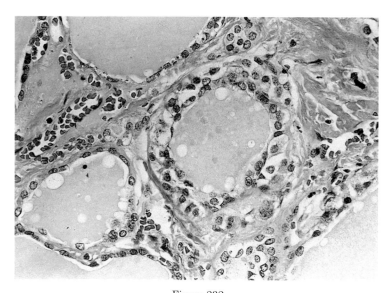

Figure 232
C CELL HYPERPLASIA ASSOCIATED WITH MEN IIA
C cells form a circumferential proliferation around follicular cells.

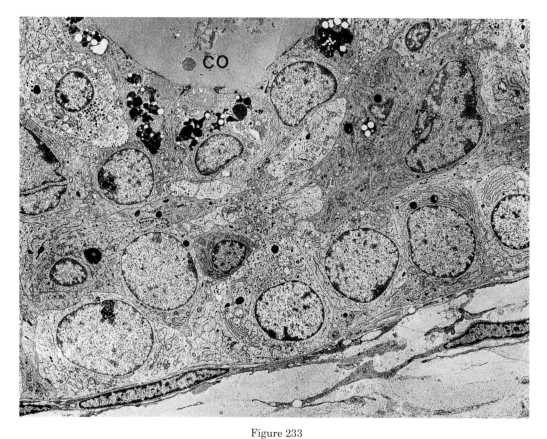

Figure 233
NODULAR C CELL HYPERPLASIA ASSOCIATED WITH MEN IIA

Ultrastructurally, a small amount of colloid (CO) is present within the center of the follicle. The C cells are separated from the interstitium by the follicular basal lamina. X3354.(Fig. 3 from DeLellis RA, Nunnemacher G, Wolfe HJ. C-cell hyperplasia: an ultrastructural analysis. Lab Invest 1977;36:237–48.)

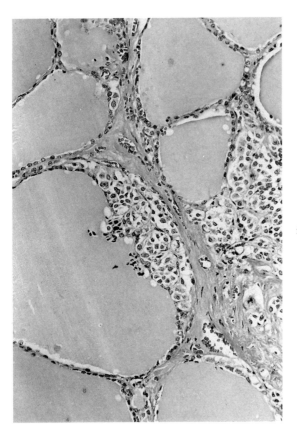

Figure 234
C CELL HYPERPLASIA ASSOCIATED WITH MEN IIA
C cells form an eccentric intrafollicular proliferation in this field.

Figure 235
C CELL HYPERPLASIA WITH EARLY MEDULLARY
CARCINOMA ASSOCIATED WITH MEN IIA
A group of C cells has extended into the interstitium.

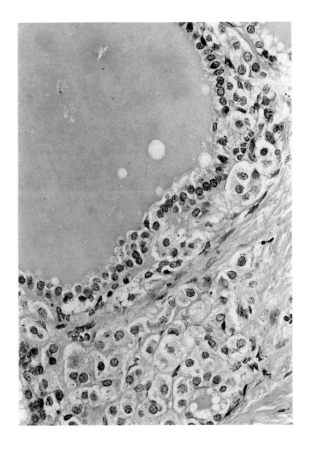

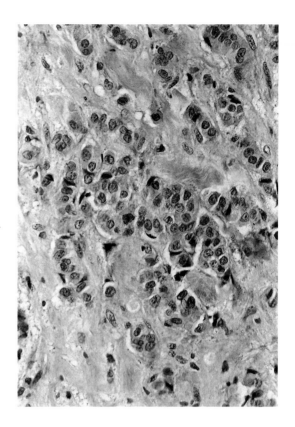

Figure 236
EARLY MEDULLARY THYROID CARCINOMA
ASSOCIATED WITH MEN IIA
Groups of neoplastic C cells infiltrate the interstitium as columns of cells.

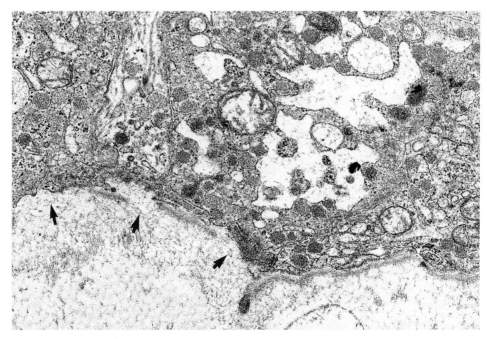

Figure 237
C CELL HYPERPLASIA IN MEN IIA
This C-cell filled follicle was seen in a patient with early medullary thyroid carcinoma associated with MEN IIA. The basal lamina shows multiple gaps (arrows). X18,000. (Fig. 19 from DeLellis RA, Wolfe HJ. The pathobiology of the human calcitonin (C)-cell: a review. Pathol Annual 1981;16 (Pt. 2):25–52.)

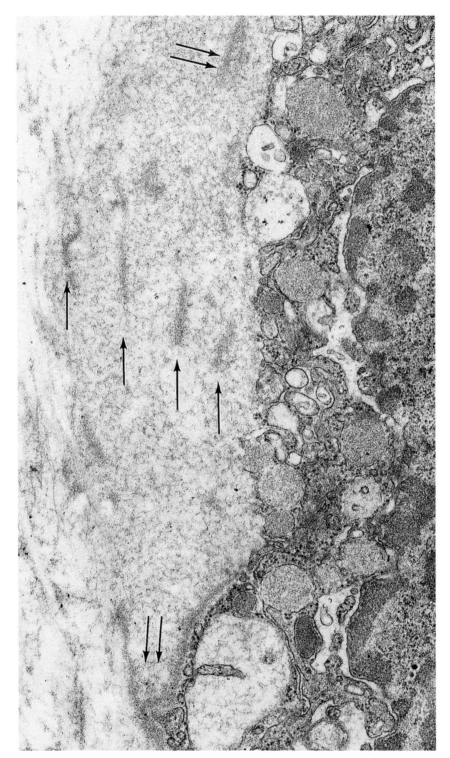

Figure 238
C-CELL HYPERPLASIA IN MEN IIA
This C-cell filled follicle shows splitting (double arows) and areas of reduplication (single arrows) of the basal lamina. (Fig. 10 from DeLellis RA, Nunnemacher G, Wolfe HJ. C-cell hyperplasia: an ultrastructural analysis. Lab Invest 1977;36:237–48.)

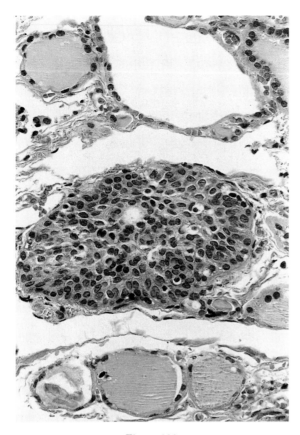

Figure 239
SQUAMOUS METAPLASIA
This thyroid contains a focus of squamous metaplasia.

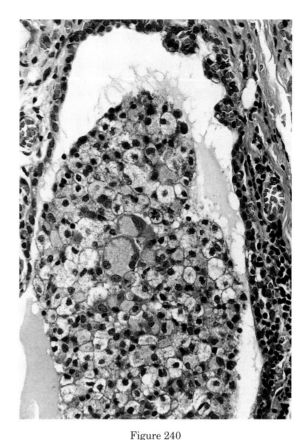

Figure 240
PALPATION THYROIDITIS
This illustration shows a thyroid with a focus of palpation thyroiditis.

of normal follicles. Squamous metaplasia in the thyroid has been noted in a variety of inflammatory and neoplastic states (see page 195) (24). Foci of squamous metaplasia of the inflammatory type are particularly evident in nodular goiter and chronic thyroiditis of the Hashimoto type (fig. 239). The studies of Vollenweider and Hedinger (30) have suggested that the epidermoid nests found in Hashimoto thyroiditis more closely resemble solid cell nests than foci of follicular cell metaplasia, as seen in nodular goiters. The origin of the epidermoid nests in chronic thyroiditis, however, is unknown. It is likely that they do not bear any ontogenic relationship to the true solid cell nests as described by Yamaoka (24). Solid cell nests are discussed on page 12.

Occasional remnants of thymus may be found within the thyroid gland (see page 282) (pl. XXXII-C). The epithelial cells of such thymic nests resemble the cells of the solid cell nests; however, remnants of thymic epithelium are typically associated with abundant lymphoid elements. Parathyroid nests are composed principally of chief cells with associated stromal fat.

Palpation thyroiditis refers to a trauma-induced change characterized by the accumulation of intrafollicular histiocytes, lymphocytes, plasma cells, and giant cells (7). Affected follicles typically show a focal loss of the epithelial lining (figs. 240, 241). In some instances, the histiocytes encircle the inner aspect of the follicle in a pattern similar to that of early phases of C cell hyperplasia. In contrast to C cells, the histiocytes generally have eosinophilic vacuolated cytoplasm that may be positive for iron. Foci of palpation thyroiditis are typically negative for calcitonin but show positive staining for lysozyme (fig. 241).

Tangential cuts of follicles may occasionally be extremely difficult to distinguish from foci of

PLATE XXXII

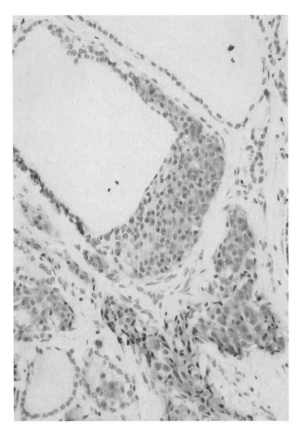 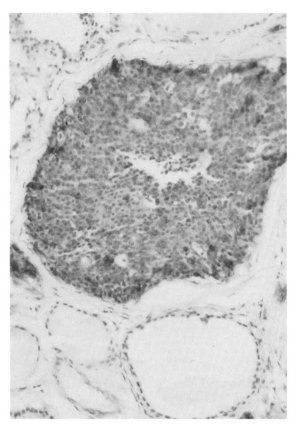

A. C CELL HYPERPLASIA IN A
PATIENT WITH MEN IIA

C cells are present between the follicular epithelium and the follicular basement membrane. Immunoperoxidase stain for calcitonin.

B. NODULAR C CELL HYPERPLASIA
IN A PATIENT WITH MEN IIA

The follicle is replaced by C cells. Immunoperoxidase stain for calcitonin.

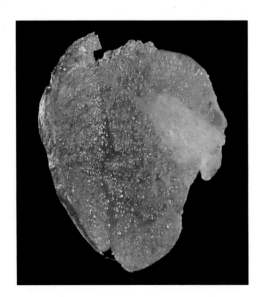

C. INTRATHYROIDAL THYMUS GLAND

This illustration shows an intrathyroidal thymus gland.

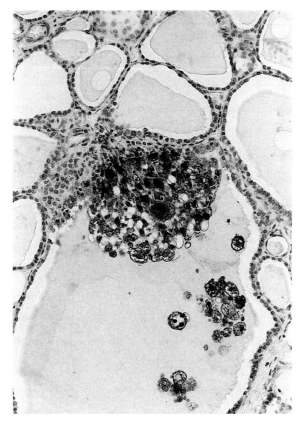

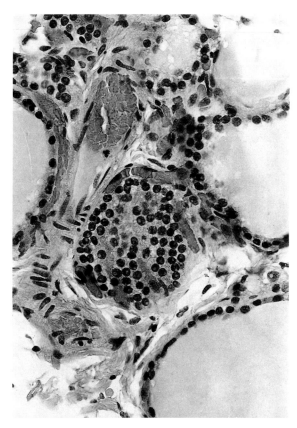

Figure 241
PALPATION THYROIDITIS
This illustration shows a thyroid with focus of palpation thyroiditis. The histiocytes within the follicle are strongly positive for lysozyme. Immunoperoxidase reaction for lysozyme.

Figure 242
NORMAL THYROID FOLLICLE
This illustration shows a tangential cut of a normal thyroid follicle.

nodular C cell hyperplasia (fig. 242); however, tangential cuts of follicles generally show polyhedral cells with well-defined cell borders and centrally placed nuclei. The cytologic characteristics of the nuclei are identical to those of the surrounding follicular cells. Serial sections will reveal a colloid-filled lumen.

Treatment and Prognosis. The optimal treatment for patients with C cell hyperplasia is total thyroidectomy. In Gagel's series of patients

with MEN IIA, 23 individuals had thyroidectomies on the basis of calcitonin abnormalities discovered by provocative testing. In this group, 13 had C cell hyperplasia alone, 9 had C cell hyperplasia together with early medullary carcinomas, and 1 had no apparent C cell abnormalities. All of the patients also had dissection of central lymph nodes at the time of thyroidectomy. None of the patients had evidence of nodal metastases, and all are considered to be disease free with an average follow-up of more than 10 years.

REFERENCES

1. Albores-Saavedra J. C-cell hyperplasia [Letter]. Am J Surg Pathol 1989;13:987–9.

2. _____, Monforte H, Nadji M, Morales AR. C-cell hyperplasia in thyroid tissue adjacent to follicular cell tumors. Hum Pathol 1988;19:795–9.

3. Al Saadi AA. Ultrastructure of C-cell hyperplasia in asymptomatic patients with hypercalcitoninemia and a family history of medullary thyroid carcinoma. Hum Pathol 1981;12:617–22.

4. Biddinger PW, Brennan MF, Rosen PP. Symptomatic C-cell hyperplasia associated with chronic lymphocytic thyroiditis. Am J Surg Pathol 1991;15:599–604.

5. Boorman GA, Hollander CF. Animal model of human disease: medullary carcinoma of the thyroid in the rat. Am J Pathol 1976;83:237–40.

6. Capen CC, Young DM. Fine structural alterations in thyroid parafollicular cells of cows in response to experimental hypercalcemia induced by vitamin D. Am J Pathol 1969;57:365–82.

7. Carney JA, Moore SB, Northcutt RC, Woolner LB, Stillwell GK. Palpation thyroiditis (multifocal granulomatous folliculitis). Am J Clin Pathol 1975;64:639–47.

8. DeLellis RA, Nunnemacher G, Wolfe HJ. C-cell hyperplasia: an ultrastructural analysis. Lab Invest 1977;36:237–48.

9. _____, Wolfe HJ. The pathobiology of the human calcitonin (C) cell: a review. Pathol Annu 1981;16:25–52.

10. Gagel RF, Tashjian AH Jr, Cummings T, et al. The clinical outcome of prospective screening for multiple endocrine neoplasia type 2a. An 18 year experience. N Engl J Med 1988;318:478–84.

11. Gibson WC, Peng T-C, Croker BP. C-cell nodules in adult human thyroid. A common autopsy finding. Am J Clin Pathol 1981;75:347–50.

12. Libbey NP, Nowakowski KJ, Tucci JR. C-cell hyperplasia of the thyroid in a patient with goitrous hypothyroidism and Hashimoto's thyroiditis. Am J Surg Pathol 1989;13:71–7.

13. Lips CJ, Leo JR, Berends MJ, et al. Thyroid C-cell hyperplasia and micronodules in close relatives of MEN-2A patients: pitfalls in early diagnosis and re-evaluation of criteria for surgery. Henry Ford Hosp Med J 1987;35:133–8.

14. LiVolsi VA, Feind CR, Lo Gerfo P, Tashjian AH Jr. Demonstration by immunoperoxidase staining of hyperplasia of parafollicular cells in the thyroid gland in hyperparathyroidism. J Clin Endocrinol Metab 1973;37:550–9.

15. Melvin KE, Miller HH, Tashjian AH Jr. Early diagnosis of medullary carcinoma of the thyroid gland by means of calcitonin assay. N Engl J Med 1971;285:1115–20.

16. O'Toole K, Fenoglio-Preiser C, Pushparaj N. Endocrine changes associated with the human aging process: III. Effect of age on the number of calcitonin immunoreactive cells in the thyroid gland. Hum Pathol 1985;16:991–1000.

17. Schürch W, Babäi F, Boivin Y, Verdy M. Light, electron microscopic and cytochemical studies on the morphogenesis of familial medullary thyroid carcinoma. Virchows Arch [A] 1977;376:29–46.

18. Scopsi L, DiPalma S, Ferrari C, Holst JJ, Rehfeld JF, Rilke F. C-cell hyperplasia accompanying thyroid diseases other than medullary thyroid carcinoma: an immunocytochemical study by means of antibodies to calcitonin and somatostatin. Mod Pathol 1991;4:297–304.

19. Sobol G, Narod SA, Nakamura T, et al. Screening for multiple endocrine neoplasia type 2a with DNA-polymorphism analysis. N Engl J Med 1989;321:996–1001.

20. Vollenweider I, Hedinger C. Solid cell nests (SCN) in Hashimoto's thyroiditis. Virchows Arch [A] 1988;412:357–63.

21. Wells SA, Ontjes DA, Cooper CW, et al. The early diagnosis of medullary carcinoma of the thyroid in patients with multiple endocrine neoplasia type II. Ann Surg 1975;182:362–70.

22. Wolfe HJ, DeLellis RA, Scott RT, Tashjian AH Jr. C-cell hyperplasia in chronic hypercalcemia in man [Abstract]. Am J Pathol 1975;78:20A.

23. _____, Melvin KE, Cervi-Skinner SJ, et al. C-cell hyperplasia preceding medullary thyroid carcinoma. N Engl J Med 1973;289:437–41.

24. Yamaoka Y. Solid cell nest (SCN) of the human thyroid gland. Acta Pathol Jpn 1973;23:493–506.

❖❖❖

SARCOMAS

Definition. A malignant tumor with mesenchymal features and of presumed mesenchymal derivation arising within the thyroid gland.

General Considerations. A priori, sarcoma of the thyroid might be thought of as a straightforward subject, both conceptually and in practice, by applying the following reasoning: 1) The thyroid, like any other organ, has a mesenchymal (stromal) component; 2) This component, like that of any other site, can undergo malignant transformation; 3) The result should be a sarcoma not differing from those arisen from analogous mesenchymal cell types in the somatic soft tissues or in other organs and therefore diagnosable according to similar criteria.

Unfortunately, this seemingly logical scheme cannot be applied as stated, because undifferentiated (anaplastic) carcinomas of this organ can resemble various sarcomas to such a degree that they render the differential diagnosis difficult or sometimes impossible. Of course, the thyroid is not the only organ in the body in which this situation arises; however, it seems to be here, more than in any other site, that the vexing antinomy between differentiation and assumed histogenesis is more sorely tested (3). This general subject is discussed at length in the section on Undifferentiated (Anaplastic) Carcinoma. It is important to remember that most malignant thyroid tumors with a sarcoma-like appearance are undifferentiated carcinomas, in the sense that they exhibit telltale signs of epithelial differentiation by either morphologic or immunohistochemical criteria. Therefore, sarcoma-like tumors of the thyroid should be regarded as undifferentiated thyroid carcinomas "in the absence of indisputable proof to the contrary," as described by the WHO Committee for the Histologic Typing of Thyroid Tumors (4). The same committee commented that the diagnosis of thyroid sarcoma should only be made in tumors lacking *all* evidence of epithelial differentiation and showing *definite* evidence of specific sarcomatous differentiation. This definition may be criticized for being too restrictive. There is no reason, for instance, why a fibrosarcoma (a tumor that does not show a specific pattern of sarcomatous differentiation) could not occur in the thyroid. However, in view of the above considerations, the WHO proposal seems logical. Perhaps another factor that needs to be added into the equation is the patient's age at the time of the diagnosis. Because undifferentiated thyroid carcinomas are exceptionally rare before the age of 50 years, the possibility of any given sarcoma-like thyroid tumor actually being a true sarcoma increases proportionally as the patient's age decreases. Another diagnostic possibility to be considered under these circumstances is that of a sarcoma of the soft tissues of the neck that has invaded the thyroid secondarily, even if this phenomenon is just as unusual as true primary thyroid sarcoma itself.

Many isolated case reports of thyroid sarcoma are on record, and the range of specific diagnoses used for them is wide. It includes *fibrosarcoma* (2,8), *liposarcoma* (1), *leiomyosarcoma* (5), *osteosarcoma* (6), *chondrosarcoma* (9), and *malignant (diffuse) hemangiopericytoma* (7). However, few of them would qualify if the WHO criteria were to be applied to them. Fortunately, the issue is of no great practical significance, inasmuch as their natural history and response to therapy do not differ significantly from those of undifferentiated carcinoma. The outstanding exception is *angiosarcoma*, a highly controversial entity that deserves to be discussed separately because of its distinct morphologic, immunohistochemical, ultrastructural, and geographic peculiarities.

ANGIOSARCOMA

Definition. A malignant tumor exhibiting endothelial cell differentiation. Theoretically, any malignant tumor of the blood vessels could be designated as angiosarcoma; however, in practice, the term is reserved for those tumors exhibiting endothelial (rather than perithelial, glomic, or smooth muscle) differentiation. Angiosarcoma is therefore synonymous with malignant hemangioendothelioma, a more specific and accurate but less popular alternative.

General Features. One of the most striking features of thyroid angiosarcoma is that nearly all reported cases are from mountainous areas, especially the Alpine regions of central Europe, where it is said to comprise as much as 16 percent of all thyroid malignancies (12). The identification of this tumor type and the heated defense about its authenticity that followed came almost exclusively from Swiss authors (17,18). Most American pathologists have been skeptical about the existence of this entity, assuming that most if not all of the reported cases were undifferentiated carcinomas with an angiosarcomatoid appearance (19). Some European pathologists have adopted a similar point of view (20). However, evidence has accumulated in recent years that a thyroid malignancy exhibiting phenotypical features of endothelial cell differentiation exists. Its predilection for mountainous regions had been linked to the iodine deficiency that existed in those areas and the goiter that followed. Indeed, thyroid angiosarcoma develops in most instances in a long-standing nodular goiter. It has been hypothesized that the marked vascularization that takes place in hyperplastic glands (and that caused enormous technical difficulties for surgeons in the past) is the milieu on which angiosarcoma arises. It should be pointed out, however, that thyroid angiosarcoma is not limited to these regions and/or goitrous glands (14,27).

Clinical Features. Most patients are elderly individuals with a history of long-standing goiter who have noticed sudden enlargement, sometimes painful, of the gland. In Egloff's series (13), the average age was 62 years. In some instances, signs due to metastatic spread, such as chest pain and hemothorax resulting from pleuropulmonary metastases, are already present at presentation.

Gross Features. The tumor is typically large, with extensive areas of necrosis and hemorrhage (pl. XXXIII-A). The latter may result in blood-filled cystic cavities resembling hematomas. Although almost always invasive, it may exhibit a nodular well-circumscribed appearance on the cut surface (11).

Microscopic Features. As in angiosarcomas elsewhere, the distinguishing feature of this tumor when it involves the thyroid is the presence of freely anastomosing channels lined by atypical endothelial cells. This may be associated with a papillary configuration resulting from a predominantly intraluminal pattern of growth (12,13). However, this may represent only a focal finding in what is otherwise a poorly differentiated neoplasm with a pre-

dominantly solid pattern of growth (fig. 243). The shape of the tumor cells varies from spindle to epithelioid; multinucleated and other bizarre cellular forms are relatively unusual. In general, the tumor cells lining the vascular spaces are plumper than those located between them. Some of the epithelioid cells may exhibit intracytoplasmic vacuoles, sometimes containing intact or fragmented red blood cells. These formations are thought to represent early formations of vascular lumina. The nuclei of the epithelioid endothelial cells are often large, vesicular, of regular outlines, and endowed with a large basophilic or amphophilic nucleolus connected by chromatin strands to the nuclear membrane (fig. 244). The eosinophilic cytoplasm is abundant in the epithelioid endothelial cells but less so in the spindle forms. Mitoses, typical and atypical, are invariably found, often in large numbers.

The pattern of growth is nearly always highly invasive. Thyroid follicles are first displaced and then destroyed by the tumor growth. On occasion, the sarcoma is seen growing within the wall of sizable intrathyroidal arteries, between the two elastic laminae. A constant feature is the presence of extensive fresh and old hemorrhage, the latter represented by conglomerates of hemosiderin-laden macrophages. Fresh tumor necrosis is usually widespread.

Immunohistochemical Features. The most constant immunohistochemical result in this tumor is strong reactivity for vimentin (pl. XXXIII-B). Unfortunately, this reactivity is shared by other types of sarcomas and undifferentiated carcinomas. The most specific reaction currently available for endothelial cells and their tumors is factor VIII–related antigen (16,22), which has been found to be expressed by the cells of thyroid angiosarcoma (pl. XXXIII-C) (23,25,26,30). Unfortunately, this is a labile antigen that is often lost in routinely processed material. Another important marker is *U. europaeus* I, although the receptor for this lectin is also expressed by epithelial cells in individuals with blood group O (pl. XXXIII-D).

In the better differentiated areas of the tumor, the formation of vascular channels includes the deposition of basement membrane, a feature that can be evidenced by the demonstration of type IV collagen or laminin (pl. XXXIV-A) (14). Finally, epithelioid angiosarcomas have been

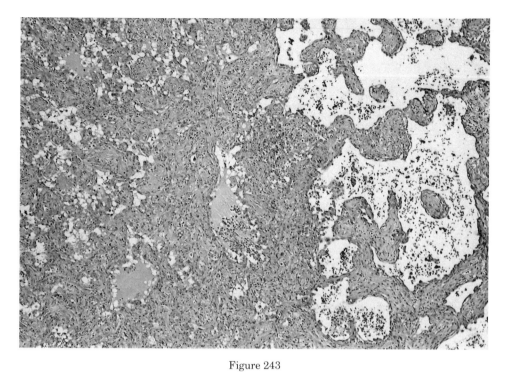

Figure 243
EPITHELIOID ANGIOSARCOMA
Foci with clear-cut anastomosing vascular channel formation (right) are adjacent to more solid and cellular areas (left).

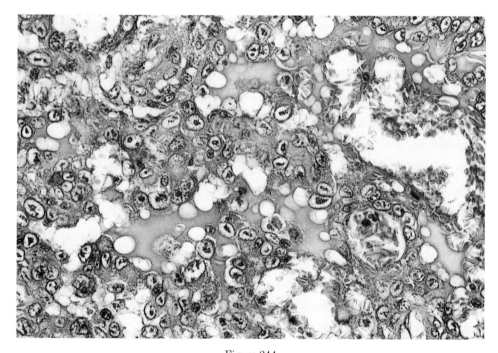

Figure 244
EPITHELIOID ANGIOSARCOMA
This high magnification shows the large vesicular nucleus and the prominent and irregularly shaped nucleolus that are typical of this tumor type. Abortive vascular lumina can be seen.

PLATE XXXIII

EPITHELIOID ANGIOSARCOMA

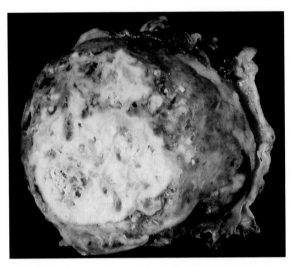

A. This tumor is characteristically necrotic and hemorrhagic. (Courtesy of Dr. Vincenzo Eusebi, Bologna, Italy.)

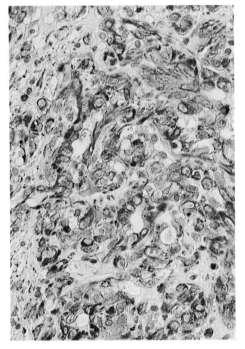

B. The tumor cells in this field are strongly immunoreactive for vimentin.

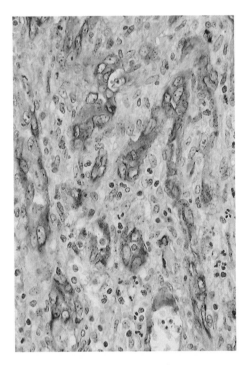

C. These plump epithelioid endothelial cells are strongly positive for factor VIII–related antigen.

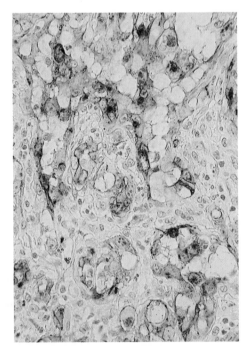

D. There is strong immunoreactivity of the neoplastic elements for *Ulex europaeus* I lectin.

PLATE XXXIV

EPITHELIOID ANGIOSARCOMA

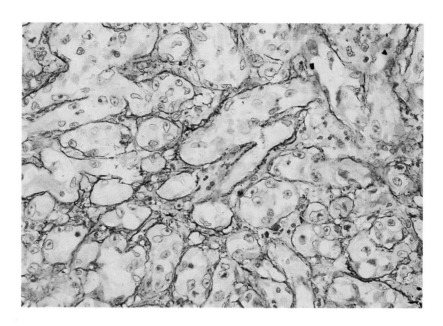

A. Immunostain for type IV collagen shows the presence of this basal lamina component around groups of tumor cells, thus highlighting the formation of primitive vascular tubules.

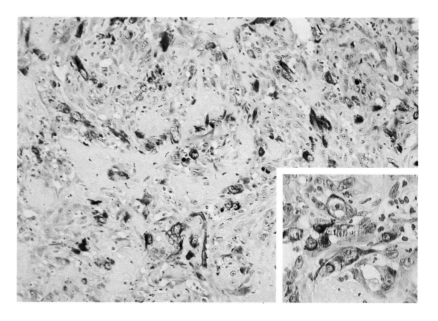

B. Many of the tumor cells are immunoreactive for keratin.

found to be immunoreactive for keratin, a feature shared with similar tumors in bone and other sites and that adds still another twist to the controversy concerning thyroid angiosarcoma versus undifferentiated carcinoma (pl. XXXIV-B) (14,15,29). This finding indicates that keratin positivity can no longer be reported as necessarily indicative of epithelial differentiation. Conversely, factor VIII–related antigen positivity may theoretically be the result in some cases of nonspecific uptake of antigen-rich serum and platelets by the tumor cells. Judging from the conclusions reached about these issues in two recent papers, the controversy is far from subsiding (21,28).

Ultrastructural Features. The better differentiated tumor cells exhibit basal lamina formation, primitive cell junctions, numerous pinocytotic vesicles, and a variable number of cytoplasmic filaments. The latter are more abundant in the epithelioid cell types. In some tumor cells, intracytoplasmic vacuoles are seen, bordered by a membrane featuring pinocytotic vesicles. These formations are analogous to those seen in neoformed normal vessels and are interpreted as the earliest sign of vascular lumen formation (24). The Weibel-Palade bodies are the only specific ultrastructural feature of endothelial cells. They are rod-shaped, membrane-bound cytoplasmic structures that contain a variable number of tubules of approximately 15 nm diameter and have been shown to be the storage site for the factor VIII–related protein (10). These structures are likely to be present in the better differentiated tumors but not in others, and their absence therefore does not rule out a diagnosis of angiosarcoma (11,14).

Differential Diagnosis. The differential diagnosis of thyroid angiosarcoma is discussed in the chapter on Undifferentiated (Anaplastic) Carcinoma (see page 135).

Spread and Metastasis; Prognosis. Thyroid angiosarcoma is an exceedingly malignant tumor. It grows rapidly, infiltrates beyond the gland, and metastasizes distantly, particularly to lung and lymph nodes. The Swiss authors have emphasized the high frequency of subpleural hemorrhagic tumor nodules, often associated with massive hemothorax (12). Response to radiation therapy or chemotherapy is poor, and the mortality rate is at least as high as that for undifferentiated carcinoma.

REFERENCES

Sarcomas

1. Andrion A, Gaglio A, Dogliani N, Bosco E, Mazzucco G. Liposarcoma of the thyroid gland. Fine-needle aspiration cytology, immunohistology, and ultrastructure. Am J Clin Pathol 1991;95:675–9.
2. Chesky VE, Hellwig CA, Welch JW. Fibrosarcoma of the thyroid gland. Surg Gynecol Obstet 1960;111:767–70.
3. Hedinger CE. Sarcomas of the thyroid gland. In: Hedinger CE, ed. Thyroid cancer. Berlin: Springer-Verlag, 1969:47–52. (UICC monograph series; Vol 12.)
4. _____. Histological typing of thyroid tumours. New York: Springer-Verlag, 1988.
5. Kawahara E, Nakanishi I, Terahata S, Ikegaki S. Leiomyosarcoma of the thyroid gland. A case report with a comparative study of five cases of anaplastic carcinoma. Cancer 1988;62:2558–63.
6. Ohbu M, Kameya T, Wada C, Okudaira M, et al. Primary osteogenic sarcoma of the thyroid gland: a case report. Surg Pathol 1989;2:67–72.
7. Proks C. Generalized hemangiopericytoma of the thyroid gland: report of a case. Neoplasma 1961;8:219–24.
8. Shin W-Y, Aftalion B, Hotchkiss E, Schenkman R, Berkman J. Ultrastructure of a primary fibrosarcoma of the human thyroid gland. Cancer 1979;44:584–91.
9. Tseleni-Balafouta S, Arvanitis D, Kakaviatos N, Paraskevakou H. Primary myxoid chondrosarcoma of the thyroid gland. Arch Pathol Lab Med 1988;112:94–6.

Angiosarcoma

10. Carstens PH. The Weibel-Palade body in the diagnosis of endothelial tumors. Ultrastruct Pathol 1981;2:315–25.
11. Chan YF, Ma L, Boey JH, Yeung HY. Angiosarcoma of the thyroid. An immunohistochemical and ultrastructural study of a case in a Chinese patient. Cancer 1986;57:2381–8.
12. Egloff B. The hemangioendothelioma. In: Hedinger CE, ed. Thyroid cancer. Berlin: Springer-Verlag, 1969:52-9. (UICC monograph series; Vol 12.)
13. _____. The hemangioendothelioma of the thyroid. Virchows Arch [A] 1983;400:119–42.
14. Eusebi V, Carcangiu ML, Dina R, Rosai J. Keratin-positive epithelioid angiosarcoma of thyroid. A report of four cases. Am J Surg Pathol 1990;14:737–47.
15. Gray MH, Rosenberg AE, Dickersin GR, Bhan AK. Cytokeratin expression in epithelioid vascular neoplasms. Hum Pathol 1990;21:212–7.
16. Guarda LA, Ordòñez NG, Smith JL Jr, Hanssen G. Immunoperoxidase localization of factor VIII in angiosarcomas. Arch Pathol Lab Med 1982;106:515–6.

17. Hedinger CE. Geographic pathology of thyroid diseases. Pathol Res Pract 1981;171:285–92.

18. _____. Zur Lehre der Struma sarcomatosa. I. Die Blutgefabendotheliome der Struma. Frankfurt Z Pathol 1909;3:487–540.

19. Klinck GH. Hemangioendothelioma and sarcoma of the thyroid. In: Hedinger CE, ed. Thyroid cancer. Berlin: Springer-Verlag, 1969:60–3. (UICC monograph series; Vol 12.)

20. Krisch K, Holzner JH, Kokoschka R, Jakesz R, Niederle B, Roka R. Hemangioendothelioma of the thyroid gland—true endothelioma or anaplastic carcinoma? Pathol Res Pract 1980;170:230–42.

21. Mills SE, Stallings RG, Austin MB. Angiomatoid carcinoma of the thyroid gland. Anaplastic carcinoma with follicular and medullary features mimicking angiosarcoma. Am J Clin Pathol 1986;86:674–8.

22. Mukai K, Rosai J, Burgdorf WH. Localization of factor VIII-related antigen in vascular endothelial cells using an immunoperoxidase method. Am J Surg Pathol 1980;4:273–6.

23. Pfaltz M, Hedinger C, Saremaslani P, Egloff B. Malignant hemangioendothelioma of the thyroid and factor VIII-related antigen. Virchows Arch [A] 1983;401:177–84.

24. Rosai J, Sumner HW, Kostianovsky M, Perez-Mesa C. Angiosarcoma of the skin. A clinicopathologic and fine structural study. Hum Pathol 1976;7:83–109.

25. Ruchti C, Gerber HA, Schaffner T. Factor VIII-related antigen in malignant hemangioendothelioma of the thyroid: additional evidence for the endothelial origin of this tumor. Am J Clin Pathol 1984;82:474–80.

26. Schäffer R, Ormanns W. Immunohistochemic detection of factor VIII antigen in malignant hemangioendotheliomas of the thyroid. A contribution to histogenesis. Schweiz Med Wochenschr 1983;113:601–5.

27. Tanda F, Massarelli G, Bosincu L, Cossu U. Angiosarcoma of the thyroid: a light, electron microscopic and histoimmunological study. Hum Pathol 1988;19:742–5.

28. Tötsch M, Dobler G, Feichtinger H, Sandbichler P, Ladurner D, Schmid KW. Malignant hemangioendothelioma of the thyroid. Its immunohistochemical discrimination from undifferentiated thyroid carcinoma. Am J Surg Pathol 1990;14:69–74.

29. van Haelst UJ, Pruszczynski M, ten Cate LN, Mravunac M. Ultrastructural and immunohistochemical study of epithelioid hemangioendothelioma of bone: coexpression of epithelial and endothelial markers. Ultrastruct Pathol 1990;14:141–9.

30. Vollenweider I, Hedinger C, Saremaslani P, Pfaltz M. Malignant hemangioendothelioma of the thyroid. Immunohistochemical evidence of heterogeneity. Pathol Res Pract 1989;184:376–81.

MALIGNANT LYMPHOMA

Definition. A malignant tumor composed of lymphoid cells involving the thyroid gland. The term is usually reserved for those cases in which the thyroid gland is the predominant, and often exclusive, site of involvement. This process should be clearly separated from involvement of the thyroid by a systemic lymphoma or leukemia, which in autopsy studies has been found to occur in approximately 10 percent of the cases (26). Primary thyroid lymphoma constitutes approximately 8 percent of all thyroid malignancies (13).

Thyroiditis and Other Antecedent Factors. In about 80 percent of the cases of thyroid lymphoma, the residual non-neoplastic gland exhibits features of autoimmune thyroiditis of either Hashimoto or lymphocytic type. As Williams (28) pointed out, the frequency of this association is clearly significant and much higher than that found between thyroiditis and thyroid carcinoma. Thus, the existence of a causal relationship between the two disorders is now widely accepted (14,17). Although it is possible that the presence of lymphoma in the thyroid may result in thyroiditis, it seems more likely that, in most cases, it is the thyroiditis that predisposes the patient to the development of the lymphoma. The situation may be analogous to that seen at several other sites, in which prolonged antigenic stimulation has been shown to favor the development of a lymphoid malignancy. One such example is the salivary gland lymphoma arising in patients with Sjogren syndrome. There are also some epidemiologic data supporting this interpretation. A comparison between populations of Iceland and northeast Scotland has shown that thyroiditis, prevalence of thyroid antibodies, and thyroid lymphoma were all considerably more common in the latter (29). To put the above facts in perspective, it should be pointed out that only an exceedingly small percentage of patients with thyroiditis will develop a malignant lymphoma of this organ.

Another possible etiopathogenetic factor for the development of thyroid lymphoma is radiation injury to the gland. A few suggestive cases have been reported, the exposure having been in the form of external radiation to the neck and/or thymic area (7). There is no convincing evidence that administration of ^{131}I results in an increased incidence of this type of malignancy.

Clinical Features. Most cases of primary thyroid lymphoma are seen in middle-aged or elderly patients. The most common age of presentation is in the sixties. The ratio of women to men ranges from 2:1 to 8:1 in the various series. The clinical presentation is in the form of thyroid enlargement, which is often firm or hard and may be fixed. The duration of the symptoms is usually short. Hoarseness, dysphagia, and/or dyspnea occur in about 25 percent, and cord paresis in about 17 percent of the patients. As expected, these symptoms are much more common in tumors exhibiting extrathyroid extension (8,24). Most patients are euthyroid, and the tumor presents as one or more cold nodules on thyroid scan (11).

Most of the reported cases of thyroid lymphoma have had only minimal staging of the disease. In a series of 11 patients published from Stanford University, 8 patients had stage I–II disease and three patients had stage III–IV disease (9).

Gross Features. The gross features vary to some extent, depending on the microscopic type of lymphoma. However, in most instances, the tumor presents as a solid mass with a homogeneous, bulging white surface featuring the classic "fish-flesh" appearance (pl. XXXV-A). The interface between the tumor and adjacent gland is usually ill defined, and encapsulation is absent. Large and/or peripherally located lesions tend to invade the thyroid capsule and extend into the surrounding soft tissue. Necrosis and hemorrhage are uncommon, in contrast with their almost universal presence in undifferentiated carcinoma.

Microscopic Features. Most primary thyroid lymphomas are of non-Hodgkin type, have a B cell phenotype, and belong to the large cell category. In the past they have often been designated as *reticulum cell sarcomas* or *histiocytic lymphomas*. The pattern of growth is almost always diffuse. Entrapment and invasion of thyroid follicles is the rule. Some of the tumor cells are present between the follicular cells, and others accumulate within the follicular lumina (figs. 245, 246). Compagno and Oertel (10) remarked on the high frequency and diagnostic importance of this follicular packing by the malignant lymphoid cells, although the change can also be seen in thyroiditis and Graves disease (18). The close intermingling of neoplastic and follicular cells and the common presence of abnormalities in the latter either as a reaction to the lymphoma or (when oncocytic) as an expression of the preexisting thyroiditis are the main reasons thyroid lymphomas are misdiagnosed as undifferentiated small cell carcinomas (13). Another source of difficulty is the fact that some of these lymphomas are associated with the formation of fibrous bands that compartmentalize the tumor cells into well-defined solid nests, a feature analogous to that sometimes seen in large cell lymphomas of lymph nodes, mediastinum, and other locations (fig. 247) (23,25). A feature of diagnostic importance is the spreading of tumor cells along the wall of blood vessels, some of which lie beneath the intima, narrowing but not obliterating the lumen (22,28).

At high magnification, the tumor cells usually have large-cleaved and noncleaved cells, the lat-

ter predominating (fig. 247). The nucleus is large, round or oval, with clumped chromatin and conspicuous basophilic nucleoli. The cytoplasm is abundant and pale eosinophilic. In formalin-fixed material, the nuclei may appear smaller and hyperchromatic, accompanied by an optically clear cytoplasm and a sharply outlined cell membrane. The same material fixed in Zenker's or B-5 solutions does not exhibit this change, which should therefore be interpreted as of artifactual nature.

The second most common thyroid lymphoma is the immunoblastic type. Less frequent varieties include the poorly differentiated lymphocytic (small-cleaved) and intermediate types (fig. 248) (21). These are recognized by the use of criteria similar to those used in lymph nodes. For the intermediate type, this includes the identification of small atypical lymphoid cells surrounding randomly distributed secondary follicles in a mantle-like fashion (4). A high percentage of the small lymphocytic tumors exhibit focal or extensive plasmacytoid features; these should not be equated with plasmacytomas. Exceptionally, the

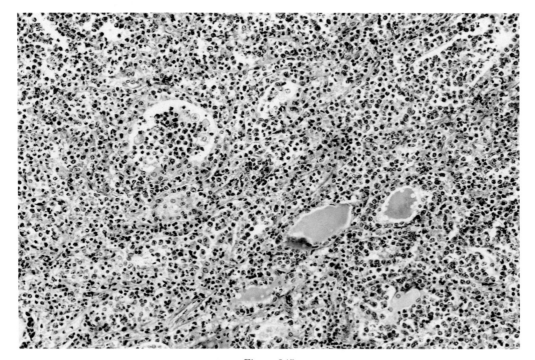

Figure 245
LARGE CELL LYMPHOMA
The tumor is growing between non-neoplastic follicles. Some of these follicles show packing of the lumina by lymphoma cells.

small-cleaved lymphomas may show focal signet-ring features and thus simulate metastatic adenocarcinoma (1).

Anscombe and Wright (2) have included thyroid lymphomas within the family of neoplasms of mucosa-associated lymphoid tissue (MALT). They base their proposal, originally advanced by Isaacson and Wright (16), on the presence of lymphoid packing of the follicles (which they regard as a form of lymphoepithelial lesion), marked plasmacytoid differentiation, tendency of the tumor to remain localized for long periods, and predilection for other sites of mucosa-associated lymphoid tissue (e.g., the gastrointestinal tract) when relapse occurs. As a corollary of this still-controversial concept, the authors have suggested that most of these tumors are not of follicular center cell origin, as originally believed, but of parafollicular B cell derivation (15).

Immunohistochemical Features. The tumor cells are positive for leukocyte-common antigen, a marker that can be detected consistently in paraffin-embedded material (pl. XXXV-B) (12). In keeping with the B cell derivation of nearly all cases,

they also exhibit immunoreactivity for pan-B markers, such as the one demonstrated by L26 monoclonal antibody, as applied to paraffin-embedded material. In addition, immunoglobulin light-chain restriction is easily demonstrable on fresh suspended cells or frozen sections and less consistently in formalin-fixed, paraffin-embedded material (5). Only exceptionally will primary thyroid lymphomas exhibit T cell markers, but such cases have been documented (20).

Stains for keratin or thyroglobulin are useful in delineating the entrapped follicles and in highlighting the close intermingling of neoplastic lymphoid cells (which are negative for these two markers) and the entrapped, atrophic, or hyperplastic follicular cells (which are highly reactive for both) (pl. XXXVI) (12). However, diffusion of thyroglobulin from the entrapped follicles may create difficulties (pl. XXXVI).

Ultrastructural Features. The electron-microscopic features are similar to those seen in malignant lymphoma elsewhere. Actually, the most important determination to be made at the

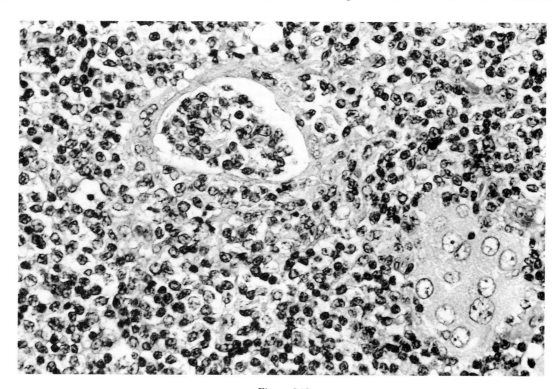

Figure 246
LARGE CELL LYMPHOMA
In this high magnification, one of the follicles shows packing of the lumen by lymphoma cells. Another, located in the right lower corner, shows large vesicular nuclei and granular acidophilic cytoplasm as a sign of a preexisting Hashimoto thyroiditis.

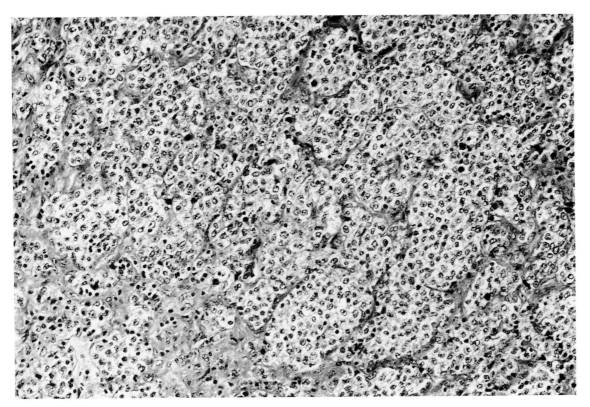

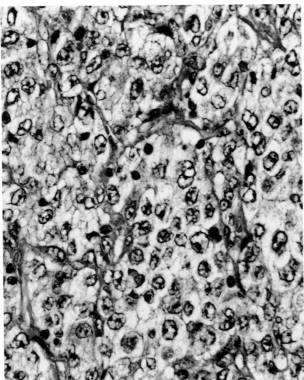

Figure 247
LARGE CELL LYMPHOMA
WITH SCLEROSIS
The presence of fibrous bands results in compartmentalization of the tumor cells and an appearance that can simulate carcinoma or paraganglioma.

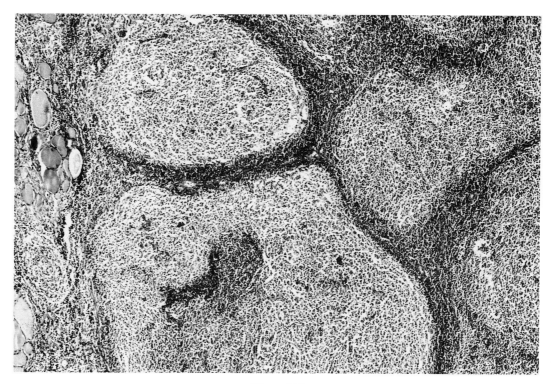

Figure 248
FOLLICULAR LYMPHOMA OF SMALL-CLEAVED TYPE
A few residual thyroid follicles can be seen in the upper left side of the field.

electron-microscopic level is to document the absence of epithelial markers such as desmosomes in the malignant cells (being careful not to misinterpret the entrapped follicular cells as neoplastic elements).

Other Special Studies. Taniwaki and co-workers (27) reported solely numerical chromosomal abnormalities in some cases of thyroid lymphoma and solely structural abnormalities in others. They claimed that patients in the first group have a higher frequency of antecedent thyroiditis and that the disease is associated with a longer clinical course. Malignant lymphomas of B and T cell type exhibit immunoglobulin and T cell receptor gene rearrangements, respectively, whereas the lymphocytes of Hashimoto thyroiditis lack both (6).

Cytologic Features. Cytologic specimens from malignant lymphomas are characterized by a monotonous population of noncohesive atypical cells. In most cases, these cells are large, with irregular

vesicular nuclei and prominent nucleoli. Karyorrhexis is often prominent (fig. 249).

The most important differential diagnosis is with Hashimoto thyroiditis. In this condition, the lymphoid population is polymorphic and accompanied by plasma cells, macrophages, and oncocytic cells. It should be remembered that Hashimoto thyroiditis and malignant lymphoma often coexist.

Spread and Metastasis. Malignant lymphoma of the thyroid invades locally until eventually most or all of the gland is replaced by tumor. At that stage, direct extension into the surrounding soft tissues is the rule. Regional lymph nodes may also be affected. When this is the case, the involvement may be only focal, as if the tumor had metastasized from the thyroid. This phenomenon is analogous to that sometimes seen with lymphomas of other organs (e.g., stomach) in relation to their respective regional nodes. When post-treatment relapse occurs, it often involves the gastrointestinal tract, sometimes exclusively (2,28).

PLATE XXXV

LARGE CELL LYMPHOMA

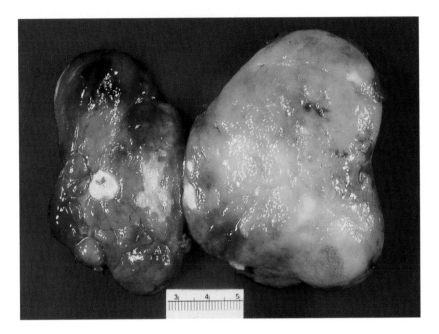

A. The typical "fish-flesh" appearance of this tumor type can be clearly appreciated in the cut surface of this gross specimen.

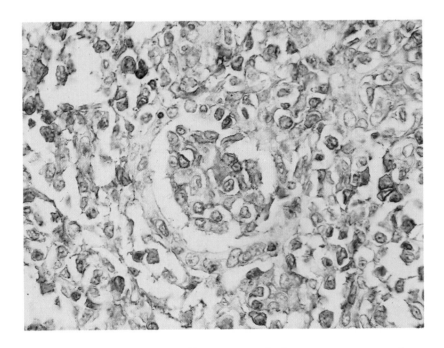

B. The tumor cells in this field are positive for leucocyte-common antigen, including those located within an entrapped follicle. The epithelial follicular cells are negative.

PLATE XXXVI

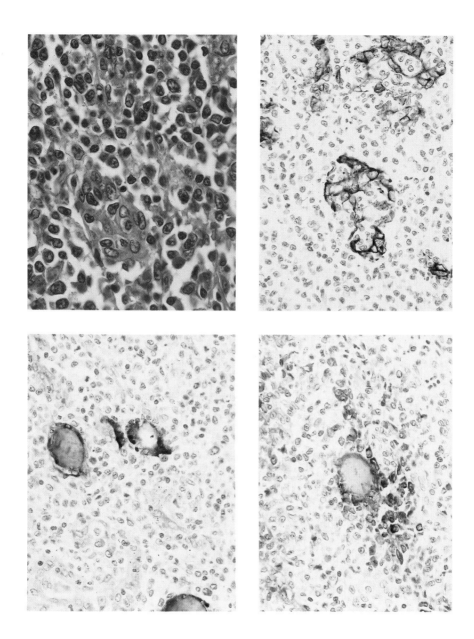

LARGE CELL LYMPHOMA

    The H&E section shows entrapment and infiltration of thyroid follicles by the tumor cells (top left). Immunostaining for keratin illustrates entrapment and distortion of epithelial follicular cells by the lymphoma (top right). Immunostaining for thyroglobulin shows several entrapped follicles (bottom left). Another area of the same tumor stained for thyroglobulin shows that the latter has diffused out from an entrapped follicle and has been absorbed by the adjacent malignant lymphoma cells. These cells have thus acquired apparent positivity for this marker (bottom right).

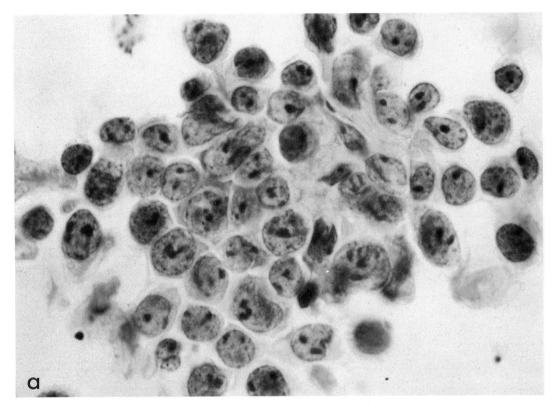

Figure 249
MALIGNANT LYMPHOMA
In this fine-needle aspiration specimen from the thyroid, there are discrete mononuclear cells with scant cytoplasm, large nuclei with open chromatin pattern, and multiple nucleoli. Papanicolaou preparation. X1000. (Fig. 12.5a from Kini SR. Thyroid. In: Kline TS, ed. Guides to clinical aspiration biopsy; Vol 3. New York:, Igaku-Shoin, 1987.)

Treatment. Although some authors have questioned the need for a thyroidectomy in primary thyroid lymphoma (24), in most institutions the therapeutic policy has been that of removing the affected gland (11). This seems to us a rather sensible approach, similar to that advocated for lymphomas of other extranodal sites. The excision should be followed by high-dose irradiation to the field, including the regional lymph nodes. Whether chemotherapy is indicated in patients with localized disease remains controversial (9). In cases with extrathyroid involvement, it seems reasonable to avoid surgical resection and proceed directly to radiation therapy, which is usually combined with chemotherapy. The latter is mandatory in patients with stage III–IV disease.

Prognosis. In older series, the most important prognostic factor in malignant lymphoma of the thyroid gland was found to be the presence or absence of extrathyroid extension, i.e., the stage of the disease (30). This feature still retains prognostic validity, although the differences are not as striking in more recent series (8,11).

The cell type is also prognostically important. Among the large cell tumors, large-cleaved and noncleaved cell lymphomas are associated with a better outcome than immunoblastic lymphomas (3). This may be related at least in part to the fact that immunoblastic lymphomas frequently present as advanced disease (19).

In a small series of stage I–II patients treated at Stanford University with high-dose regional irradiation after excision, there was an 83.3 percent survival at 3 years and a 75 percent relapse-free survival at 2 years. There was not a single instance of local recurrence in this group (9). In a series from Japan composed of 79 cases (3), the overall 5-year survival rate was 74 percent, and in a series from the Mayo Clinic composed of 103 cases, the corresponding figure for patients seen through 1979 was 50 percent (11).

OTHER LYMPHOID TUMORS

Plasmacytoma

Involvement of the thyroid gland by a plasma cell malignancy can be seen as an expression of widespread myeloma or as the only manifestation of the disease (36). When the latter is the case, the term plasmacytoma is used (31). The disease, even if localized, may be accompanied by detectable immunoglobulin abnormalities in the serum (34,35).

Plasmacytoma should be distinguished from the types of malignant lymphoma exhibiting plasmacytoid features, such as immunoblastic lymphoma, some forms of small lymphocytic lymphoma, and "pleomorphic immunocytoma." In true plasmacytoma, all of the tumor cells have the appearance of plasma cells exhibiting various degrees of immaturity or atypia, whereas in the lymphomas, the plasmacytoid elements alternate with cells of lymphoid type. Immunoglobulin light-chain restriction can be demonstrated immunohistochemically (32). Plasmacytoma may be associated with amyloid deposits and foreign-body reaction, features that may simulate the appearance of medullary carcinoma.

Primary plasmacytoma of the thyroid, like malignant lymphoma, is often accompanied by evidence of autoimmune thyroiditis in the residual portion of the gland (31). The differential diagnosis of plasmacytoma also includes *plasma cell granuloma* (see page 315).

Hodgkin Disease

It is exceptional for Hodgkin disease to involve primarily the thyroid gland. As in many other extranodal sites, most cases so diagnosed in the past would be classified otherwise today; however, indisputable cases of Hodgkin disease of the thyroid are on record. Most of the cases have been of the nodular sclerosis type, and some have shown concomitant involvement of the regional lymph nodes (pl. XXXVII; figs. 250, 251) (33).

Involvement of the thyroid in cases of systemic Hodgkin disease is also rare. It was seen in only 2 percent of the cases in the series of Shimaoka and coworkers (37).

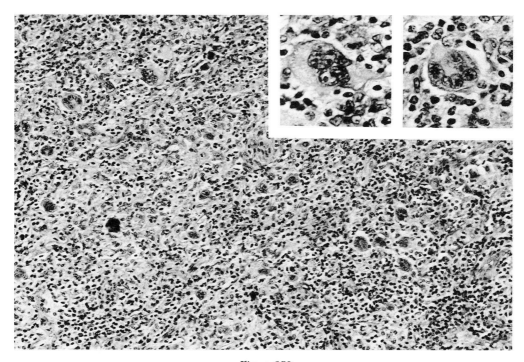

Figure 250

HODGKIN DISEASE OF NODULAR SCLEROSIS TYPE

This tumor was located in the thyroid gland. The insets in this illustration show two typical Reed-Sternberg cells. The regional lymph nodes were also involved.

PLATE XXXVII

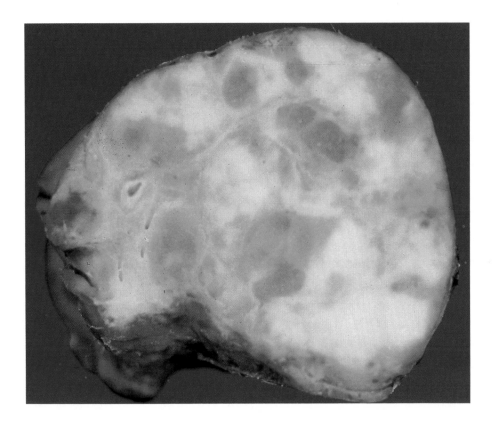

HODGKIN DISEASE OF NODULAR SCLEROSIS TYPE INVOLVING THE THYROID

Nodularity resulting from the presence of numerous fibrous bands can be seen in this gross specimen. The tumor appears variegated, with white nodules alternating with others having a reddish color.

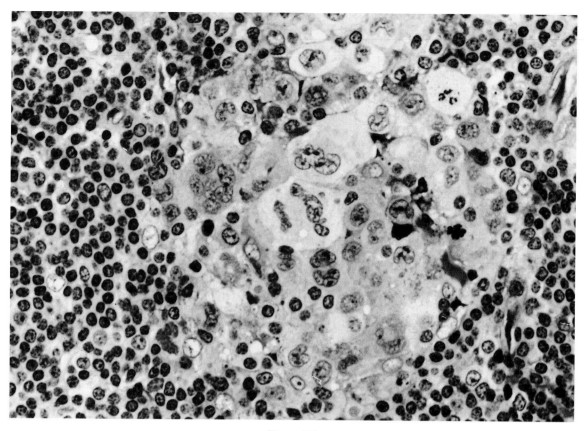

Figure 251
HODGKIN DISEASE OF NODULAR SCLEROSIS TYPE
This tumor was located in the thyroid. Note the numerous lacunar cells with typical polylobated nuclei in this plastic-embedded section. (Courtesy of Dr. Juan José Segura, San Jose, Costa Rica).

REFERENCES

Malignant Lymphoma

1. Allevato PA, Kini SR, Rebuck JW, Miller JM, Hamburger JI. Signet ring cell lymphoma of the thyroid: a case report. Hum Pathol 1985;16:1066–8.
2. Anscombe AM, Wright DH. Primary malignant lymphoma of the thyroid—a tumour of mucosa-associated lymphoid tissue: review of seventy-six cases. Histopathology 1985;9:81–97.
3. Aozasa K, Inoue A, Tajima K, Miyauchi A, Matsuzuka F, Kuma K. Malignant lymphomas of the thyroid gland. Analysis of 79 patients with emphasis on histologic prognostic factors. Cancer 1986;58:100–4.
4. _____, Inoue A, Yoshimura H, et al. Intermediate lymphocytic lymphoma of the thyroid. An immunologic and immunohistologic study. Cancer 1986;57:1762–7.
5. _____, Ueda T, Katagiri S, Matsuzuka F, Kuma K, Yonezawa T. Immunologic and immunohistologic analysis of 27 cases with thyroid lymphomas. Cancer 1987;60:969–73.
6. Ben-Ezra J, Wu A, Sheibani K. Hashimoto thyroiditis lacks detectable clonal immunoglobulin and T cell receptor gene rearrangements. Hum Pathol 1988;19:1444–8.
7. Bisbee AC, Thoeny RH. Malignant lymphoma of the thyroid following irradiation. Cancer 1975;35:1296–9.
8. Burke JS, Butler JJ, Fuller LM. Malignant lymphomas of the thyroid: a clinical pathologic study of 35 patients including ultrastructural observations. Cancer 1977;39:1587–602.
9. Chak LY, Hoppe RT, Burke JS, Kaplan HS. Non-Hodgkin's lymphoma presenting as thyroid enlargement. Cancer 1981;48:2712–6.
10. Compagno J, Oertel JE. Malignant lymphoma and other lymphoproliferative disorders of the thyroid gland. A clinicopathologic study of 245 cases. Am J Clin Pathol 1980;74:1–11.
11. Devine RM, Edis AJ, Banks PM. Primary lymphoma of the thyroid: a review of the Mayo Clinic experience through 1978. World J Surg 1981;5:33–8.

12. Fauré P, Chittal S, Woodman-Mémeteau W, et al. Diagnostic features of primary malignant lymphomas of the thyroid with monoclonal antibodies. Cancer 1988;61:1852–61.
13. Heimann R, Vannineuse A, De Sloover C, Dor P. Malignant lymphomas and undifferentiated small cell carcinoma of the thyroid: a clinicopathological review in the light of the Kiel classification for malignant lymphomas. Histopathology 1978;2:201–13.
14. Holm LE, Blomgren H, Löwhagen T. Cancer risks in patients with chronic lymphocytic thyroiditis. N Engl J Med 1985;312:601–4.
15. Hyjek E, Isaacson PG. Primary B cell lymphoma of the thyroid and its relationship to Hashimoto thyroiditis. Hum Pathol 1988;19:1315–26.
16. Isaacson PG, Wright DH. Extranodal malignant lymphoma arising from mucosa-associated lymphoid tissue. Cancer 1984;53:2515–24.
17. Kato I, Tajima K, Suchi T, et al. Chronic thyroiditis as a risk factor of B-cell lymphoma in the thyroid gland. Jpn J Cancer Res 1985;76:1085–90.
18. Matias-Guiu X, Esquius J. Lymphoepithelial lesion in the thyroid. A non-specific histological finding. Pathol Res Pract 1991;187:296–300.
19. Maurer R, Taylor CR, Terry R, Lukes RJ. Non-Hodgkin lymphomas of the thyroid. A clinico-pathological review of 29 cases applying the Lukes-Collins classification and an immunoperoxidase method. Virchows Arch [A] 1979;383:293–317.
20. Mizukami Y, Matsubara F, Hashimoto T, et al. Primary T-cell lymphoma of the thyroid. Acta Pathol Jpn 1987;37:1987–95.
21. _____, Michigishi T, Nonomura A, et al. Primary lymphoma of the thyroid: a clinical, histological and immunohistochemical study of 20 cases. Histopathology 1990;17:201–9.
22. Oertel JE, Heffess CS. Lymphoma of the thyroid and related disorders. Semin Oncol 1987;14:333–42.
23. Perrone T, Frizzera G, Rosai J. Mediastinal diffuse large-cell lymphoma with sclerosis. A clinicopathologic study of 60 cases. Am J Surg Pathol 1986;10:176–91.
24. Rasbach DA, Mondschein MS, Harris NL, Kaufman DS, Wang C-A. Malignant lymphoma of the thyroid gland. Surgery 1985;98:1166–70.
25. Rosas-Uribe A, Rappaport H. Malignant lymphoma, histiocytic type with sclerosis (sclerosing reticulum cell sarcoma). Cancer 1972;29:946–53.
26. Shimaoka K, Sokal JE, Pickren JW. Metastatic neoplasms in the thyroid gland. Cancer 1962;15:557–65.
27. Taniwaki M, Nishida K, Misawa S, et al. Correlation of chromosome abnormalities with clinical characteristics in thyroid lymphoma. Cancer 1989;63:873–6.
28. Williams ED. Malignant lymphoma of the thyroid. Clin Endocrinol Metab 1981:10:379–89.
29. _____, Doniach I, Bjarnason O, Michie W. Thyroid cancer in an iodide rich area—a histopathological study. Cancer 1977;39:215–22.
30. Woolner LB, McConahey WM, Beahrs OH, Black BM. Primary malignant lymphoma of the thyroid. Review of forty-six cases. Am J Surg 1966;111:502–23.

Other Lymphoid Tumors

31. Aozasa K, Inoue A, Yoshimura H, Miyauchi A, Matsuzuka F, Kuma K. Plasmacytoma of the thyroid gland. Cancer 1986;58:105–10.
32. _____, Ueda T, Katagiri S, Matsuzuka F, Kuma K, Yonezawa T. Immunologic and immunohistologic analysis of 27 cases with thyroid lymphomas. Cancer 1987;60:969–73.
33. Feigin GA, Buss DH, Paschal B, Woodruff RD, Myers RT. Hodgkin's disease manifested as a thyroid nodule. Hum Pathol 1982;13:774–6.
34. Ottó S, Péter I, Végh S, Juhos E, Besznyák I. Gamma-chain heavy-chain disease with primary thyroid plasmacytoma. Arch Pathol Lab Med 1986;110:893–6.
35. Rubin J, Johnson JT, Killeen R, Barnes L. Extramedullary plasmacytoma of the thyroid associated with a serum monoclonal gammopathy. Arch Otolaryngol Head Neck Surg 1990;116:855–9.
36. Shimaoka K, Gailani S, Tsukada Y, Barcos M. Plasma cell neoplasm involving the thyroid. Cancer 1978;41:1140–6.
37. _____, Sokal JE, Pickren JW. Metastatic neoplasms in the thyroid gland. Cancer 1962;15:557–65.

❖❖❖

MISCELLANEOUS TUMORS

PARATHYROID TUMORS

Although parathyroid tumors do not represent primary thyroid neoplasms, those located within the thyroid gland certainly appear as such to the surgeon and can even present interpretative problems at the microscopic level. True intrathyroidal parathyroid glands are rare (~ 0.2 percent) compared with the high frequency of these glands abutting the thyroid gland (1). These intra- or perithyroidal parathyroid structures can be affected by primary or secondary chief cell hyperplasia, adenoma, or carcinoma (3). The formation of follicles with colloid-like material in the lumen can closely simulate the appearance of a thyroid follicular neoplasm. Furthermore, the occurrence of tumor cells with clear or oncocytic cytoplasm can lead to confusion with clear cell and oncocytic thyroid neoplasms, respectively.

At the light-microscopic level, features that, according to LiVolsi (2), favor a parathyroid origin are a more delicate vascular pattern, more pronounced nesting pattern, smaller size of the individual cells, and thinner quality of the trabeculae. Cytoplasmic glycogen, as evidenced by PAS staining, is generally more abundant in parathyroid than in thyroid clear cells. Obviously, clinical and laboratory evidence of hyperparathyroidism is also important in this differential diagnosis.

For the cases in which the distinction cannot be made on morphologic grounds, immunocytochemical stains for thyroglobulin and parathyroid hormone should settle the issue in nearly every instance.

PARAGANGLIOMA

A handful of cases of primary paraganglioma of the thyroid gland have been reported (4–8), one of them behaving aggressively (fig. 252) (8). Some are probably authentic; in particular, the case in which an intrathyroidal paraganglioma was found in association with bilateral paragangliomas of the carotid body seems incontrovertible (6). The probable source for these tumors is small paraganglia located in or immediately beneath the thyroid capsule (10). However, it is important before accepting a diagnosis of primary thyroid paraganglioma to consider the following three alternatives:

- Paraganglioma of the carotid body or other cervical paraganglion that has grown in close proximity or even extended into the thyroid. The distinction is entirely dependent on the surgical and gross findings, inasmuch as their microscopic, ultrastructural, and immunohistochemical features are identical.
- Hyalinizing trabecular adenoma of thyroid. The nesting pattern of this tumor can result in a striking paraganglioma-like appearance, to the point that the term *paraganglioma-like adenoma of the thyroid* has been proposed for it (see page 31). Presence of trabeculae, occasional follicles, immunoreactivity for thyroglobulin, and overall negativity for chromogranin and other neuroendocrine markers should establish the distinction with ease.
- Medullary thyroid carcinoma with a nesting (paraganglioma-like) pattern of growth (see page 237). This distinction may be difficult or impossible to achieve because of the numerous features that these two types of neuroendocrine tumor share. The most important criterion in favor of medullary carcinoma is the immunohistochemical demonstration of calcitonin and/or calcitonin gene–related peptide (see page 219). Features supportive of paraganglioma are the immunohistochemical demonstration of opioid peptides and the detection by either electron microscopy or immunohistochemistry (S-100 protein staining) of sustentacular cells at the edges of the tumor nests (pl. XXXVIII) (9). Unfortunately, none of these features can be regarded as absolute, in the sense that calcitonin can be undetectable for technical or other reasons in medullary thyroid carcinomas and occasionally present in paragangliomas, that opioid peptides have been found in some thyroid medullary carcinomas, and that sustentacular cells have been described in neuroendocrine neoplasms other than paragangliomas, such as pulmonary carcinoid tumors.

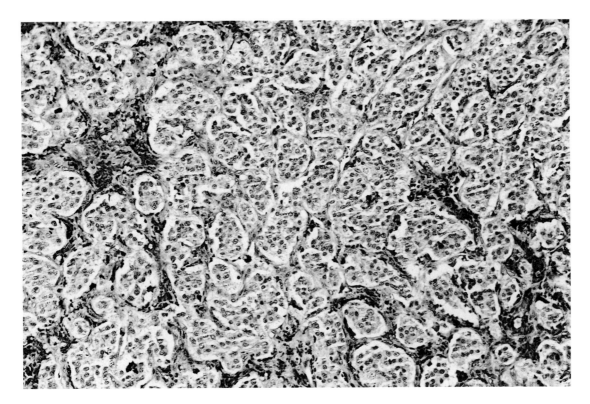

Figure 252
INTRATHYROIDAL PARAGANGLIOMA
The tumor is characterized by distinct nesting ("Zellballen"). The tumor cells are relatively uniform and have a moderately abundant granular basophilic cytoplasm.

TERATOMA

The neck is not an unusual site for the occurrence of teratomas in neonates and infants (11). They are usually located in the midneck and can reach huge dimensions (20,22–24). In some instances, emergency surgery is needed because of symptoms resulting from compression of the upper respiratory tract (14). At the gross level, most of these tumors have a multiloculated cystic appearance, which may be combined with smaller solid areas. Microscopically, the usual haphazard admixture of tissues derived from all three germ layers (including neural tissue) is identified (fig. 253). Nearly all of the reported cases in this age group have been entirely mature microscopically and have followed a benign clinical course.

Many of these cervical teratomas partially involve the thyroid gland, and that is why they are included in this section. They differ in no way from those cervical teratomas that are found to be anatomically separate from the thyroid.

Teratomas of the thyroid developing in adults differ from the above, in the sense that most have shown microscopic features of malignancy and have run an aggressive clinical course (12,13, 15,16,19–21). It is our impression that many and perhaps most of the reported cases do not qualify as true examples of germ cell neoplasia. For instance, we would interpret the lesion reported by Kimler and Muth (17), as well as two nearly identical cases we have observed, as *malignant primitive neuroepithelial tumors* and ascribe the cartilage present in them to the fact that much of the mesenchyme of the neck is of neural crest derivation. As for the cases of malignant teratoma of the thyroid reported by Kingsley and coworkers (18) and Murao and coworkers (19), we have reinterpreted them as neoplasms showing thymic or related branchial pouch differentiation (see page 282).

PLATE XXXVIII

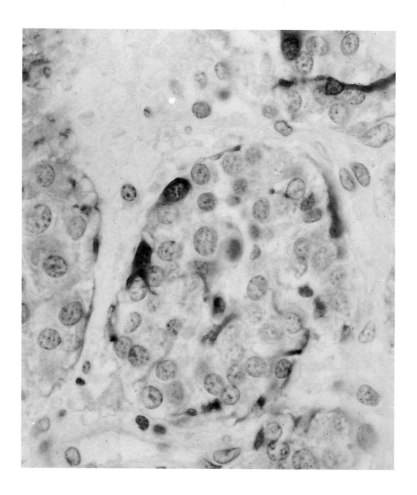

PARAGANGLIOMA OF THE THYROID

The cells positive for S-100 protein, which are located at the periphery of the "Zellballen" in this field, are thought to represent sustentacular cells.

BENIGN SOFT TISSUE–TYPE TUMORS

Isolated cases of *hemangioma* (28), *lymphangioma* (27), *neurilemoma* (25,26), and *leiomyoma* (25) of the thyroid have been reported.

TUMORS WITH THYMIC OR RELATED BRANCHIAL POUCH DIFFERENTIATION

There is a family of cervical tumors that have features consistent with an origin from branchial pouch derivatives and exhibit differentiation toward thymic tissue. Although not of thyroid origin, a brief mention of these lesions is appropriate, not only because they can be found adjacent to or even within the thyroid but also

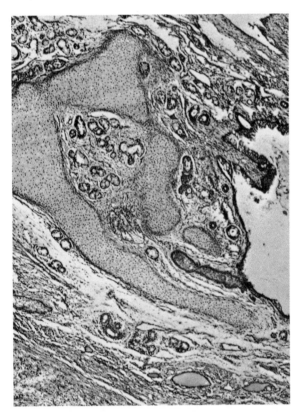

Figure 253
TERATOMA OF THE THYROID
This lesion was present in a newborn infant. At the bottom of the field, there are a few follicles of normal thyroid compressed by the large benign tumor. This teratoma contained cartilage, several types of epithelium, and neural tissue. (Fig. 54 from Series II, Fascicle 4.)

because the microscopic appearance of some of them bears a resemblance to some forms of primary thyroid carcinoma.

We have divided these lesions into four distinctive categories, which are listed below.

Ectopic Cervical Thymoma

This is the easiest lesion in the group to recognize, in the sense that its microscopic appearance mirrors that of its most common counterpart in the mediastinum. The usual location is the anterolateral neck, generally deep to the sternomastoid muscle. It can be subjacent to or inside the lower pole of the thyroid gland. When this is the case, the clinical diagnosis of primary thyroid nodule is usually made. Residual ectopic thymic tissue is often found at the periphery. As in the mediastinum, the tumor can be encapsulated or invasive, but the former is more common. Microscopically, there is a dual composition of neoplastic epithelial thymic cells and non-neoplastic lymphocytes, as classically encountered in mediastinal thymoma (fig. 254) (29,30,36,40,42).

Ectopic Hamartomatous Thymoma

This tumor is not likely to be confused with a primary thyroid neoplasm on the basis of either location or microscopic appearance. It is mentioned here only for the sake of completeness.

The typical location is the supraclavicular or suprasternal region. Microscopically, a proliferation of bland-looking spindle cells simulating mesenchymal or schwannian elements is seen admixed with solid or cystic epithelial islands and mature adipose tissue (figs. 255, 256). The spindle cells have an epithelial phenotype ultrastructurally (desmosomes and tonofibrils) and immunohistochemically (keratin positivity). The behavior has invariably been benign (30,32,41).

Spindle Epithelial Tumor with Thymus-Like Differentiation (SETTLE)

We have proposed the acronym SETTLE (30) for a tumor that was previously reported as thyroid spindle cell tumor with mucous cysts (33) and malignant teratoma of the thyroid (35,39). It occurs in children and young adults (mean age 15 years) and typically presents as a thyroid nodule.

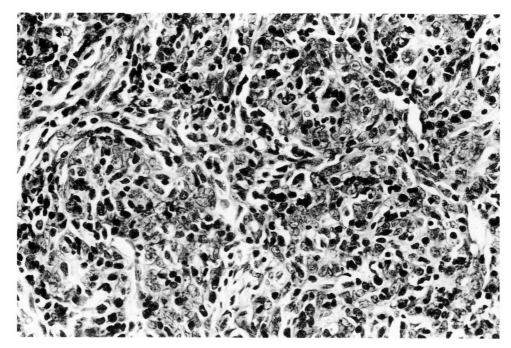

Figure 254
INTRATHYROIDAL THYMOMA
The typical dual composition of plump epithelial cells and small lymphocytes can be seen.

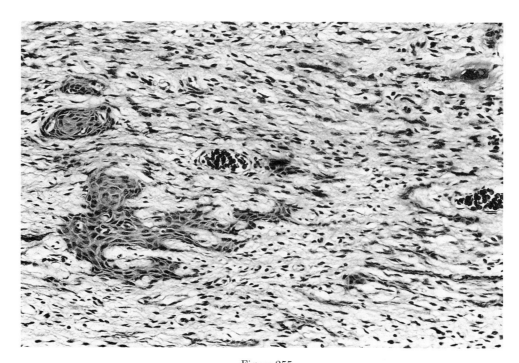

Figure 255
ECTOPIC HAMARTOMATOUS THYMOMA
The predominant element in this field is a spindle cell of mesenchymal-like appearance. This merges with islands with an obvious squamous pattern of differentiation.

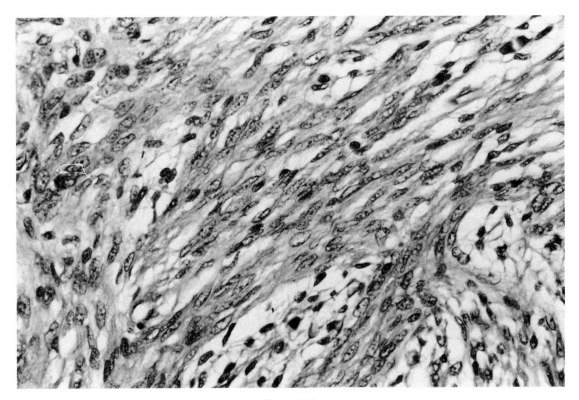

Figure 256
ECTOPIC HAMARTOMATOUS THYMOMA
The spindle cells of this tumor, which are epithelial, simulate mesenchymal or peripheral nerve elements.

At the gross level, the lesion can be encapsulated, partially circumscribed, or infiltrative. The cut surface is firm, grayish white to tan, and vaguely whorled; small cysts might be visible. Residual thyroid is often identified at the periphery.

Microscopically, the tumor is highly cellular and traversed by sclerotic bands that result in the formation of incompletely demarcated nodules. The diagnostic feature is represented by the merging of compact, relatively monotonous spindle cells, with plumper cells showing obvious epithelial differentiation. Interstitial accumulation of mucin is a constant feature, and vascular invasion may be present (fig. 257).

The spindle cells show ultrastructural and immunohistochemical features of epithelial cells, similar to those of ectopic hamartomatous thymoma. The cells with a clear-cut epithelial appearance at the light-microscopic level may appear in the form of complex narrow tubules, small papillae, trabecular islands, and solid sheets, all of these blending imperceptibly with the predominant spindle cell component. In addition, in many of the cases, there are branching cystic glands lined by mucinous or respiratory-type epithelium with basally located nuclei.

The natural history of this tumor is characterized by the occasional development of late distant metastases to lung, mediastinum, or kidney (as late as 25 years after resection of the original tumor).

Carcinoma Showing Thymus-Like Differentiation (CASTLE)

This tumor, which we have designated CASTLE and which was first described by Miyauchi and coworkers (38) as intrathyroidal epithelial thymoma, occurs in adults (mean age 48.5 years) and presents as a thyroid mass (30,31, 34,37,38). At the gross level, it involves predominantly the lower lobe of the thyroid and often extends to the juxtathyroid soft tissue. It is hard and lobulated, and its cut surface is gray to pinkish gray.

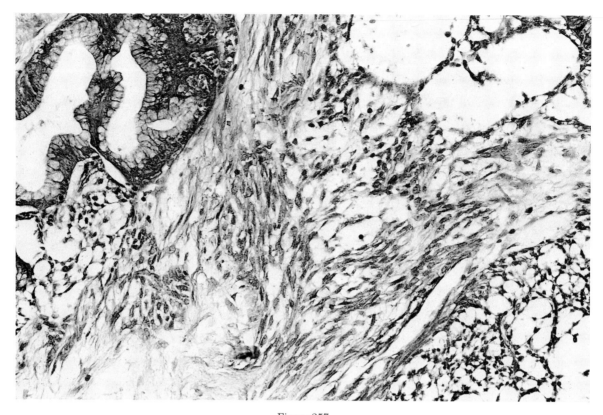

Figure 257
SPINDLE EPITHELIAL TUMOR WITH THYMUS-LIKE DIFFERENTIATION (SETTLE)
An admixture of spindle elements with a mesenchymal-like appearance and well-differentiated glandular epithelium is seen in this illustration. The spindle component had epithelial features at the immunohistochemical level.

Microscopically, the tumor is divided into irregularly shaped lobules and cords by fibrous septa infiltrated by lymphocytes and plasma cells (fig. 258). The tumor cells have large vesicular nuclei, prominent nucleoli, relatively abundant cytoplasm, and indistinct cell borders (fig. 259). The overall appearance is similar to that of lymphoepithelioma-like thymic carcinoma. Mitotic activity is relatively scanty. Foci of definite squamous differentiation may be present, and there may be perivascular spaces containing lymphocytes.

Immunohistochemically, the tumor cells are reactive for cytokeratin and negative for thyroglobulin and calcitonin. Ultrastructurally, they exhibit elongated cell processes, tonofilaments, and numerous desmosomes. The natural history is generally characterized by slow evolution and a tendency for late local recurrence (as long as 17 years after the initial diagnosis) (37).

The differential diagnosis of CASTLE includes primary undifferentiated and/or squamous cell thyroid carcinoma and metastatic carcinoma (particularly from upper aerodigestive tract, lung, and mediastinum). Features favoring the diagnosis of CASTLE include a lobulated pattern of expansile growth, lymphocytic infiltration, perivascular spaces, low mitotic count, and paucity of neutrophils (30).

SALIVARY GLAND–TYPE TUMORS

Lange (43) reported a case of *pleomorphic adenoma* of the thyroid with features analogous in all regards to those of the homonymous salivary gland tumor, including the presence of myoepithelial cells and cartilage.

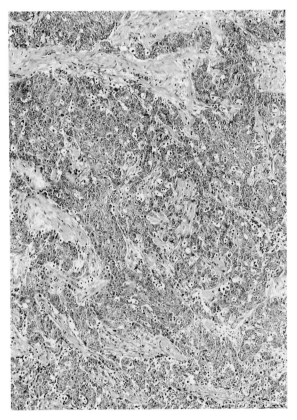

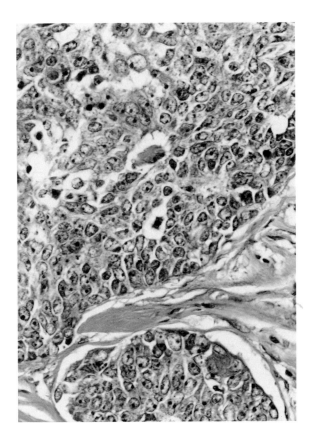

Figure 258
CARCINOMA SHOWING THYMUS-LIKE
DIFFERENTIATION (CASTLE)
This tumor, which was located within the thyroid, shows irregularly shaped lobules separated by fibrous septa infiltrated by lymphocytes. The pattern of growth is solid.

Figure 259
CARCINOMA SHOWING THYMUS-LIKE
DIFFERENTIATION (CASTLE)
At high magnification, a sharply defined tumor lobule composed of cells with large vesicular nuclei and prominent nucleoli is seen. The appearance is indistinguishable from that of thymic carcinoma.

REFERENCES

Parathyroid Tumors

1. Akerström G, Malmaeus J, Bergström R. Surgical anatomy of human parathyroid glands. Surgery 1984;95: 14–21.
2. LiVolsi VA. Surgical pathology of the thyroid. In: Bennington JL, ed. Major problems in pathology; Vol 22. Philadelphia: WB Saunders, 1990.
3. Sawady J, Mendelsohn F, Sirota RL, Taxy JB. The intrathyroidal hyperfunctioning parathyroid gland. Mod Pathol 1989;2:652–7.

Paraganglioma

4. Banner B, Morecki R, Eviatar A. Chemodectoma in the mid-thyroid region. J Otolaryngol 1979;8:271–3.
5. Buss DH, Marshall RB, Baird FG, Myers RT. Paraganglioma of the thyroid gland. Am J Surg Pathol 1980;4:589–93.
6. Haegert DG, Wang NS, Ferrer PA, Seemayer TA, Thelmo W. Non-chromaffin paragangliomatosis manifesting as a cold thyroid nodule. Am J Clin Pathol 1974;61: 561–70.
7. Kay S, Montague JW, Dodd RW. Nonchromaffin paraganglioma (chemodectoma) of thyroid region. Cancer 1975;36:582–5.
8. Mitsudo SM, Grajower MD, Balbi H, Silver C. Malignant paraganglioma of the thyroid gland. Arch Pathol Lab Med 1987;111:378–80.
9. Schroder HD, Johannsen L. Demonstration of S-100 protein in sustentacular cells of pheochromocytomas and paragangliomas. Histopathology 1986;10:1023–33.
10. Zak F, Lawson W. Glomic (paraganglionic) tissue in the larynx and capsule of the thyroid gland. M Sinai J Med 1972;39:82–90.

Teratoma

11. Bale GF. Teratoma of the neck in the region of the thyroid gland. A review of the literature and report of four cases. Am J Pathol 1950;26:565–79.
12. Buckley NJ, Burch WM, Leight GS. Malignant teratoma of the thyroid gland in an adult: a case report and a review of the literature. Surgery 1986;100:932–7.
13. Buckwalter JA, Layton JM. Malignant teratoma in the thyroid gland of an adult. Ann Surg 1954;139:218–23.
14. Fisher JE, Cooney DR, Voorhess ML, Jewett TC Jr. Teratoma of thyroid gland in infancy: review of the literature and two case reports. J Surg Oncol 1982;21:135–40.
15. Hajdu SI, Hajdu EO. Malignant teratoma of the neck. Arch Pathol 1967;83:567–70.
16. Kier R, Silverman PM, Korobkin M, Wain S, Leight G, Burch W Jr. Malignant teratoma of the thyroid in an adult: CT appearance. J Comput Assisted Tomogr 1985;9:174–6.
17. Kimler SC, Muth WF. Primary malignant teratoma of the thyroid: case report and literature review of cervical teratomas in adults. Cancer 1978;42:311–7.
18. Kingsley DP, Elton A, Bennett MH. Malignant teratoma of the thyroid. Case report and review of the literature. Br J Cancer 1968;22:7–11.
19. Murao T, Nakanishi M, Toda K, Konishi H. Malignant teratoma of the thyroid gland in an adolescent female. Acta Pathol Jpn 1979;29:109–17.
20. Newstedt JR, Shirkey HC. Teratoma of the thyroid region. Am J Dis Child 1964;107:88–95.
21. O'Higgins N, Taylor S. Malignant teratoma in the adult thyroid gland. Br J Clin Pract 1975;29:237–8.
22. Silberman R, Mendelson IR. Teratoma of the neck. Report of two cases and review of the literature. Arch Dis Child 1960;35:159–70.
23. Stone HH, Henderson WD, Guidio FA. Teratomas of the neck. Am J Dis Child 1967;113:222–4.
24. Weitzner S. Benign teratoma of the neck in an infant. Am J Dis Child 1964;107:84–7.

Benign Soft Tissue–Type Tumors

25. Andrion A, Bellis D, Delsedime L, Bussolati G, Mazzucco G. Leiomyoma and neurilemoma: report of two unusual non-epithelial tumours of the thyroid gland. Virchows Arch [A] 1988;413:367–72.
26. Delaney WE, Fry KE. Neurilemoma of the thyroid gland. Ann Surg 1964;160:1014–6.
27. Gardner DF, Frable WJ. Primary lymphangioma of the thyroid gland. Arch Pathol Lab Med 1989;113:1084–5.
28. Pickleman JR, Lee JF, Straus FH II, Paloyan E. Thyroid hemangioma. Am J Surg 1975;129:331–6.

Tumors with Thymic or Related Branchial Pouch Differentiation

29. Bothra R, Dahiya SL, Treisman E, Goodman P. Cervical thymoma. Int Surg 1975;60:301–2.
30. Chan JK, Rosai J. Tumors of the neck showing thymic or related branchial pouch differentiation: a unifying concept. Hum Pathol 1991;22:349–67.
31. Damiani S, Filotico M, Eusebi V. Carcinoma of the thyroid showing thymoma-like features. Virchows Arch [A] 1991;418:463–6.
32. Fetsch JR, Weiss SW. Ectopic hamartomatous thymoma: clinicopathologic, immunohistochemical, and histogenetic considerations in four new cases. Hum Pathol 1990;21:662–8.
33. Harach HR, Day Saravia E, Franssila KO. Thyroid spindle cell tumor with mucous cysts. An intrathyroid thymoma? Am J Surg Pathol 1985;9:525–30.
34. Kakudo K, Mori I, Tamaoki N, Watanabe K. Carcinoma of possible thymic origin presenting as a thyroid mass: a new subgroup of squamous cell carcinoma of the thyroid. J Surg Oncol 1988;138:187–92.
35. Kingsley DP, Elton A, Bennett MH. Malignant teratoma of the thyroid, case report and a review of the literature. Br J Cancer 1968;22:7–11.
36. Martin JM, Randhawa G, Temple WJ. Cervical thymoma. Arch Pathol Lab Med 1986;110:354–7.
37. Miyauchi A, Ishikawa H, Maeda M, et al. Intrathyroidal epithelial thymoma: a report of 6 cases with immunohistochemical and ultrastructural studies. Endocr Surg 1989;6:289–95 (in Japanese, with English abstract).
38. _____, Kuma K, Matsuzuka F, et al. Intrathyroidal epithelial thymoma: an entity distinct from squamous cell carcinoma of the thyroid. World J Surg 1985; 9:128–35.
39. Murao T, Nakanishi M, Toda K, Konishi H. Malignant teratoma of the thyroid gland in an adolescent female. Acta Pathol Jpn 1979;29:109–17.
40. Ridenhour CE, Henzel JH, DeWeese MS, Kerr SE. Thymoma arising from undescended cervical thymus. Surgery 1970;67:614–9.
41. Rosai J, Limas C, Husband EM. Ectopic hamartomatous thymoma. A distinctive benign lesion of the lower neck. Am J Surg Pathol 1984;8:501–13.
42. Yamashita H, Murakami N, Noguchi S, et al. Cervical thymoma and incidence of cervical thymus. Acta Pathol Jpn 1983;33:189–94.

Salivary Gland–Type Tumors

43. Lange MJ. Pleomorphic adenoma of the thyroid containing salivary gland cells with pseudocartilage and myoepithelial cells. Int Surg 1974;59:178–9.

❖❖❖

SECONDARY TUMORS

The thyroid gland may be involved by direct extension from carcinomas of pharynx, larynx, trachea, and esophagus, as well as from metastatic lesions in adjacent cervical lymph nodes. It is said that postcricoid and subglottic laryngeal tumors have a particular tendency to extend into the thyroid via the thyroidal cartilages (5). Most of these tumors are of squamous cell type, and the fact that the thyroid involvement is secondary is usually obvious on clinical grounds. In view of the rarity of primary squamous cell carcinoma of the thyroid, the possibility of a metastasis should be considered whenever such a tumor type is present in a thyroid biopsy, particularly if the tumor is well to moderately well differentiated (see page 197).

Blood-borne metastases to the thyroid are not uncommon at autopsy in patients with widespread malignancy, particularly malignant melanoma and carcinomas of lung, gastrointestinal tract, head and neck region, breast, and kidney (pl. XXXIX-A; figs. 260–263). In one large series, metastases to the thyroid were found in 9.5 percent of 1980 patients who died of malignancy in other organs (11). However, these metastases are the cause of clinically detectable thyroid enlargement or functional disturbances in only 25 percent or less of all cases (11). Occasionally, cancer metastatic to the thyroid is accompanied by hyperthyroidism, presumably as a result of tumor destruction of the follicles and massive release of thyroid hormones (12). We have seen a case of breast carcinoma metastasizing into a thyroid papillary carcinoma (pl. XXXIX-B) and a renal cell carcinoma metastasizing into a follicular adenoma (figs. 264, 265). Mizukami and coworkers (8) reported a case of lung carcinoma metastatic to a microfollicular thyroid adenoma.

At the gross level, the secondary deposits are more frequently multiple than single. Microscopically, they show a predominantly interstitial pattern of infiltration; the follicles are surrounded and deformed by the tumor but rarely

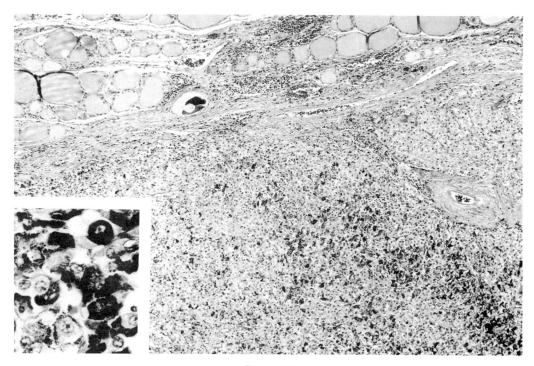

Figure 260
MALIGNANT MELANOMA METASTATIC TO THE THYROID
The inset shows malignant melanocytes, many of which are deeply pigmented.

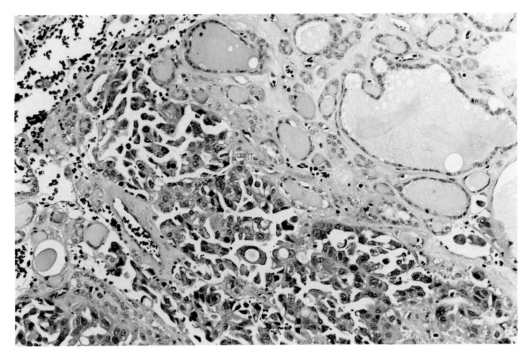

Figure 261
POORLY DIFFERENTIATED ADENOCARCINOMA OF LUNG METASTATIC TO A
MEDIASTINAL THYROID GLAND WITH NODULAR HYPERPLASIA
This case was originally misinterpreted as a primary undifferentiated carcinoma of the thyroid.

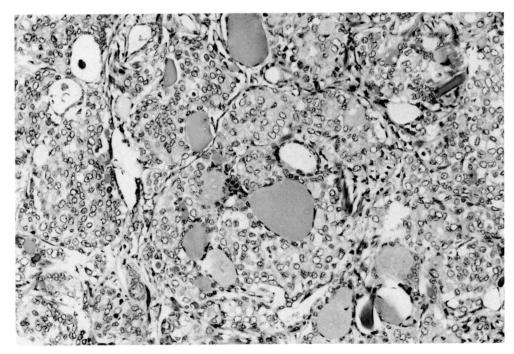

Figure 262
LOBULAR CARCINOMA OF THE BREAST METASTATIC TO THE THYROID
An intimate intermingling of metastatic malignant cells and entrapped thyroid follicles can be seen.

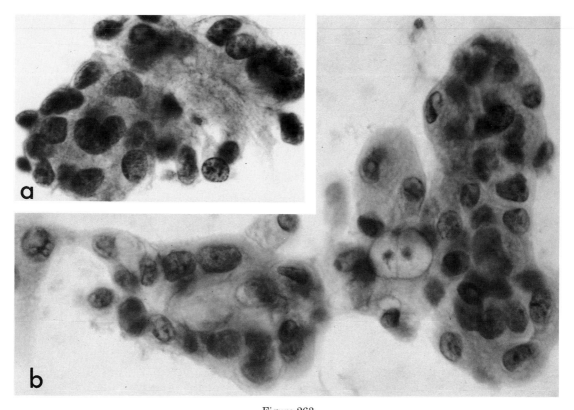

Figure 263
COLONIC ADENOCARCINOMA METASTATIC TO THE THYROID
In A, the typical "picket-fence" arrangement of the nuclei can be seen. Papanicolaou preparation. X630. Syncytial-type
tissue fragments of carcinoma cells with an acinar pattern can be seen in B. Papanicolaou preparation. X630. (Fig. 13.7
from Kini SR. Thyroid. In: Kline TS, ed. Guides to clinical aspiration biopsy; Vol 3. New York: Igaku-Shoin, 1987.)

infiltrated. Occasionally, however, there is an extensive infiltration of the follicles, the pattern thus simulating that of a primary neoplasm.

For the surgical pathologist, the most important type of thyroid metastasis is one that presents as a thyroid mass while the original source remains occult, thus simulating a primary tumor or a thyroiditis (3,12). Of these, the most common are renal cell carcinoma, large bowel adenocarcinoma, and malignant melanoma (2,6,7,13). We have seen a carcinoid tumor of the lung metastasizing to the thyroid and simulating a medullary carcinoma of the organ (fig. 266). A similar event was reported by Nesland and coworkers (9).

Metastatic renal cell carcinoma deserves special mention. It may present as a thyroid mass while the primary renal tumor is totally silent or as long as 22 years after nephrectomy (1,4). The thyroid nodule may be solitary or multiple, and the microscopic appearance is usually that of a

clear cell carcinoma. This being the case, the obvious differential diagnosis is with primary thyroid neoplasms exhibiting clear cell changes (see page 183).

Features favoring a diagnosis of metastatic renal cell carcinoma are multiplicity of tumor nodules; marked vascularization with presence of sinusoidal vessels, "follicles" (in reality, glandular lumina) packed with red blood cells, and a prominent water-clear appearance of the cytoplasm with little if any granularity. The latter feature is particularly useful because the cells of thyroid follicular clear cell tumors usually maintain a certain degree of cytoplasmic granularity, which becomes even more noticeable in PAS-stained slides (figs. 264, 265) (1).

The PAS stain is otherwise of only limited use in this differential diagnosis. Absence of glycogen points against a diagnosis of metastatic renal cell carcinoma, but its presence, even in large

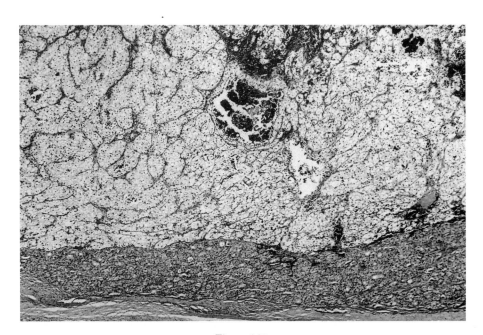

Figure 264
(Figures 264 and 265 are from the same patient)
RENAL CELL CARCINOMA METASTATIC TO
THYROID FOLLICULAR ADENOMA
The clear cell appearance of the metastatic tumor is well appreciated.

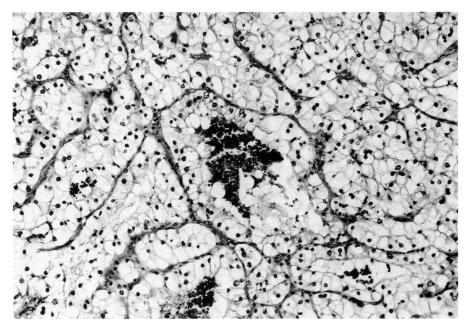

Figure 265
RENAL CELL CARCINOMA METASTATIC TO
THYROID FOLLICULAR CARCINOMA
In this high magnification of the same case as fig. 264, the cytoplasm is abundant and completely clear, without the fine granularity that is seen in most cases of primary thyroid tumor with clear cell changes. The central gland shows filling of the lumen with red blood cells, another important feature in the differential diagnosis with primary clear cell neoplasms of thyroid.

amounts, does not rule out the alternative possibility of a primary thyroid tumor. Similar considerations apply to lipid stains (pl. XXXIX-C). The most useful technique in this situation is an immunohistochemical reaction for thyroglobulin. This marker is negative in metastatic tumors and usually positive (at least focally) in the primary neoplasms. The interpretation requires caution for two reasons. Primary clear cell tumors of the thyroid may contain very small amounts of this marker (1). Conversely, entrapment of normal follicles followed by thyroglobulin diffusion and absorption by the metastatic cells may occur and be misinterpreted as

a positive result (pl. XL-A) (1). A similar phenomenon can occur with tumors metastatic from other sites (pl. XL-B).

Just as it is important to single out the secondary tumors that are more likely to simulate primary neoplasms, mention should be made of the opposite situation. Primary thyroid tumors for which the danger of misinterpretation in this regard is particularly high include those with clear cell, mucinous (including signet ring) and squamous changes, columnar cell carcinoma, and the group of tumors showing thymic or related branchial pouch differentiation (see page 282) (10).

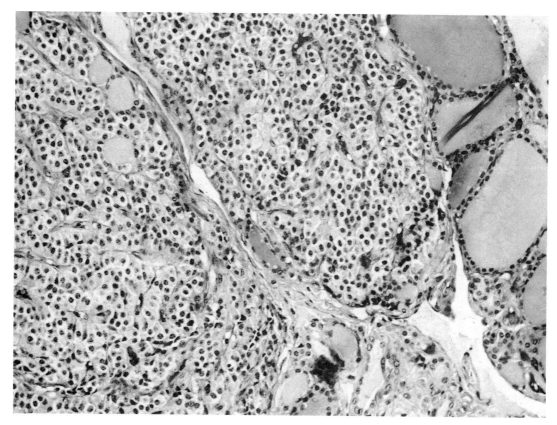

Figure 266

PULMONARY CARCINOID TUMOR
METASTATIC TO THYROID

There is a well-defined nesting pattern and a remarkable uniformity in the appearance of the cells of this tumor. Some entrapped follicles are evident. It is practically impossible to distinguish this tumor from medullary carcinoma on the basis of routinely stained sections.

PLATE XXXIX

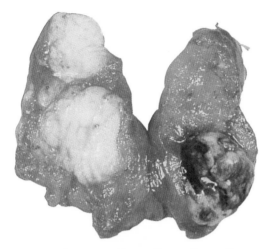

A. METASTATIC MALIGNANT MELANOMA IN THE THYROID

Three independent tumor nodules are present in this gland, one of which is pigmented. The primary tumor was located in the skin. (Plate III-A from Fascicle 4, Second Series.)

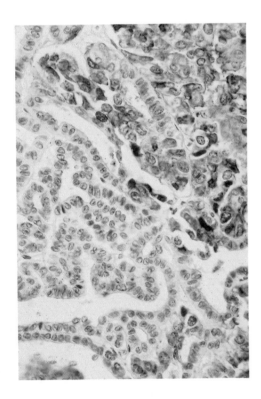

B. BREAST CARCINOMA METASTATIC TO A PAPILLARY THYROID CARCINOMA

The metastatic carcinoma is positive for EMA, whereas the papillary carcinoma is completely negative for this marker.

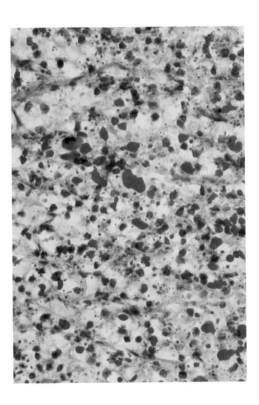

C. RENAL CELL CARCINOMA METASTATIC TO THYROID

There is strong Oil Red O positivity, indicative of neutral fat in the cytoplasm.

PLATE XL

A. RENAL CELL CARCINOMA METASTATIC TO THYROID

Some of the thyroglobulin from the entrapped follicles located in the upper left field has diffused out and been nonspecifically absorbed by the adjacent tumor cells, which have thus acquired an apparent positivity for this marker.

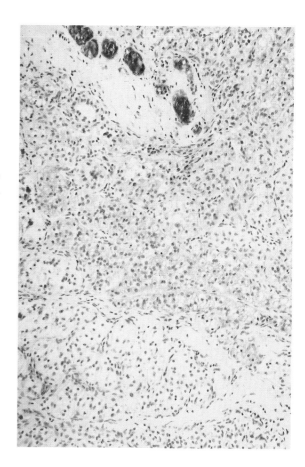

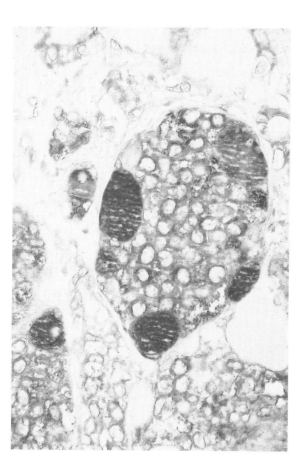

B. MAMMARY LOBULAR CARCINOMA METASTATIC TO THYROID

There is strong positivity for thyroglobulin in the entrapped thyroid and in many of the tumor cells, probably resulting from diffusion of the marker. This artifactual staining may result in a mistaken diagnosis of primary thyroid carcinoma.

REFERENCES

1. Carcangiu ML, Sibley RK, Rosai J. Clear cell change in primary thyroid tumors. A study of 38 cases. Am J Surg Pathol 1985;9:705–22.
2. Czech JM, Lichtor TR, Carney JA, van Heerden JA. Neoplasms metastatic to the thyroid gland. Surg Gynecol Obstet 1982;155:503–5.
3. Elliott RH Jr, Kneeland Frantz V. Metastatic carcinoma masquerading as primary thyroid cancer: a report of authors' 14 cases. Ann Surg 1960;151:551–61.
4. Green LK, Ro JY, Mackay B, Ayala AG, Luna MA. Renal cell carcinoma metastatic to the thyroid. Cancer 1989;63:1810–5.
5. Harrison DF. Thyroid gland in the management of laryngopharyngeal cancer. Arch Otolaryngol 1973;97:301–2.
6. Ivy HK. Cancer metastatic to the thyroid: a diagnostic problem. Mayo Clin Proc 1984;59:856–9.
7. McCabe DP, Farrar WB, Petkov TM, Finkelmeier W, O'Dwyer P, James A. Clinical and pathologic correlations in disease metastatic to the thyroid gland. Am J Surg 1985;150:519–23.
8. Mizukami Y, Saito K, Nonomura A, et al. Lung carcinoma metastatic to microfollicular adenoma of the thyroid. A case report. Acta Pathol Jpn 1990;40:602–8.
9. Nesland JM, Sobrinho-Simões MA, Holm R, Johannessen JV. Organoid tumor in the thyroid gland. Ultrastruct Pathol 1985;9:65–70.
10. Rigaud C, Bogomoletz WV, Delisle MJ, Diebold MD, Caulet T. Metastatic cancers of the thyroid gland. Diagnostic difficulties. Bull Cancer (Paris) 1987;74:117–27.
11. Shimaoka K, Sokal JE, Pickren JW. Metastatic neoplasms in the thyroid. Cancer 1962;15:557–65.
12. Tibaldi JM, Shapiro LE, Mahadevia PS. Thyroiditis mimicked by metastatic carcinoma to the thyroid [Letter]. Mayo Clin Proc 1986;61:399–400.
13. Wychulis AR, Beahrs OH, Woolner LB. Metastases of carcinoma to the thyroid gland. Ann Surg 1964;160:169–77.

TUMOR-LIKE CONDITIONS

Listed in this section is a heterogeneous group of non-neoplastic thyroid disorders that can simulate a neoplastic process at a gross or microscopic level. Some aspects of some of these conditions have already been discussed in other chapters.

NODULAR HYPERPLASIA

Nodular hyperplasia (nodular or multinodular goiter, adenomatoid goiter, adenomatous hyperplasia) is a common thyroid disease. The form known as endemic goiter is due to low iodine content of the water and soil, and it can be largely prevented by adding iodine to common salt. The deficiency in thyroid hormone production induced by the iodine deficiency leads to an increase in thyroid-stimulating hormone secretion, which results initially in a hyperplastic gland with tall follicular epithelium and small amounts of colloid *(parenchymatous goiter)* and later in follicular atrophy with abundant storage of colloid *(colloid goiter)*.

The form known as sporadic nodular goiter is by far the most common seen in the United States. Some cases are associated with lymphocytic or Hashimoto thyroiditis and can be viewed as the nodular forms of these immune-mediated inflammatory diseases. The incidence in the general adult population is 3 to 5 percent clinically and about 50 percent at autopsy (2,4). Thyroid growth-stimulating immunoglobulins have been implied in its pathogenesis. These have been found in some series in up to 70 percent of the cases (3,5).

Clinically, most patients are euthyroid and present with a multinodular gland that may become very large, cause tracheal obstruction, and produce considerable disfigurement. In cases with a single, firm, dominant nodule, the clinical distinction from a true neoplasm may become impossible. Hemorrhage within a nodule can cause sudden enlargement and pain. Cases associated with hyperfunction are referred to as *toxic nodular hyperplasia*. Some cases of thyroid nodular hyperplasia are located substernally and enter in the differential diagnosis with superior mediastinal tumors.

At the gross level, the thyroid is enlarged and its shape is distorted; one lobe may be larger than the other (fig. 267). Cases weighing over 2000 g have been recorded. The thyroid capsule may be stretched but is intact. On cross section, multiple nodules are seen, some partially encapsulated. Secondary changes in the form of hemorrhage, calcification, and cystic degeneration are common (pl. XLI-A; figs. 268, 269). Microscopically, there is a wide range of appearances. Some nodules are composed of very dilated follicles lined

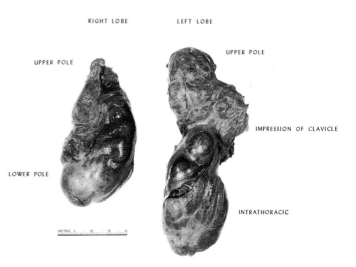

Figure 267
NODULAR HYPERPLASIA
This gross specimen of nodular hyperplasia shows intrathoracic extension and characteristic bilateral nodularity. Asymmetrical enlargement is the rule in this disorder. (Fig. 21 from Fascicle 4, Second Series.)

297

by flattened epithelium, others are extremely cellular, and still others are composed predominantly or exclusively of oncocytes or clear cells (fig. 270). Some of the dilated follicles have a conglomerate of small active follicles at one pole "Sanderson polsters" (fig. 271). Rupture of follicles may lead to a granulomatous reaction to the colloid, with appearance of histiocytes and foreign-body–type giant cells. Areas of fresh and old hemorrhage, coarse fibrous trabeculation, and foci of calcification are common. Occasionally, osseous metaplasia is seen. Greatly thickened vessels with calcified media may be present at the periphery. A variable number of chronic inflammatory cells are present in the stroma in many of the cases, indicating the existence of a coexisting chronic thyroiditis. It has been noted that autolytic changes occur more rapidly in hyperplastic than in normal glands. In rare cases, the follicular cells may exhibit clear cell changes (fig. 272), and the stroma may undergo focal adipose metaplasia (fig. 273).

Nodular hyperplasia can simulate malignancy via several mechanisms, i.e., hypercellularity of some of the nodules, focal presence of vesicular (ground-glass–like) nuclei, occurrence of papillary formations, and development of parasitic nodules (see page 320). The papillae that can be seen in this condition tend to be located within cystically dilated follicles, their tips pointing toward the center of that follicle. As with the papillae accompanying diffuse hyperplasia, they are characteristically lined by a columnar or tall cuboidal epithelium with basally located nuclei that lack the features of those of papillary carcinoma (figs. 274–276). Furthermore, it has been shown that the apical surface of the benign papillae of nodular hyperplasia stain slightly or not at all with Alcian blue or epithelial membrane antigen (EMA), whereas that in the papillae of papillary carcinoma usually reacts strongly (1). The criteria for distinguishing nodular hyperplasia from follicular adenoma are discussed on page 30.

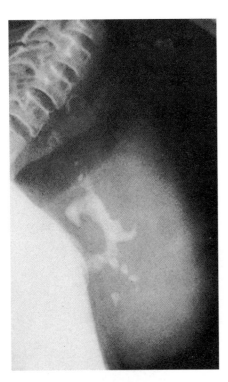

Figure 268
NODULAR HYPERPLASIA
This X-ray view of a large nodular hyperplasia shows central calcification secondary to regressive changes. (Fig. 24 from Fascicle 4, Second Series.)

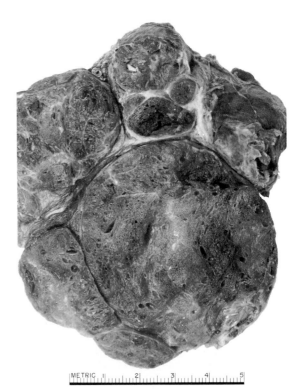

Figure 269
NODULAR HYPERPLASIA
This cut surface of a thyroid gland with nodular hyperplasia shows numerous poorly circumscribed nodules of various sizes. (Fig. 22 from Fascicle 4, Second Series.)

298

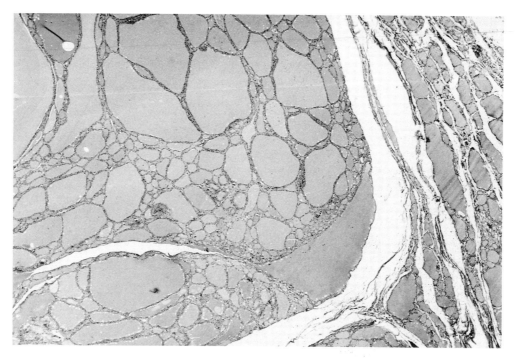

Figure 270
NODULAR HYPERPLASIA
At low magnification, this hyperplastic nodule contains variously sized but predominantly large follicles. There is no capsule separating it from the rest of the gland.

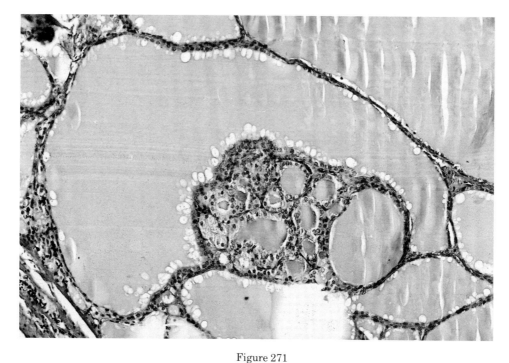

Figure 271
"SANDERSON POLSTER" IN NODULAR HYPERPLASIA
This structure is formed by a cluster of small follicles protruding into a large dilated follicle. The polster is covered by columnar epithelium. There are numerous reabsorption vacuoles.

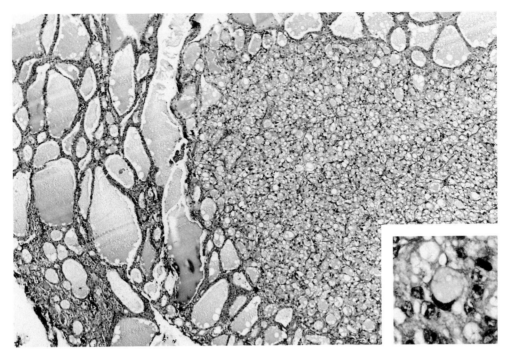

Figure 272
NODULAR HYPERPLASIA
This illustration shows nodular hyperplasia with a hypercellular focus exhibiting clear cell changes.
The inset shows the signet-ring configuration of some of the clear cells.

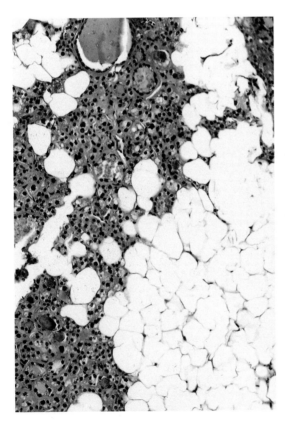

Figure 273
NODULAR HYPERPLASIA
In this case of nodular hyperplasia adipose
metaplasia of the stroma can be seen.

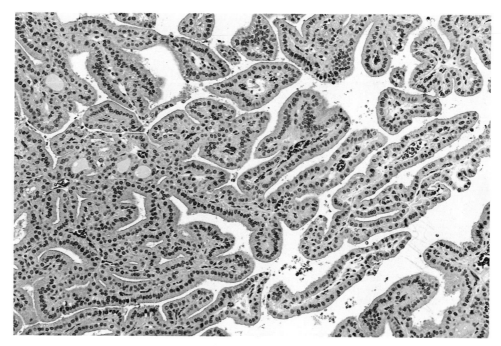

Figure 274
(Figures 274 and 275 are from the same patient)
DIFFUSE HYPERPLASIA
This example of diffuse hyperplasia (Graves disease) shows a markedly hyperplastic nodule that features well-developed papillae.

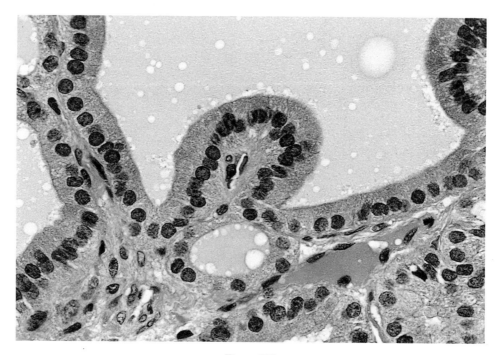

Figure 275
DIFFUSE HYPERPLASIA
In this high magnification of the case in figure 274, the follicular cells lining the papillae are tall columnar. The nuclei are basally located, small, and hyperchromatic.

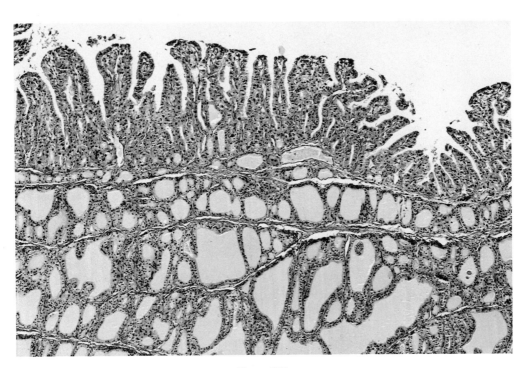

Figure 276

PAPILLARY AREA IN NODULAR HYPERPLASIA

The papillae face the center of a cystically dilated cavity. The nuclear changes of papillary carcinoma are absent.

DIFFUSE HYPERPLASIA

The diffusely hyperplastic gland of Graves disease may simulate malignancy on three grounds: 1) through the presence of well-developed papillary formations, 2) through the occurrence of large vesicular nuclei in the follicular epithelium, and 3) through the occasional extension of the hyperplastic process outside the confines of the thyroid gland. The nuclear clearing is not nearly as well developed as that seen in papillary carcinoma and is even less pronounced than that sometimes associated with Hashimoto thyroiditis. The benign nature of the papillary formations can be recognized because of their widespread occurrence in relation to clearly hyperplastic follicles, lack of fibrous stromal response, and the fact that they are usually lined by columnar follicular cells with basally located normo- or hyperchromatic nuclei.

In some cases of Graves disease, the follicular cells can proliferate into the adjacent perithyroid soft tissue. Perhaps this represents not invasion from the thyroid gland itself but rather concom-itant hyperplasia of preexisting thyroid follicles embedded in the skeletal muscle of the neck, a microscopic finding often seen in normal individuals (6). Whatever the mechanism, infiltration of skeletal muscle fibers by this highly cellular thyroid tissue may result in a mistaken diagnosis of malignancy (fig. 277). If the patient's hyperthyroid status is known and it is realized that the morphologic changes in the extrathyroid tissue are those of diffuse hyperplasia (and therefore not different from those present inside the gland) this error should be avoidable. It should also be remembered that striated muscle is occasionally included within the normal thyroid gland (see page 6).

DYSHORMONOGENETIC GOITER

This group of genetically determined thyroid hyperplasias result from the lack of one or another of the enzymes involved in the synthesis of thyroid hormones. The absence of feedback to the pituitary gland leads to a continuous hypersecretion of thyroid-stimulating hormone

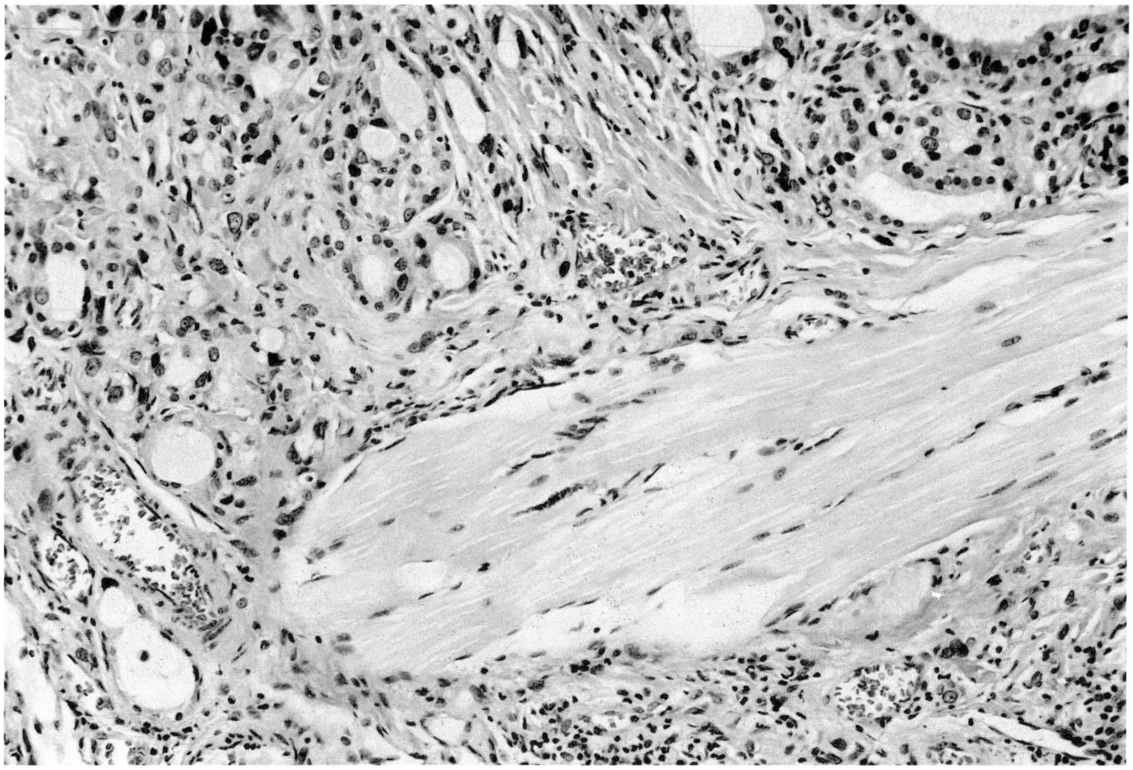

Figure 277
DIFFUSE HYPERPLASIA
Hyperplastic small follicles and skeletal muscle are closely intermingled in this case of Graves disease. This should not be interpreted as a sign of malignancy.

and a markedly hyperactive thyroid gland (pl. XLI-B). The hypercellularity can be extreme and is often accompanied by bizarre (large, hyperchromatic, and/or misshapen) nuclear forms (figs. 278, 279). Encapsulated nodules may develop, and the capsule may appear focally violated by the hyperplastic process (fig. 280) (9–11).

It should be apparent from this description that to make a diagnosis of malignancy developing against such a background is a difficult task, to the point that some observers have stated that it can only be made if metastases have occurred. We regard this position as unreasonably restrictive and have made a diagnosis of malignancy (particularly of papillary carcinoma) if the required cytoarchitectural features of this entity are present (see page 49) (7,12). In any event, well-documented cases associated with distant metastases are on record (8).

HASHIMOTO THYROIDITIS

Hashimoto disease usually presents as a bilateral diffuse enlargement of the gland (pl. XLI-C). It can simulate a malignant thyroid neoplasm on several grounds. The nuclei of scattered oncocytic follicular cells may show marked enlargement, hyperchromasia, and abnormal shape, a feature that they share with oncocytes of several other organs and that is not to be taken as a sign of malignancy or even of neoplastic transformation. Conversely, these nuclei may be vesicular and slightly overlapping, their appearance thus approaching that of the ground-glass nuclei of papillary carcinoma (fig. 281).

Papillary formations may appear in Hashimoto thyroiditis when the disease is associated with the changes of diffuse hyperplasia ("Hashitoxicosis") or nodular hyperplasia (nodular Hashimoto

Tumors of

(figs. 284, 285) (17,18). It should be distinguished from the spindle cell type of undifferentiated (anaplastic) carcinoma, which exhibits obvious cytologic atypia, high mitotic rate, and necrosis; from the desmoplastic reaction that may accompany papillary carcinoma, which in some instances may be extremely florid and acquire a nodular fasciitis-like quality (16); and from large cell malignant lymphoma with sclerosis.

We have seen several cases of a thyroid disorder characterized by innumerable microscopic foci of stellate-shaped fibrosis composed of cellular fibroblastic tissue that may entrap a few thyroid follicles in the center. At low magnification, the individual lesions appear similar to the form of papillary carcinoma classically known as occult sclerosing carcinoma and recently renamed papillary microcarcinoma (see page 96), from which it is distinguished by the absence of cytoarchitectural features of papillary carcinoma in the epithelial component, if such a component is present (figs. 286–288). Furthermore, although a given thyroid gland may harbor more than one papillary microcarcinoma, we are not aware of the latter condition ever presenting in the widespread fashion that characterizes this entity.

The etiology and pathogenesis of this process are not known. The appearance is suggestive of a multifocal injury that has led to follicular loss and replacement by a scar-like tissue. It is possible that the process is of inflammatory nature, in which case a term such as *multifocal fibrosing thyroiditis* may be justified.

MALAKOPLAKIA

Malakoplakia has been described as involving the thyroid gland and mimicking a malignant neoplasm clinically (19). The disease is recognized by the presence of an inflammatory infiltrate rich in histiocytes, some of which contain Michaelis-Guttmann bodies.

RADIATION CHANGES

Exposure of the thyroid gland to external radiation, whether accidental or therapeutic, is known to result in a variety of morphologic alterations. It has been estimated that low-dose radiation (<1500 rads), which has been used in the past for a variety of benign conditions, has a marked potential for inducing thyroid alterations

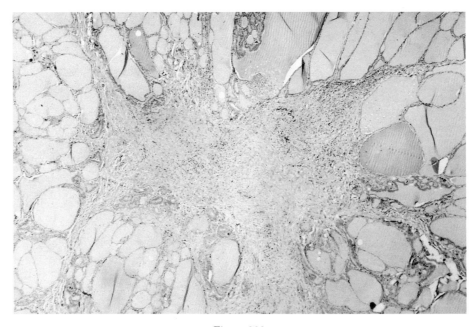

Figure 286
(Figures 286 and 287 are from the same patient)
MULTIFOCAL FIBROSING THYROIDITIS
The stellate appearance of the scar closely resembles that seen in papillary microcarcinoma.

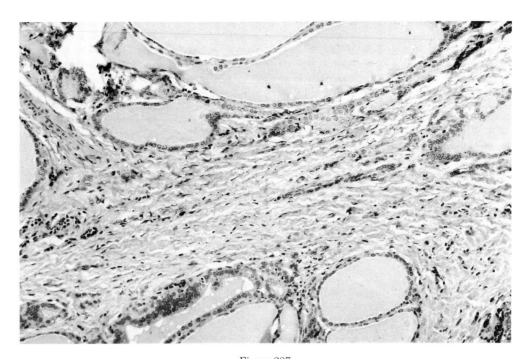

Figure 287
MULTIFOCAL FIBROSING THYROIDITIS
In a closer view of the case in figure 286, the follicles within the scar are irregularly shaped, but they lack the cytoarchitectural features of papillary carcinoma.

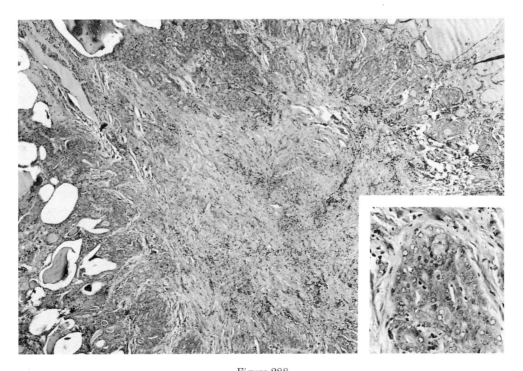

Figure 288
PAPILLARY MICROCARCINOMA
This papillary microcarcinoma is shown for comparison. Its appearance at low magnification is similar to that of multifocal fibrosing thyroiditis, but examination at high magnification shows typical features of papillary carcinoma at the periphery (inset).

on a long-term basis. The most common abnormality is nodular hyperplasia, which reached 16.5 percent in one population (21). It has been shown that similar changes can occur after high-dose irradiation, such as that administered for Hodgkin disease (20). In both instances, the hyperplastic nodules can be extremely hypercellular and exhibit marked cytologic atypia, characterized by nuclear enlargement, vesicular changes with nucleolar prominence, nuclear crowding, and hyperchromasia (fig. 289). It is typical for this atypia to be distributed in a random fashion within the various nodules. The combination of radiation-induced nuclear atypia and papillary hyperplastic changes can result in a very disturbing microscopic picture (fig. 290). Other abnormalities often seen in these glands include fibrosis, hyalinization, and chronic inflammation.

Systemic administration of radioactive iodine for therapeutic purposes can induce changes of similar type but usually of much lesser degree (22). Whether this therapy results in an increased incidence of malignancy in the thyroid or other sites remains to be established.

AMYLOID GOITER

Amyloid goiter is the term given to the form of thyroid amyloidosis accompanied by clinical enlargement of the gland (pl. XLII-A). It may be unilateral or bilateral, and it is commonly associated with a foreign-body–type giant cell reaction. In most cases, the disease is accompanied by amyloid deposition in other organs.

Microscopically, the amyloid deposits are in the vessel walls and other interfollicular (particularly perifollicular) sites, sometimes massively and diffusely (fig. 291). They are often accompanied by the presence of mature adipose tissue. The ultrastructural appearance and histochemical reactivity are typical of amyloid in general (pl. XLII-B). The amyloid being deposited is of AA type (24). The differential diagnosis includes amyloid deposition in medullary carcinoma, amyloidosis associated with multiple myeloma (in which the amyloid is of AL type) (23), and conditions resulting in heavy hyalinization (such as hyalinizing trabecular adenoma) (see page 31).

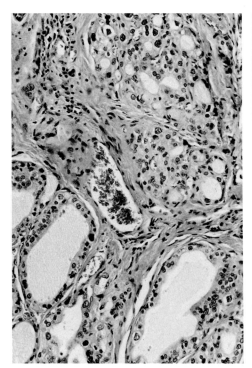 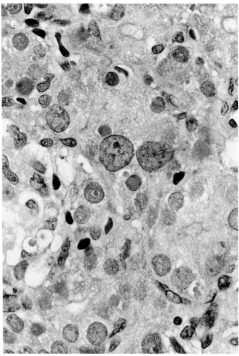

Figure 289
RADIATION CHANGES
Bizarre nuclear changes after radiation therapy are seen in this hyperplastic thyroid.

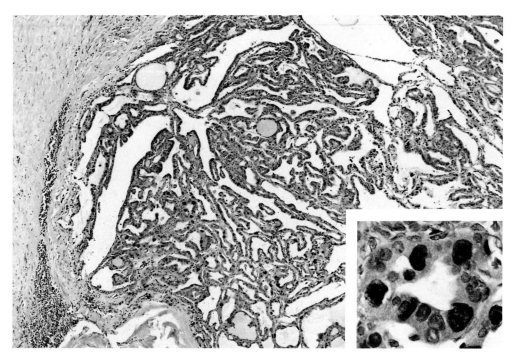

Figure 290
RADIATION CHANGES
This illustration shows papillary changes and marked nuclear atypicality in a case of hyperplastic thyroid after radiation treatment.

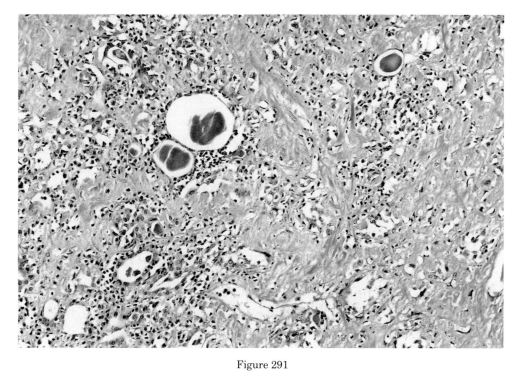

Figure 291
LOCALIZED AMYLOIDOSIS OF THE THYROID
Amyloid material accompanied by inflammatory cells permeates the stroma and surrounds atrophic follicles.

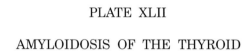

PLATE XLII

AMYLOIDOSIS OF THE THYROID

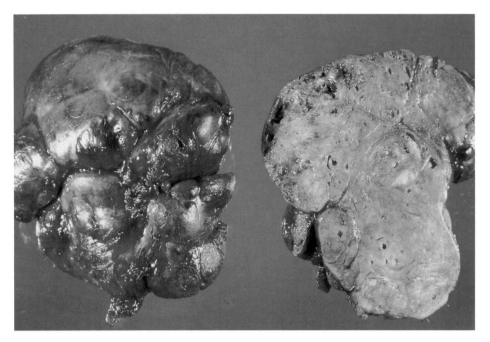

A. This illustration shows the outer aspect and cut surface of localized amyloidosis of the thyroid gland (amyloid tumor). The gland is enlarged and bosselated and exhibits a salmon color on cross section.

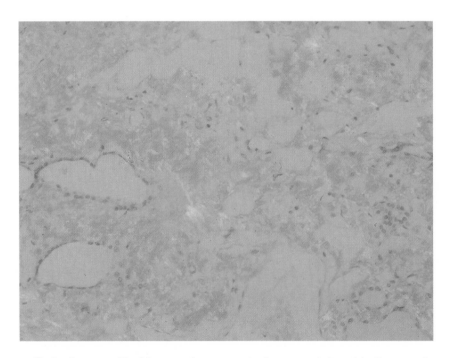

B. Apple green birefringence is apparent when examining this Congo red–stained slide of amyloidosis of the thyroid under polarized light.

HISTIOCYTOSIS X

Histiocytosis X (eosinophilic granuloma, Langerhans cell histiocytosis) involves the thyroid gland exceptionally (28). One such case, apparently limited to the gland, was initially misdiagnosed as a malignancy (25). Two other cases were seen in association with papillary carcinoma (26,27), and we have seen two cases associated with Hashimoto thyroiditis. The microscopic features are similar to those seen elsewhere, and the diagnosis rests on the identification of Langerhans cells against the appropriate background.

SINUS HISTIOCYTOSIS WITH MASSIVE LYMPHADENOPATHY

Two cases of thyroid involvement by sinus histiocytosis with massive lymphadenopathy (Rosai-Dorfman disease) have been reported. In one, this was thought to probably represent secondary extension from adjacent lymph nodes (29). In the other, the involved thyroid was moderately and diffusely enlarged and markedly tender, resulting in a clinical picture simulating subacute thyroiditis (30).

PLASMA CELL GRANULOMA

Plasma cell granuloma is the term used for a tumor-like condition of inflammatory nature and unknown etiology in which plasma cells predominate. As in other organs in which this process occurs (e.g., lung or oral cavity), it is distinguished from plasmacytoma by the mature appearance of all the plasma cells, the presence of Russell bodies (sometimes in large numbers), the admixture with other inflammatory cells, the conspicuous fibrosis, and, most important, the demonstration of light-chain polyclonality on immunohistochemical evaluation (31,33). The case reported by Mizukama and coworkers (32) as pseudolymphoma of the thyroid may be viewed as the expression of a pathogenetically similar phenomenon.

REFERENCES

Nodular Hyperplasia

1. Damiani S, Fratamico F, Lapertosa G, Dina R, Eusebi V. Alcian blue and epithelial membrane antigen are useful markers in differentiating benign from malignant papillae in thyroid. Virchows Arch [A] 1991;419: 131–5.
2. Mortensen JD, Woolner LB, Bennett WA. Gross and microscopic findings in clinically normal thyroid glands. J Clin Endocrinol Metab 1955;15:1270–80.
3. Smyth PA, Smith DF, McKenna TJ. Studies on the natural history of toxic nodular goitre. In: Drexhage HA, Wiersinga WM, eds. The thyroid and autoimmunity: Proceedings of the international symposium on thyroid and autoimmunity, Amsterdam, 19-21 March 1986. Excerpta Medica International Congress Series no. 711. Amsterdam: Elsevier, 1986:227–8.
4. Tunbridge WM, Evered DC, Hall R, et al. The spectrum of thyroid disease in a community: the Whickham survey. Clin Endocrinol (Oxf) 1977;7:481–93.
5. van der Gaag RD, Drexhage HA, Wiersinga WM, et al. Further studies on thyroid growth-stimulating immunoglobulins in euthyroid nonendemic goiter. J Clin Endocrinol Metab 1985;60:972–9.

Diffuse Hyperplasia

6. Hanson GA, Komorowski RA, Cerletty JM, Wilson SD. Thyroid gland morphology in young adults: normal subjects versus those with prior low-dose neck irradiation in childhood. Surgery 1983;94:984–8.

Dyshormonogenetic Goiter

7. Abs R, Verhelst J, Schoofs E, De Somer E. Hyperfunctioning metastatic follicular thyroid carcinoma in Pendred's syndrome. Cancer 1991;67:2191–3.
8. Cooper DS, Axelrod L, DeGroot LJ, Vickery AL Jr, Maloof F. Congenital goiter and the development of metastatic follicular carcinoma with evidence for a leak of nonhormonal iodide: clinical, pathological, kinetic, and biochemical studies and a review of the literature. J Clin Endocrinol Metab 1981;52:294–306.
9. Kennedy JS. The pathology of dyshormonogenetic goitre. J Pathol 1969;99:251–64.
10. Milles G. Structural features of goiters in sporadic cretins. Am J Pathol 1955;31:997–1003.
11. Smith JF. The pathology of the thyroid in the syndrome of sporadic goitre and congenital deafness. Q J Med New Series 1960;29:297–303.
12. Vickery AL Jr. The diagnosis of malignancy in dyshormonogenetic goiter. Clin Endocrinol Metab 1981;10:317–35.

Hashimoto Thyroiditis

13. Chan JK, Albores-Saavedra J, Battifora H, Carcangiu ML, Rosai J. Sclerosing mucoepidermoid carcinoma with eosinophilia. A distinctive low-grade thyroid malignancy arising from the metaplastic follicles of Hashimoto's thyroiditis. Am J Surg Pathol 1991;15: 438–48.
14. Louis DN, Vickery AL Jr, Rosai J, Wang CA. Multiple branchial cleft-like cysts in Hashimoto's thyroiditis. Am J Surg Pathol 1989;13:45–9.

15. Vollenweider I, Hedinger C. Solid cell nests (SCN) in Hashimoto's thyroiditis. Virchows Arch [A] 1988;412: 357–63.

Other Forms of Thyroiditis

16. Chan JK, Carcangiu ML, Rosai J. Papillary carcinoma of thyroid with exuberant nodular fasciitis-like stroma. Report of three cases. Am J Clin Pathol 1991;95:309–14.
17. Harach HR, Williams ED. Fibrous thyroiditis—an immunopathological study. Histopathology 1983;7:739–51.
18. Schwaegerle SM, Bauer TW, Esselstyn CB Jr. Riedel's thyroiditis. Am J Clin Pathol 1988;90:715–22.

Malakoplakia

19. Katoh R, Ishizaki T, Tomichi N, Yagawa K, Kurihara H. Malacoplakia of the thyroid gland. Am J Clin Pathol 1989;92:813–20.

Radiation Changes

20. Carr RF, LiVolsi VA. Morphologic changes in the thyroid after irradiation for Hodgkin's and non-Hodgkin's lymphoma. Cancer 1989;64:825–9.
21. Favus MJ, Schneider AB, Stachura ME, et al. Thyroid cancer occurring as a late consequence of head-and-neck irradiation. N Engl J Med 1976;294:1019–25.
22. Kennedy JS, Thomson JA. The changes in the thyroid gland after irradiation with ^{131}I or partial thyroidectomy for thyrotoxicosis. J Pathol 1974;112:65–81.

Amyloid Goiter

23. Hirota S, Miyamoto M, Kasugai T, Kitamura Y, Morimura Y. Crystalline light-chain deposition and amyloidosis in the thyroid gland and kidneys of a patient with myeloma. Arch Pathol Lab Med 1990;114:429–31.

24. Kanoh T, Shimada H, Uchino H, Matsumura K. Amyloid goiter with hypothyroidism. Arch Pathol Lab Med 1989;113:542–4.

Histiocytosis X

25. Coode PE, Shaikh MU. Histiocytosis X of the thyroid masquerading as thyroid carcinoma. Hum Pathol 1988; 19:239–41.
26. Goldstein N, Layfield LJ. Thyromegaly secondary to simultaneous papillary carcinoma and histiocytosis X. Acta Cytol 1991;35:422–6.
27. Schofield JB, Alsanjari NA, Davis J, Maclennan KA. Eosinophilic granuloma of lymph nodes associated with metastatic papillary carcinoma of the thyroid. Histopathology 1992;20:181–3.
28. Teja K, Sabio H, Langdon DR, Johanson AJ. Involvement of the thyroid gland in histiocytosis X. Hum Pathol 1981;12:1137–9.

Sinus Histiocytosis with Massive Lymphadenopathy

29. Carpenter RJ III, Banks PM, McDonald RJ, Sanderson DR. Sinus histiocytosis with massive lymphadenopathy (Rosai-Dorfman disease): report of a case with respiratory tract involvement. Laryngoscope 1978;88:1963–9.
30. Larkin DF, Dervan PA, Munnelly J, Finucane J. Sinus histiocytosis with massive lymphadenopathy simulating subacute thyroiditis. Hum Pathol 1986;17:321–4.

Plasma Cell Granuloma

31. Holck S. Plasma cell granuloma of the thyroid. Cancer 1981;48:830–2.
32. Mizukami Y, Ikuta N, Hashimoto T, et al. Pseudolymphoma of the thyroid. Acta Pathol Jpn 1988;38:1329–36.
33. Yapp R, Linder J, Schenken JR, Karrer FW. Plasma cell granuloma of the thyroid. Hum Pathol 1985;16:848–50.

THYROID TISSUE IN ABNORMAL LOCATIONS

There are several situations in which benign thyroid tissue can be found outside the anatomic confines of and separate from the thyroid gland It is important to be aware of them to avoid an overdiagnosis of metastatic thyroid carcinoma.

ECTOPIA

A migration failure along the pathway of the thyroglossal duct (see page 1) can result in the presence of ectopic thyroid tissue anywhere between the foramen caecum at the base of the tongue and the site of the normal gland (fig. 292) (1,7,13). The most common sites are 1) at the base of the tongue (lingual thyroid), 2) beneath the tongue (sublingual thyroid), and 3) in or around the hyoid bone (as a component of thyroglossal duct cyst). On occasion, the opposite phenomenon occurs, in which the thyroglossal duct migrates excessively, resulting in a mediastinal thyroid. It is likely, however, that most substernal glands with features of nodular hyperplasia were once in the normal cervical position and were pulled down by the hyperplastic nodular transformation that occurred in them.

Lingual thyroid is rare as a clinical problem but relatively common as an incidental microscopic finding. In one series, almost 10 percent of tongues examined at autopsy had remnants of thyroid tissue in them (2). When voluminous, lingual thyroid may result in dysphagia, bleeding, and severe respiratory distress (13,20). In most instances, the diagnosis is made during adolescence, and a preponderance in women has been noted (2,10,16). In over 75 percent of the cases, the migration failure is total, in the sense that no thyroid tissue is present in the normal location; however, some follicles may be found in the hyoid region (16,27,28).

Microscopically, the ectopic thyroid follicles usually have a normal appearance, but the irregular interface with the surrounding skeletal muscle fibers and the hypercellularity may result in a pseudomalignant appearance (fig. 293) (30). True malignancy arising in lingual thyroid is rare. About 25 cases have been reported, but not all of them are convincing (6,16,24).

Thyroglossal duct cyst is nearly always connected with the hyoid bone (1). Upward movement of the mass on swallowing is characteristic of this condition. Most cysts measure from 1 to 2 cm in diameter (fig. 294). The original lining epithelium of the duct is cuboidal ("transitional") or columnar and often ciliated. However, it tends to become squamous or to disappear altogether as a result of secondary inflammatory changes (fig. 295) (26). Thyroid tissue is found in the wall in over half of the cases, usually in the form of irregular aggregates.

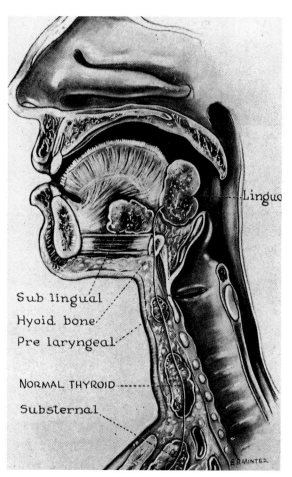

Figure 292
SITES OF THYROID ECTOPIA
This diagram shows the most common sites of thyroid ectopia. (Fig. 1 from Lemmon WT, Paschal GW Jr. Lingual thyroid. Am J Surg 1941;52:82–85.)

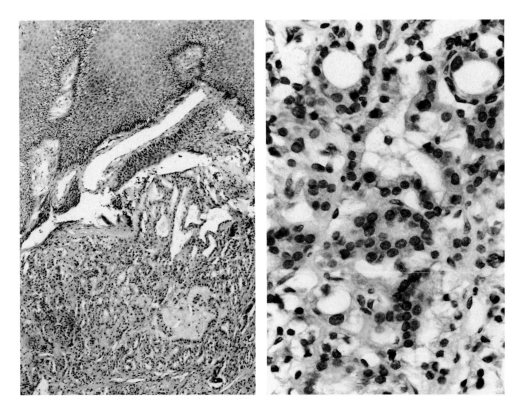

Figure 293
LINGUAL THYROID
The ectopic thyroid tissue is located beneath the squamous epithelium of the tongue. At high magnification, it has a hypercellular appearance and microfollicular pattern that may result in a mistaken diagnosis of malignancy. Radioiodine scan in this case showed absence of thyroid in its normal location in the neck.

The treatment of thyroglossal duct cyst is surgical. It includes the removal of the middle third of the hyoid bone and the suprahyoid tract up to the foramen cecum (25). This extended operation will prevent most recurrences of this condition, although a few will still develop (5).

The thyroid tissue in thyroglossal duct cyst may have a normal appearance, it may exhibit inflammatory or hyperplastic nodular changes, or it may be the site of a malignancy (fig. 296). The latter event is an unusual but well-documented complication of this condition. Nearly all of the reported cases have been papillary carcinomas, but there are scattered reports of other tumor types, including follicular carcinoma and undifferentiated and/or squamous carcinoma (8,9,14,15,17,22,29). The outstanding exception is medullary carcinoma, and this can be explained by the fact that C cells have a different embryologic source. The papillary carcinoma arising in a thyroglossal duct cyst is morphologically

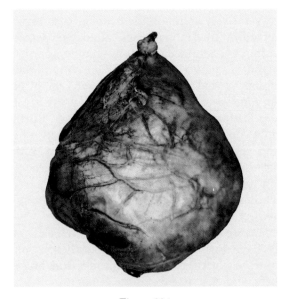

Figure 294
THYROGLOSSAL DUCT CYST
Typical gross appearance of a thyroglossal duct cyst.
(Fig. 1 from Fascicle 14, First Series.)

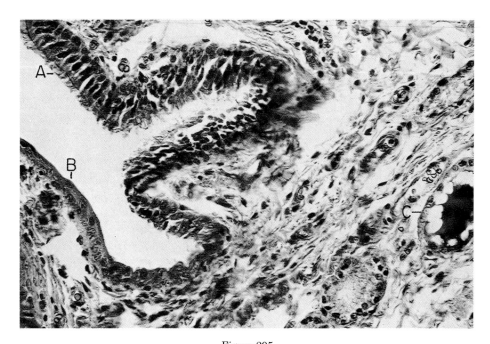

Figure 295
THYROGLOSSAL DUCT CYST
Microscopic examination of a thyroglossal duct cyst reveals that the lining is composed of ciliated epithelium (A) and stratified squamous epithelium (B). Thyroid follicles are present in the wall (C). (Fig. 20 from Fascicle 4, Second Series.)

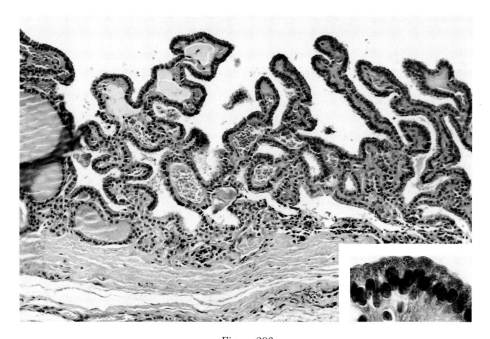

Figure 296
PAPILLARY CHANGES IN NODULAR HYPERPLASIA OCCURRING
IN A THYROGLOSSAL DUCT CYST
The papillae face the lumen of the cyst. The inset shows the columnar shape of the cells and the basal location of the hyperchromatic nuclei.

identical to its homologue in the orthotopic gland, and its behavior is similar. Removal of the cyst containing the tumor is usually curative. The possibility of an independent papillary carcinoma in the thyroid itself is remote, and there is therefore no need for a prophylactic thyroidectomy if the gland is normal on palpation and scintigraphic examination.

It should be noted that all instances of ectopic thyroid related to the thyroglossal duct appear as midline lesions, in keeping with the path of descent of this embryologic structure. Thyroid tissue located laterally in the neck may still be of benign nature but cannot be ascribed to the developmental abnormality discussed here.

Other sites of ectopic thyroid tissue have been documented. They include larynx, trachea, aortic arch, heart and pericardium, mediastinal esophagus, diaphragm, gallbladder, common bile duct, retroperitoneum, vagina, sella turcica, and inguinal region (3,4,11,12,18,19,21). There is also a report of ectopic thyroid tissue in the lung, but it is difficult to rule out the alternative possibility of a well-differentiated metastasis, in view of the fact that the patient had a small carcinoma within the thyroid gland itself (23).

MECHANICAL IMPLANTATION

Normal or abnormal thyroid tissue disrupted mechanically from the main gland can lodge in the soft tissues of the neck, survive, and thereby result in the formation of a discrete nodule, usually of microscopic size. The most common mechanism for this event is a previous operation. In such instance, the implanted thyroid tissue is likely to be surrounded by a fibrous reaction, and suture material may be detected nearby (31–33).

Implantation of thyroid tissue can also be the result of accidental trauma. We know of a patient with a thyroid adenoma who had a crush injury to the neck. Months later, an operation disclosed numerous little nodules of adenomatous thyroid tissue scattered throughout the region (Williams ED, personal communication). The event seems analogous to that referred to in the spleen as splenosis, and it may therefore be designated thyroidosis.

PARASITIC NODULE

A parasitic sequestered nodule represents the focal expression of a nodular hyperplasia (adenomatoid goiter) in which one of the most peripherally located nodules is anatomically separate from the main gland, or so it appears to the surgeon (figs. 297, 298). It is a much more common process than suggested by the meager number of reports on the subject (35,36). Many pathologists and surgeons do not know of its existence and, as a result, often label a perfectly innocuous condition as malignant. Many of the cases labeled *aberrant lateral thyroid* in the past are examples of parasitic nodules. Others represent metastatic well-differentiated carcinoma in a cervical lymph node (see page 323). The parasitic nodule is probably the result of nodular enlargement of thyroid tissue located outside the capsule of the gland, a relatively common microscopic finding in normal glands (34).

At the time of surgery, a thin pedicle may be found in some cases, joining the nodule to the thyroid. In other cases, the original connection with the main organ may have been lost, and a new vascular supply may have been acquired. Whatever the situation, the result is a detached thyroid nodule. The clue to the diagnosis is provided by the fact that the microscopic appearance is that of a benign hyperplastic process throughout and that the orthotopic gland, if it has been removed or sampled, shows similar morphologic features. No lymph node remnants should be found around the nodule, which should also be devoid of any of the cytoarchitectural features that characterize conventional papillary carcinoma or its follicular variant.

A particularly treacherous variant of this phenomenon occurs when the parasitic nodule is seen in the context of a nodular Hashimoto thyroiditis. In such a case, the nodule is likely to feature a prominent lymphoid component that may simulate residual lymph node and the nuclear features that often accompany Hashimoto thyroiditis, such as partial nuclear clearing or the opposite phenomenon of bizarre hyperchromatic nuclei. Here, too, comparison with the orthotopic gland and realization that the changes present in it are the same as those in the nodule should lead to a correct interpretation of the lesion (figs. 299, 300).

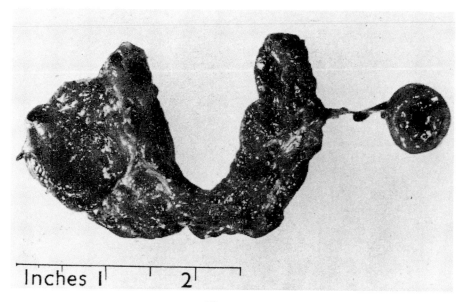

Figure 297
PARASITIC NODULE
As seen in this gross view, the nodule is connected to the thyroid gland by a thin, fibrous strand.
(Fig. 6 from Sisson JC, Schmidt RW, Beierwaltes WH. Sequestered nodular goiter. N Engl J Med
1964;270:927–32.)

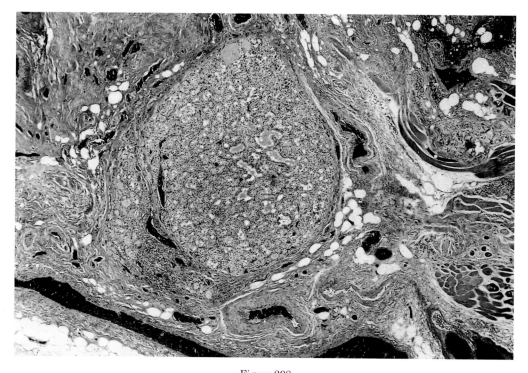

Figure 298
PARASITIC NODULE IN NODULAR HYPERPLASIA
The small hyperplastic nodule is surrounded by fibroadipose tissue and muscle and is anatomically
separate from the thyroid gland.

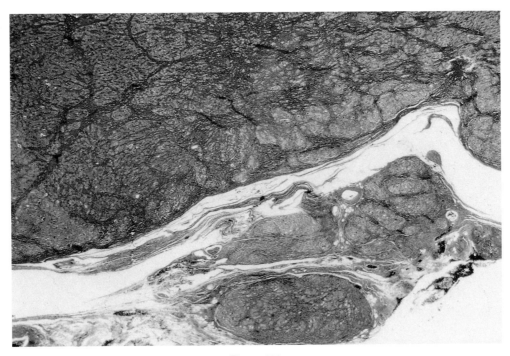

Figure 299
(Figures 299 and 300 are from the same patient)
PARASITIC NODULES IN HASHIMOTO THYROIDITIS
The parasitic nodules show the same microscopic abnormalities as those present in the thyroid gland.

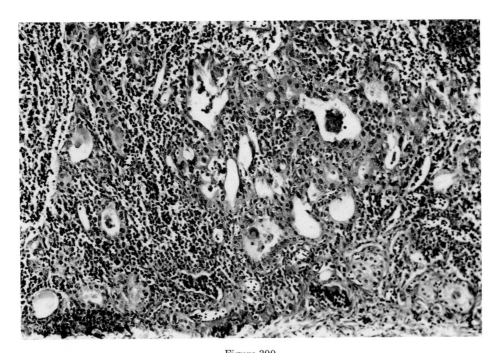

Figure 300
PARASITIC NODULES IN HASHIMOTO THYROIDITIS
At high magnification, this parasitic nodule shows irregularly shaped follicles lined by oncocytic epithelium and a heavy lymphocytic infiltration. The changes were identical to those seen in the thyroid gland.

Parasitic thyroid nodules are not restricted to the neck. They can also occur in the anterosuperior mediastinum, here also as a result of nodular hyperplasia (mediastinal goiter) and through a mechanism analogous to the one described above (pl. XLIII).

THYROID INCLUSIONS IN LYMPH NODES

This controversial issue concerns the alleged presence of normal thyroid follicles within the confines of a cervical lymph node. Some authors deny their occurrence, claiming that all of these formations represent metastatic foci from an occult thyroid primary, regardless of how well differentiated they might appear (37,40). There is no question that metastatic thyroid cancer may present initially in a cervical node in the absence of an obvious thyroid nodule and that the microscopic appearance of this metastasis may closely resemble non-neoplastic thyroid tissue. For this reason, the criteria for benign thyroid inclusions need to be stringent. In any case in which the thyroid tissue has replaced one third or more of the node, or in which several nodes are affected, the diagnosis of metastasis should be preferred. This is also true whenever the intranodal thyroid tissue shows any of the cytoarchitectural features of papillary carcinoma (e.g., abortive papillae or ground-glass nuclei). Presence of psammoma bodies is almost a guarantee that the process is metastatic, no matter how benign its microscopic appearance. For intranodal thyroid tissue to be regarded as a possible benign inclusion, it should be restricted to a few small follicles located in or immediately beneath the nodal capsule, and these follicles should have an unremarkable microscopic appearance (fig. 301) (38).

The best evidence in favor of the existence of this abnormality was provided by Meyer and Steinberg (39). The authors identified five cases at autopsy in which one of the cervical nodes contained thyroid tissue and serially sectioned the entire thyroid gland in those cases to search for a possible primary. Only one primary was found, and this was located in the contralateral lobe.

The fact that this phenomenon occurs should not be surprising. Well-documented examples of ectopic benign tissue in lymph node are plentiful.

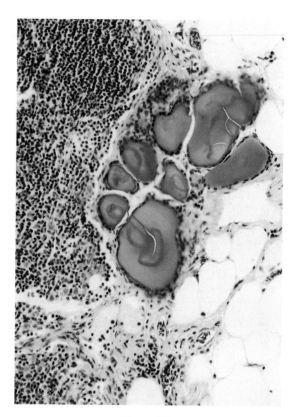

Figure 301
ECTOPIC THYROID FOLLICLES
IN A CERVICAL LYMPH NODE
The follicles, which have a normal architectural and cytologic appearance, are present as a small cluster in the capsule of the node.

They include salivary gland, müllerian epithelium, breast, and nevus cells.

THYROID AS A COMPONENT OF TERATOMA

Thyroid tissue is a relatively common component of ovarian teratomas, but it is seen only infrequently in teratomas at other sites. The thyroid tissue may appear normal or exhibit diffuse or nodular hyperplastic changes. Cases of hyperthyroidism resulting from hyperfunction of teratoma-based thyroid tissue are on record (42,47).

In some instances, the thyroid tissue is the predominant or sole component of the ovarian lesion, a process interpreted as a monodermal

PLATE XLIII

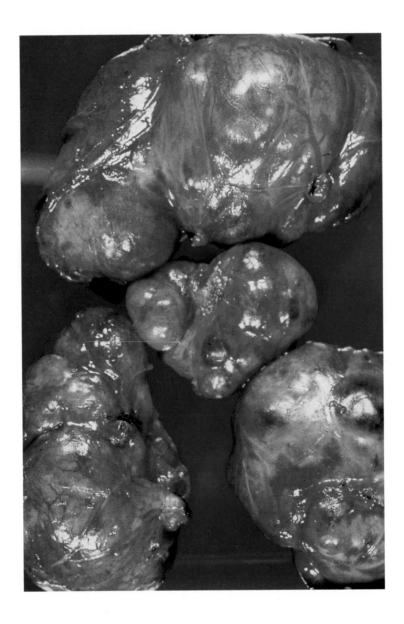

MEDIASTINAL THYROID GLAND WITH NODULAR HYPERPLASIA

Several anatomically separate nodules can be appreciated.

form of teratoma and designated as *struma ovarii* (47). A very intriguing variation on that type is represented by *strumal carcinoid*, an ovarian neoplasm in which thyroid tissue coexists with a carcinoid tumor, usually in the absence of other teratomatous elements (44). It has been suggested that the tumor represents a medullary carcinoma arising from C cells located in the thyroid tissue, but this seems unlikely. The neoplasm rarely contains amyloid, it is usually negative for calcitonin, and its morphologic appearance is more in keeping with a trabecular carcinoid of pulmonary or gastrointestinal type.

Malignant neoplasms of obvious thyroid type developing in struma ovarii are rare (42,43,45–47). Most of the reported cases are in the older literature, and have been diagnosed as follicular carcinomas. It is not always easy to decide on the basis of the description and illustrations how these neoplasms would be classified if current criteria were applied. At least some of them seem to correspond to the follicular variant of papillary carcinoma (41).

REFERENCES

Ectopia

1. Allard RH. The thyroglossal cyst. Head Neck Surg 1982;5:134–46.
2. Baughman RA. Lingual thyroid and lingual thyroglossal tract remnants. A clinical and histopathologic study with a review of the literature. Oral Surg 1972;34:781–99.
3. Bone RC, Biller HF, Irwin TM. Intralaryngotracheal thyroid. Ann Otol Rhinol Laryngol 1972;81:424–8.
4. Donegan JO, Wood MD. Intratracheal thyroid—a familial occurrence. Laryngoscope 1985;95:6–8.
5. Ein SH, Shandling B, Stephens CA, Mancer K. The problem of recurrent thyroglossal duct remnants. J Pediatr Surg 1984;19:437–9.
6. Fish J, Moore RM. Ectopic thyroid tissue and ectopic thyroid carcinoma. Ann Surg 1963;157:212–22.
7. Guimaraes SB, Uceda JE, Lynn HB. Thyroglossal duct remnants in infants and children. Mayo Clin Proc 1972;47:117–20.
8. Jaques DA, Chambers RG, Oertel JE. Thyroglossal tract carcinoma. A review of the literature and addition of eighteen cases. Am J Surg 1970;120:439–46.
9. Joseph TJ, Komorowski RA. Thyroglossal duct carcinoma. Hum Pathol 1975;6:717–29.
10. Kansal P, Sakati N, Rifai A, Woodhouse N. Lingual thyroid. Diagnosis and treatment. Arch Intern Med 1987;147:2046–8.
11. Kaplan M, Kauli R, Lubin E, Grunebaum M, Laron Z. Ectopic thyroid tissue. A clinical study of 30 children and review. J Pediatr 1978;92:205–9.
12. Kurman RJ, Prabha AC. Thyroid and parathyroid glands in the vaginal wall. Am J Clin Pathol 1973;59:503–7.
13. Larochelle D, Arcand P, Belzile M, Gagnon NB. Ectopic thyroid tissue—a review of the literature. J Otolaryngol 1979;8:523–30.
14. LiVolsi VA, Perzin KH, Savetsky L. Carcinoma arising in median ectopic thyroid (including thyroglossal duct tissue). Cancer 1974;34:1303–15.
15. Mobini J, Krouse TB, Klinghoffer JF. Squamous cell carcinoma arising in a thyroglossal duct cyst. Am Surg 1974;40:290–4.
16. Nienas FW, Gorman CA, Devine KD, Woolner LB. Lingual thyroid. Clinical characteristics of 15 cases. Ann Intern Med 1973;79:205–10.
17. Nussbaum M, Buchwald RP, Ribner A, Mori K, Litwins J. Anaplastic carcinoma arising from median ectopic thyroid (thyroglossal duct remnant). Cancer 1981;48:2724–8.
18. Pollice L, Caruso G. Struma cordis. Ectopic thyroid goiter in the right ventricle. Arch Pathol Lab Med 1986;110:452–3.
19. Rahn J. Über eine eigenartige Heterotopie von Schilddrüsengewebe. Zentarbl Allg Pathol Pathol Anat 1958;99:80–6.
20. Reaume CE, Sofie VL. Lingual thyroid. Review of the literature and report of a case. Oral Surg Oral Med Oral Pathol 1978;45:841–5.
21. Reuchti C, Balli-Antunes H, Gerber HA. Follicular tumor in the sellar region without primary cancer of the thyroid. Heterotopic carcinoma? Am J Clin Pathol 1987;87:776–80.
22. Ruppmann E, Georgsson G. Squamous carcinoma of the thyroglossal duct. Ger Med Mon 1966;11:442–7.
23. Simon M, Baczako K. Thyroid inclusion in the lung. Metastasis of an occult papillary carcinoma or ectopia? Pathol Res Pract 1989;184:263–7.
24. Smithers DW. Carcinoma associated with thyroglossal duct anomalies. In: Smithers D, ed. Tumours of the thyroid gland. Edinburgh: Livingstone, 1970:155–65.
25. Solomon JR, Rangecroft L. Thyroglossal-duct lesions in childhood. J Pediatr Surg 1984;19:555–61.
26. Soucy P, Penning J. The clinical relevance of certain observations on the histology of the thyroglossal tract. J Pediatr Surg 1984;19:506–9.
27. Strickland AL, Macfie JA, Van Wyk JJ, French FS. Ectopic thyroid glands simulating thyroglossal duct cysts. JAMA 1969;208:307–10.
28. Talib H. Lingual thyroid. Br J Clin Pract 1966;20:322–3.
29. Villet WT, Kemp CB. Thyroglossal duct carcinoma. A case report and a review of the literature. S Afr Med J 1981;60:795–6.
30. Wapshaw H. Lingual thyroid. Br J Surg 1974;30:160–5.

Mechanical Implantation

31. Block MA, Wylie JH, Patton RB, Miller JM. Does benign thyroid tissue occur in the lateral part of the neck? Am J Surg 1966;112:476–81.
32. Klopp CT, Kirson SM. Therapeutic problems with ectopic non-cancerous follicular thyroid tissue in the neck: 18 case reports according to etiological factors. Ann Surg 1966;163:653–64.
33. Moses DC, Thompson NW, Nishiyama RH, Sisson JC. Ectopic thyroid tissue in the neck. Benign or malignant. Cancer 1976;38:361–5.

Parasitic Nodule

34. Hanson GA, Komorowski RA, Cerletty JM, Wilson SD. Thyroid gland morphology in young adults: normal subjects versus those with prior low-dose neck irradiation in childhood. Surgery 1983;96:984–8.
35. Hathaway BM. Innocuous accessory thyroid nodules. Arch Surg 1965;90:222–7.
36. Sisson JC, Schmidt RW, Beierwaltes WH. Sequestered nodular goiter. N Engl J Med 1964;270:927–32.

Thyroid Inclusions in Lymph Nodes

37. Block MA, Wylie JH, Patton RB, Miller JM. Does benign thyroid tissue occur in the lateral part of the neck? Am J Surg 1966;112:476–81.
38. Frantz VK, Forsythe R, Hanford JM, Rogers WM. Lateral aberrant thyroids. Ann Surg 1942;115:161–83.
39. Meyer JS, Steinberg LS. Microscopically benign thyroid follicles in cervical lymph nodes. Serial section study of lymph node inclusions and entire thyroid gland in 5 cases. Cancer 1969;24:302–11.
40. Ward R. Relation of tumors of lateral aberrant thyroid tissue to malignant disease of the thyroid gland. Arch Surg 1940;40:606–15.

Thyroid as a Component of Teratoma

41. Brunskill PJ, Rollason TP, Nicholson HO. Malignant follicular variant of papillary struma ovarii. Histopathology 1990;17:574–6.
42. Kempers RD, Dockerty MB, Hoffman DL, Bartholomew LG. Struma ovarii—ascitic, hyperthyroid, and asymptomatic syndromes. Ann Intern Med 1970;72:883–93.
43. Pardo-Mindan FJ, Vazquez JJ. Malignant struma ovarii. Light and electron microscopic study. Cancer 1983;51:337–43.
44. Robboy SJ, Scully RE. Strumal carcinoid of the ovary: an analysis of 50 cases of a distinctive tumor composed of thyroid tissue and carcinoid. Cancer 1980;46:2019–34.
45. Rosenblum NG, LiVolsi VA, Edmonds PR, Mikuta JJ. Malignant struma ovarii. Gynecol Oncol 1989;32:224–7.
46. Willemse PH, Oosterhuis JW, Aalders JG, et al. Malignant struma ovarii treated by ovariectomy, thyroidectomy, and 131I administration. Cancer 1987;60:178–82.
47. Woodruff JD, Rauh JT, Markley RL. Ovarian struma. Obstet Gynecol 1966;27:194–202.

✧✧✧

THYROID TUMORS—GENERAL CONSIDERATIONS

INCIDENCE OF THYROID CARCINOMA

Thyroid carcinoma is by far the most common type of endocrine gland malignancy; however, it represents only about 1 percent of all cancers diagnosed in the United States. The annual incidence in this country is about 10,000 (or 40/1,000,000 people), and the annual death rate is approximately 1000 (or 4/1,000,000).

CLINICAL AND LABORATORY EVALUATION OF THYROID TUMORS

Approximately 4 percent of the people in the United States between the ages of 30 and 60 years have one or more palpable thyroid nodules. Because most of these nodules are benign and most are not even neoplastic, the clinician evaluating them should be as selective as possible in the recommendation for surgical removal while avoiding missing the malignant tumors.

Evaluation of the nodule includes the following considerations:

- **Demographics**
  Age (the incidence of malignancy is higher in children and the elderly), sex (the incidence of malignancy is higher in males), and geographic location (in reference to iodine-deficient areas).

- **Family history**
  A strong family history (unrelated to dietary iodine deficiency) suggests the diagnosis of either dyshormonogenetic goiter or medullary carcinoma.

- **History of Hashimoto thyroiditis**
  The possibility that a thyroid nodule is malignant is probably the same regardless of whether the patient has a documented history of Hashimoto thyroiditis or not.

- **Rate of growth**
  Most adenomas are very slow growing, but this is also true for most well-differentiated follicular or papillary carcinomas. Rapid enlargement of a preexisting indolent nodule may signify the emergence of an undifferentiated malignant component or simply the spontaneous development of hemorrhage within the nodule.

- **Palpation**
  Solitary nodules are more likely to be malignant than multiple ones. It should be remembered that approximately one third of clinically solitary nodules are shown to be multiple on scan and an even higher number on pathologic examination. Unusually prominent, hard, or irregular nodules that occur in a multinodular gland should be regarded as suspicious. Fixation of the thyroid gland, failure to move freely on swallowing, or vocal cord paralysis should heighten the suspicion of malignancy, although some of these signs can also be seen in some forms of thyroiditis.

  Presence of an associated ipsilateral adenopathy is the strongest clinical indicator that a malignancy is present, particularly if there is no evidence of an apparent infection.

- **Isotopic imaging study**
  This test, traditionally performed with ^{131}I, is now more commonly done with either ^{123}I or ^{99}Tc pertechnetate because of reduced radiation exposure (2,8). Thyroid nodules are classified as hyperfunctional (hot), when trapping the isotope with greater avidity than (and sometimes to the exclusion of) the rest of the gland; functional (cool or warm), when trapping the isotope with the same avidity as the rest of the gland; and hypofunctional (cold), when failing to trap the isotope (fig. 302). A minimum diameter of 1 cm is necessary for a cold nodule to be detectable with this technique (5). Hyperfunctional nodules are practically always benign, and this is also true for most functional nodules. The incidence of carcinoma is notably higher for the hypofunctional nodules, even though most of them (~80 percent) will still be benign.

- **Ultrasonography**
  Solid nodules are more likely to be malignant than cystic ones, particularly if they have been found to be hypofunctioning by isotopic imaging study. Only 1 to 3 percent of the nodules found to be cystic by this technique will prove to be malignant on pathologic examination.

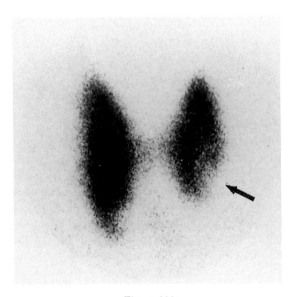

Figure 302
RADIOACTIVE THYROID SCAN
The arrow points to a cold nodule located in the lower pole of the right lobe. This lesion was excised and proved to be a papillary carcinoma.

- **Computerized tomography (CT) and magnetic resonance imaging (MRI)**
  The role of these two techniques is still limited but growing. MRI is said to be superior to CT for the evaluation of metastatic, retrotracheal, or mediastinal lesions (2).

- **Serum thyroglobulin levels**
  These levels are often elevated in patients with papillary and follicular carcinoma (particularly the latter), whereas they remain normal in patients with medullary or undifferentiated carcinoma. However, because a similar elevation can also accompany follicular adenoma, this measurement cannot be used to distinguish benign from malignant tumors before surgery. This technique is particularly useful in monitoring patients after removal of a papillary or follicular carcinoma, especially if the excision was followed by radioactive iodine therapy. As a matter of fact, it has been stated that repeated total-body scans can be omitted in patients with such tumors if the serum thyroglobulin levels are undetectable, unless a strong clinical indication exists (1,6,7,9).

- **Needle biopsy**
  This increasingly popular technique currently provides the most accurate way of determining whether a thyroid nodule is malignant, short of surgical intervention. The method usually employed is cytologic examination of material obtained through fine-needle aspiration. This is discussed further in the section on Fine-Needle Aspiration Biopsy in this chapter. The alternative procedure of histologic evaluation of a tissue core obtained through a large-needle biopsy procedure has never acquired popularity and is currently used with some frequency in only a few institutions in this country (4). It is more useful for the study of diffuse inflammatory diseases (e.g., Hashimoto thyroiditis) and in confirming the diagnosis of advanced malignant neoplasms (e.g., undifferentiated carcinoma) than in the evaluation of a solitary thyroid nodule. Some of the reluctance to use this technique for the latter stems from the small but definite risk of complications, such as bleeding, nerve injury, tracheal perforation, or tumor implantation (3).

THYROID TUMORS IN CHILDHOOD

The appearance of the thyroid tumors and tumor-like conditions developing in infants and children does not differ significantly from that of the corresponding lesions in adults; however, their relative frequency does. The most important difference is the higher frequency of carcinoma, to the point that, in some recent series, the malignant tumors surpass the benign processes (11,15). It has been estimated that the risk of malignancy in a solitary thyroid nodule is about 50 percent in patients under 25 years of age and 75 percent in patients under 15 years of age.

Among the malignancies, papillary carcinoma comprises most of the cases, and its relative frequency is even higher than in adults (10,19). This is followed by the familial form of medullary carcinoma and by oncocytic neoplasms (12). In some older series, there is also a fair number of follicular carcinomas, but we suspect that most of them would be regarded as follicular variants of papillary carcinoma by current criteria (16,21). In the series of Sierk and coworkers (19), not a single case of nononcocytic follicular carcinoma was found on review of 32 patients. Undifferentiated and poorly differentiated carcinomas are practically nonexistent in this age group.

The papillary carcinomas occurring in children tend to have extensive solid and/or squamous areas. They are associated with a higher frequency of cervical lymph node and lung metastases than their adult counterparts, but their overall prognosis is still very good (13,17,18). A single case interpreted as congenital papillary carcinoma has been reported (14). In recent series, history of previous irradiation to the neck was present in about 25 percent of the cases; this figure is substantially lower than in series before 1970, in some of which it was as high as 80 percent (19). Some of the reported cases have been seen in children who had undergone successful multimodal management of malignant tumors such as acute leukemia or Wilms tumor (20). As for the adult cases, presence of aneuploidy in pediatric thyroid malignancies does not seem to correlate with either extent of the disease at diagnosis or patient outcome (20).

THYROID TUMORS AND RADIATION EXPOSURE

During the first half of this century, low-dose radiation therapy to the head and neck region of children and adolescents was a common form of therapy for disorders such as "thymic enlargement," tonsillar hypertrophy, tuberculous adenitis, hemangiomas, nevi, eczema, or acne. The average dose was about 600 rads. In the United States, it is estimated that approximately 1,000,000 people were subjected to this treatment, which has been found to result in a variety of thyroid diseases later in life, particularly in women. Approximately one fourth of the population at risk will develop thyroid nodules. The risk is substantially greater if the radiation was given before the age of 7 years (31,33). Most of these nodules (~75 percent) are benign and consist of nodular hyperplasia, follicular adenoma (rare), lymphocytic thyroiditis, oncocytic change, focal fibrosis, and atrophy (26,27,29,30,38). The treatment for these benign follicular nodules is the same as for those seen in the general population, i.e., lobectomy or subtotal thyroidectomy, depending on their size and number. The incidence of recurrence after surgery, which is similar to that seen in nonirradiated patients, is substantially decreased if thyroid hormone is given postoperatively to suppress thyroid-stimulating hormone secretion (25).

There is also an increased occurrence of carcinoma in this population, irradiation actually being the most clearly documented etiologic factor for thyroid malignancy. Most of the tumors are papillary carcinomas (28,33–35). The incidence of this tumor type among irradiated patients having a thyroid operation has ranged from 20 to over 50 percent in the various series, and it may partially depend on the extent of the operation and thoroughness of the pathologic examination (23,40). The median latency for the development of malignancy has been approximately 20 years. Many of these papillary carcinomas show evidence of multicentricity and/or intraglandular spread and of cervical lymph node involvement, perhaps more than in those occurring in the general population, but their long-term prognosis has been just as good (31).

Other structures in the region are also subject to radiation-induced neoplasia. Benign and (less commonly) malignant tumors of salivary gland, parathyroid, bone, and soft tissues have been reported in this population, emphasizing the need for continued surveillance (36,37). Isolated examples of postradiation thyroid lymphoma have also been reported (22). Thyroid carcinoma and other thyroid abnormalities can also result from high-dose radiation to the region, such as that administered for Hodgkin disease and other malignant neoplasms (24,29, 32,39).

FINE-NEEDLE ASPIRATION BIOPSY

Fine-needle aspiration has become an extremely popular technique in recent years for the evaluation of thyroid diseases, particularly solitary nodules (50,53,54,56,57). Its appeal is that it is quick and inexpensive, it can be carried out in the physician's office, and the risk of complications (including tumor implantation) is minimal (43,51). Several large series report a sensitivity and specificity of over 90 percent, leading some authors to recommend fine-needle aspiration as the initial test in the evaluation of any thyroid nodule (41,56,58). Most papillary carcinomas and several other types of malignancy can be identified with ease. Most forms of thyroiditis are also readily detectable (44). The main difficulty resides in the identification of well-differentiated follicular carcinoma, a task that is often impossible with this method in view of the nature of the diagnostic criteria required (48). Most cytology reports done for solitary nodules fall into one of the following three categories:

- *Probable benign nodule*, when the material is composed mostly of colloid, histiocytes, and a few normal-looking follicular cells. This is an indication for a conservative approach unless the clinical data indicate otherwise.
- *Follicular neoplasm*, when cellularity is higher than that found in the usual hyperplastic nodule, but the nuclear features of papillary carcinoma are absent. The diagnosis of oncocytic neoplasm will usually fall into this category (47). The diagnosis of follicular neoplasm is an indication for removal of the nodule unless this is contraindicated for medical reasons (52).
- *Papillary carcinoma*, when the characteristic cytoarchitectural features of this tumor type are present. The cytologic diagnosis of papillary carcinoma is obviously an indication for therapeutic intervention.

Performance of fine-needle aspiration may result in partial or complete infarct of the tumor, with only a thin rim of tissue preserved at the periphery. This complication is more common with oncocytic tumors (46), and it may result in transient elevation of the serum levels of thyroglobulin (49). It may also lead to papillary endothelial hyperplasia secondary to hemorrhage or thrombosis, a change that should not be confused with angiosarcoma (42).

A short description of the cytologic findings in the specific tumor types is provided in the respective chapters. For a more detailed and authoritative discussion of the indications and limitations of the technique and an in-depth description of the results, we refer the readers to several excellent textbooks and reviews (43,45,48,55).

FROZEN-SECTION EXAMINATION

The role of frozen section in the management of thyroid nodules has greatly diminished after the widespread adoption of the fine-needle biopsy procedure (61). Lesions that are usually identifiable on frozen section are the conventional type of papillary carcinoma, widely invasive follicular carcinoma, poorly differentiated (insular) carcinoma, undifferentiated (anaplastic) carcinoma, and medullary carcinoma. Cases of thyroiditis clinically simulating tumors and of nodular hyperplasia (adenomatoid goiter) are also recognizable without difficulty in most instances (66).

The main problem (and unfortunately a frequent one) is represented by the single encapsulated nodule with a follicular pattern of growth, in which the differential diagnosis includes follicular adenoma, minimally invasive follicular carcinoma, and the encapsulated follicular variant of papillary carcinoma. This is by far the most significant factor for the relatively low sensitivity of frozen-section diagnosis of thyroid carcinomas (67). Factors contributing to the difficulty are the focal nature of the capsular and/or vascular invasion in minimally invasive follicular carcinoma, and the fact that ground-glass nuclei, one of the most important hallmarks of the follicular variant of papillary carcinoma, are seen poorly or not at all in frozen-section material (fig. 303) (62).

For this type of lesion, we believe that freezing of a maximum of three blocks including the capsule is adequate, regardless of the size of the nodule. If no capsular and/or vascular invasion is detected and if the cytoarchitectural features of the follicular variant of papillary carcinoma are not detectable, we think it is justifiable to make a diagnosis of *follicular lesion —diagnosis deferred to permanent sections*. Because we believe that most follicular adenomas, minimally invasive follicular carcinomas, and the encapsulated follicular variant of papillary carcinoma can be treated similarly (i.e., by the performance of either a lobectomy with isthmusectomy or a subtotal thyroidectomy), we do not regard the diagnostic deferral at the time of frozen section to be of great practical consequence. This has also been the experience of others (59,63,65). Of 359 patients with thyroid nodules studied by fine-needle biopsy and intraoperative frozen sections that were analyzed by Hamburger and Hamburger (60), it was found that the frozen-section diagnosis decisively influenced the surgical procedure in only 3 cases, i.e., less than 1 percent. A similar experience was recounted by Kopald and coworkers (64).

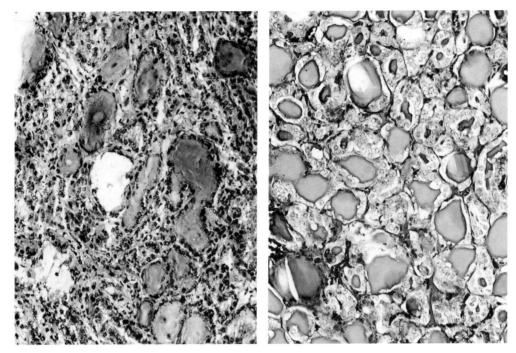

Figure 303
PAPILLARY CARCINOMA, FOLLICULAR VARIANT
The photograph on the left is from a frozen section in a case of follicular variant of papillary carcinoma.
The ground-glass nuclear features are not appreciable. The photograph on the right is from a permanent
section from the same case. The typical nuclear features of this tumor entity are now obvious.

PROCEDURE FOR PATHOLOGIC EXAMINATION

Described below is a set of guidelines for the handling, description, and microscopic sampling of surgical specimens from the thyroid gland. Only some general statements can be made in a section of this sort. The specific features of the individual specimen often call for a modification or even a substantial departure from these recommendations.

Handling

- Weigh the specimen, and measure it in three dimensions.

- Orient the specimen, if feasible (help from the surgeon may be necessary).

- Search for parathyroid glands and lymph nodes in the surrounding fat.

- Paint the outer aspect of the specimen with india ink or similar dye.

- Make parallel longitudinal cuts, 3 to 5 mm apart, either in the fresh state or after formalin fixation.

Note, if searching for papillary microcarcinoma (a lesion measuring ≤1 cm, by definition), we recommend slicing the specimen into 2- or 3-mm–thick sections and transilluminating them. Any sharply localized area with a fibrotic appearance should be regarded as suspicious, especially if it has a stellate shape.

Description

- Indicate the type of specimen received: nodulectomy (an operation that has been abandoned in most institutions), lobectomy, lobectomy with isthmusectomy, subtotal thyroidectomy, or total thyroidectomy. For specimens other than the last one, indicate the side from which most or all of the specimen was obtained.

- State the weight, dimensions, shape, color, and consistency of the specimen.

- Examine the cut surface for color and appearance. Note whether or not it is homogeneous and whether it is smooth or nodular.

- When one or more nodules are present, note the number, size, shape, color; whether they are solid or cystic, calcified, hemorrhagic, or necrotic; and whether or not they are encapsulated. If a capsule is present, note whether it is thin or thick and regular or irregular. Note whether it is apparently intact or violated by tumor growth. Calculate the shortest distance from the edge of the nodule to the line of resection.

Sections for Histology

- For diffuse and/or inflammatory lesions, take three sections from each lobe and one from isthmus.

- For solitary encapsulated nodules measuring up to 6 cm in diameter, submit the entire central slice. Each block should have a portion of the capsule and adjacent thyroid tissue, if present. For a nodule measuring exactly 6 cm in diameter, six blocks will usually have to be made.

- For larger encapsulated nodules, submit one additional block for each centimeter over 6 cm (i.e., 7 blocks for a 7-cm nodule, or 10 blocks for a 10-cm nodule).

- For multinodular thyroid glands, submit a minimum of one section for each nodule (up to five nodules), including rim and adjacent gland. Submit additional sections for the nodules that are larger than and/or grossly different from the others.

- For known papillary or medullary carcinoma, submit the entire gland and (separately) the line of resection, if the specimen is other than a total thyroidectomy.

- For grossly invasive carcinoma other than papillary or medullary, submit a minimum of three blocks from the tumor, three of non-neoplastic gland (if present), and one from the line of resection (if other than total thyroidectomy).

- For all cases, submit all parathyroid glands and lymph nodes whenever found on gross inspection.

Example of Gross Description

Received in the fresh state is a specimen of right lobectomy with isthmusectomy. A black suture is present at the isthmusectomy margin. The specimen weighs 30 g and measures 6.5 x 4.0 x 3.0 cm. The outer surface is smooth, and the consistency is homogeneously firm. An ill-defined bulging is noted in the lower pole of the lobe. No parathyroid glands or lymph nodes are identified.

Parallel longitudinal sections of the specimen reveal a round nodule in the lower lobe measuring 2.5 cm in diameter. It is entirely surrounded by a very thin fibrous capsule that shows no gross evidence of invasion. The cut surface of the nodule is solid, slightly bulging, and tan, with punctate areas of fresh hemorrhage. The capsule of the nodule is 0.5 cm distant from the thyroid capsule and 1.2 cm distant from the surgical margin at the isthmus. The rest of the thyroid shows no gross abnormalities.

Sections are submitted as follows:

A1, A2:	*nodule*
B1, B2:	*remainder of right lobe*
C:	*surgical margin at the isthmus*

STAGING AND GRADING OF THYROID CARCINOMA

Clinical Staging. The clinical staging system recommended by the International Union Against Cancer (UICC) in the fourth edition of their manual is detailed below (69). This system has also been adopted by the American Joint Committee on Cancer (68).

T—Primary Tumor (as determined by physical examination, endoscopy, and imaging)

TX	Primary tumor cannot be assessed
T0	No evidence of primary tumor
T1	Tumor 1 cm or less in greatest dimension, limited to the thyroid
T2	Tumor more than 1 cm but not more than 4 cm in greatest dimension, limited to the thyroid
T3	Tumor more than 4 cm in greatest dimension, limited to the thyroid
T4	Tumor of any size extending beyond the thyroid capsule

Note: All categories may be subdivided into
  a) solitary tumor
  b) multifocal tumor

N—Regional Lymph Nodes (cervical and upper mediastinal, as determined by physical examination and imaging)

NX Regional lymph nodes cannot be assessed
N0 No regional lymph node metastasis
N1 Regional lymph node metastasis
N1a Metastasis in ipsilateral cervical lymph node(s)
N1b Metastasis in bilateral, midline, or contralateral cervical or mediastinal lymph node(s)

M—Distant Metastasis (as determined by physical examination and imaging)

MX Presence of distant metastasis cannot be assessed
M0 No distant metastasis
M1 Distant metastasis

Note: Category M1 may be further specified according to the following notation:

PUL	Pulmonary	MAR	Bone marrow
OSS	Osseous	PLE	Pleura
HEP	Hepatic	PER	Peritoneum
BRA	Brain	SKI	Skin
LYM	Lymph nodes	OTH	Other

Pathologic Staging. The pathologic staging of thyroid carcinoma uses terminology and categories similar to the above-listed clinical staging. In this scheme, the pT, pN, and pM categories substitute for the T, N, and M categories, respectively.

Stage Grouping

Papillary or Follicular Carcinoma
(patient <45 years old)

Stage I	any T	any N	M0
Stage II	any T	any N	M1

Papillary or Follicular Carcinoma
(patient ≥45 years old)

Stage I	T1	N0	M0
Stage II	T2 or T3	N0	M0
Stage III	T4	N0	M0
	any T	N1	M0
Stage IV	any T	any N	M1

Medullary Carcinoma

Stage I	T1	N0	M0
Stage II	T2, T3, or T4	N0	M0
Stage III	any T	N1	M0
Stage IV	any T	any N	M1

Undifferentiated Carcinoma

Stage IV	any T	any N	any M

(This tumor type is regarded as stage IV by definition, regardless of size or extent of spread.)

Microscopic Grading. The UICC recommends that all carcinomas of head and neck sites (including thyroid) be graded microscopically as follows:

GX	Grade cannot be assessed
G1	Well differentiated
G2	Moderately well differentiated
G3	Poorly differentiated
G4	Undifferentiated

It should be understood that this grading system was proposed mainly on the basis of the squamous cell carcinomas of the upper aerodigestive tract, for which it works quite well. In the thyroid, instead, most tumors arising from follicular cells belong to either the well-differentiated or the undifferentiated types. The former includes nearly all the minimally invasive follicular carcinomas (including those of oncocytic type) and the papillary carcinomas of either conventional or follicular variant types, whereas the undifferentiated grade is synonymous with the undifferentiated (anaplastic) type of carcinoma. We have proposed the term insular carcinoma for poorly differentiated tumors of either follicular or papillary type that exhibit an insular pattern of growth associated with mitotic activity and necrosis and believe that this category can be expanded to include other poorly differentiated tumors of follicular cell origin that do fit the insular pattern (see page 128). No grading system has been proposed for medullary carcinoma, even though the small cell variant of this tumor could be regarded as its poorly differentiated member.

TREATMENT OF THYROID TUMORS

Some general considerations about the therapy of thyroid tumors are made here. Specific considerations are discussed with the corresponding tumor types.

The initial therapeutic approach is usually surgical. The standard types of operation are lobectomy (often coupled with resection of the isthmus for cosmetic reasons), subtotal thyroidectomy, and total thyroidectomy (71,74,75,78). Nodulectomy (i.e., enucleation of a nodule) has been abandoned in most centers because of the definite risk of recurrence if the lesion is malignant. The morbidity associated with lobectomy and with subtotal thyroidectomy is comparable and of minimal magnitude (<1 percent). In contrast, significant morbidity in the form of permanent hypoparathyroidism or recurrent laryngeal nerve paralysis has been reported to occur in about 10 percent of patients subjected to total thyroidectomy, even when performed by experienced surgeons. This operation should therefore be avoided whenever possible. Although controversy persists, most authors, ourselves included, do not believe it is indicated for most of the well-differentiated follicular and papillary carcinomas (71). This issue is discussed in more detail in connection with the treatment of papillary carcinoma (see page 94).

The performance of a neck dissection in the presence of clinically negative nodes has been largely abandoned. A modified form of neck dissection is generally carried out if the nodes are thought to be involved either clinically or at the time of thyroidectomy. This allows the preservation of the spinal accessory nerve, jugular vein, and sternocleidomastoid muscle, leading to a cosmetically superior result.

Postoperative oral administration of thyroid hormone on a long-term basis in a quantity sufficient to suppress thyroid-stimulating hormone activity is used routinely for follicular and papillary carcinomas, and with some frequency even for benign nodules, under the assumption that it results in a decrease in the incidence of clinical recurrence (73). However, a study by Cady and coworkers (72) showed no statistically significant improvement in survival with use of thyroid hormone in differentiated thyroid carcinoma when the patients were categorized by risk group and pathologic type.

Administration of radioactive iodine is another mainstay of thyroid cancer therapy (77). It is based on the principles that 1) functioning thyroid tissue concentrates iodine, 2) most thyroid carcinomas are well differentiated enough to function, and 3) if a primary tumor takes up iodine, its metastases should be expected to behave similarly. We and others believe that use of radioactive iodine should be selective rather than routine and that it should be generally restricted to nonresectable and metastatic well-differentiated carcinomas (76).

External radiation therapy is reserved for tumors showing surgically uncontrollable local spread. In most series, its efficacy has been relatively modest (70). The post-therapy monitoring includes (besides physical examination and chest X rays) radioactive scan and measurement of serum thyroglobulin levels for tumors of follicular cells and measurement of serum levels of calcitonin, CEA, and chromogranin A for tumors of C cells.

Treatment of metastatic thyroid disease includes surgical excision (for local recurrence, lymph node metastases, or isolated distant metastases), radioactive iodine (highly effective for well-differentiated tumors), and external radiation therapy (76). In general, chemotherapy has proved of little benefit.

PROGNOSIS OF THYROID TUMORS

Most of the clinical and pathologic factors related to prognosis are discussed with the specific tumor types. Generally, the most important prognostic indicators are age and sex of the patient, microscopic type, and tumor stage (see page 95). These and other factors sometimes have been combined in prognostic scoring indexes, such as those proposed by the Mayo Clinic (AGES score), the Lahey Clinic (AUES system), and the European Organization for Research on Treatment of Cancer (EORTC) (79,83,84).

Cady and coworkers (81) have divided their patients with well-differentiated (papillary or follicular) carcinomas into two categories with notably different survival rates: 1) low risk (men ≤40 years of age and women ≤50 years of age) and 2) high risk (men >40 years of age and women >50 years of age). We have confirmed the great practical utility of this division for papillary carcinomas and found that, in our series, the prognostic difference was even more striking if the low-risk group was defined as including men 40 years of age and under and women 60 years of age and under (82).

Recently, Cady and Rossi (80) proposed a modified version of their risk-group definition by incorporating some of the factors from the EORTC system.

Their new low-risk group was defined as:

A. All younger patients without distant metastases (men, <41 years; women, <51 years)
B. All older patients with:
1. Intrathyroidal papillary cancer or minor tumor capsular involvement follicular carcinoma, *and*
2. Primary cancers <5 cm in diameter, *and*
3. No distant metastases.
This group constituted 89 percent of all cases, and the death rate was 1.8 percent.

The high-risk group was defined as:

A. All patients with distant metastases
B. All older patients with:
1. Extrathyroidal papillary cancer or major tumor capsular involvement follicular carcinoma, *and*
2. Primary cancers 5 cm in diameter or larger regardless of extent of disease.
This group made up 11 percent of cases but carried a 46 percent mortality rate. Thus, a mortality ratio of 26:1 existed between the two groups.

In terms of microscopic type, most deaths from thyroid epithelial malignancies result from undifferentiated, poorly differentiated, oncocytic, and medullary carcinomas, despite the fact that the sum of all of these types represents less than 25 percent of all carcinomas.

THYROID TUMORS IN ANIMALS

Spontaneous thyroid tumors have been observed in fishes, birds, and mammals; most of these have been carcinomas (95). Interestingly, most of the cases have been seen in species that frequently exhibit goiter, presumably due to iodine deficiency.

Numerous cases of thyroid carcinoma in dogs are on record, and a few have been documented in cats, sheep, horses, cattle, and swine. Many of the canine tumors are of the medullary carcinoma type (93). Among wild animals, thyroid carcinoma has been documented in foxes, wolves, bears, lions, tigers, and raccoons.

Whereas spontaneous thyroid tumors are uncommon in rats and mice, they can be induced experimentally in these species by a variety of techniques: single or multiple exposure to radioiodine (89,94), external irradiation (90), low-iodine diets (85), long-term administration of goitrogenous agents (91,92), partial administration of thyroid-stimulating hormone (96), and partial thyroidectomy (86). Many of these methods initially result in hyperplasia of the follicular epithelium, which is then followed by a neoplastic growth. Most tumors have been diagnosed as follicular carcinomas, but papillary and undifferentiated (spindle cell) types also occur. Fortner and coworkers (87) showed that induced thyroid tumors in the hamster are of follicular type and associated with hyperplasia, whereas the spontaneous ones lack an accompanying hyperplasia and could be of either papillary, follicular, or undifferentiated (spindle cell) type.

The induced follicular neoplasms resemble their human counterparts in their capacity to concentrate radioiodine, to produce thyroid hormones, and to exhibit progressive growth. Invasion of local structures and distant metastases both occur.

Goitrogen-induced tumors in animals are initially dependent on thyroid-stimulating hormone stimulation for their continued growth. With serial transplants, however, many of them become hormonally independent (88).

REFERENCES

Clinical and Laboratory Evaluation of Thyroid Tumors

1. Ericsson UB, Tegler L, Lennquist S, Christensen SB, Stahl E, Thorell JI. Serum thyroglobulin in differentiated thyroid carcinoma. Acta Chir Scand 1984;150: 367–75.
2. Friedman M, Toriumi DM, Mafee MF. Diagnostic imaging techniques in thyroid cancer. Am J Surg 1988; 155:215–23.
3. Hawk WA, Crile G Jr, Hazard JB, Barrett DL. Needle biopsy of thyroid gland. Surg Gynecol Obstet 1966; 122:1053–65.
4. Lo Gerfo P, Colacchio T, Caushaj F, Weber C, Feind C. Comparison of fine-needle and coarse-needle biopsies in evaluating thyroid nodules. Surgery 1982;92:835–8.
5. Noyek AM, Greyson ND, Steinhardt MI, et al. Thyroid tumor imaging. Arch Otolaryngol 1983;109:205–24.
6. Ramanna L, Waxman AD, Brachman MB, et al. Correlation of thyroglobulin measurements and radioiodine scans in the follow-up of patients with differentiated thyroid cancer. Cancer 1985;55:1525–9.
7. Shlossberg AH, Jacobson JC, Ibbertson HK. Serum thyroglobulin in the diagnosis and management of thyroid carcinoma. Clin Endocrinol (Oxf) 1979;10:17–27.
8. Shulkin BI, Shapiro B. The role of imaging tests in the diagnosis of thyroid carcinoma. Endocrinol Metab Clin North Am 1990;19:523–44.
9. van Herle AJ, Uller RP. Elevated serum thyroglobulin. A marker of metastases in differentiated thyroid carcinomas. J Clin Invest 1975;56:272–7.

Thyroid Tumors in Childhood

10. Goepfert H, Dichtel WJ, Samaan NA. Thyroid cancer in children and teenagers. Arch Otolaryngol 1984;110:72–5.
11. Gorlin JB, Sallan SE. Thyroid cancer in children. Endocrinol Metab Clin North Am 1990;19;649–62.
12. Hayles AB, Kennedy RL, Beahrs OH, Woolner LB. Carcinoma of the thyroid gland in children. Am J Dis Child 1955;90:705–15.
13. Lamberg BA, Karkinen-Jaaskelainen M, Franssila KO. Differentiated follicle-derived thyroid carcinoma in children. Acta Paediatr Scand 1989;78:419–25.
14. Mills SE, Allen MS Jr. Congenital occult papillary carcinoma of the thyroid gland. Hum Pathol 1986;17:1179–81.
15. Raju U, Kini S. Neoplasms of thyroid follicular epithelium in children and adolescents [Abstract]. Lab Invest 1988;58:8A.
16. Root AW. Cancer of the thyroid in childhood and adolescence. Am J Med Sci 1963;246:734–49.
17. Samuel AM, Sharma SM. Differentiated thyroid carcinomas in children and adolescents. Cancer 1991;67: 2186–90.
18. Schlumberger M, De Vathaire F, Travagli JP, et al. Differentiated thyroid carcinoma in childhood: long term follow-up of 72 patients. J Clin Endocrinol Metab 1987;65:1088–94.
19. Sierk A, Askin FB, Reddick RL, Thomas CG Jr. Pediatric thyroid cancer. Pediatr Pathol 1990;10:877–93.
20. Vane D, King DR, Boles ET Jr. Secondary thyroid neoplasms in pediatric cancer patients: increased risk with improved survival. J Pediatr Surg 1984;19:855–60.
21. Winship T, Rosvoll RV. Childhood thyroid carcinoma. Cancer 1961;14:734–43.

Thyroid Tumors and Radiation Exposure

22. Bisbee AC, Thoeny RH. Malignant lymphoma of the thyroid following irradiation. Cancer 1975;35:1296–9.
23. Calandra DB, Shah KH, Lawrence AM, Paloyan E. Total thyroidectomy in irradiated patients. A twenty-year experience in 206 patients. Ann Surg 1985;202: 356–60.
24. Carr RF, LiVolsi VA. Morphologic changes in the thyroid after irradiation for Hodgkin's and non-Hodgkin's lymphoma. Cancer 1989;64:825–9.
25. Fogelfeld L, Wiviott MB, Shore-Freedman E, et al. Recurrence of thyroid nodules after surgical removal in patients irradiated in childhood for benign conditions. N Engl J Med 1989;320:835–40.
26. Fjälling M, Tisell L-E, Carlsson S, Hansson G, Lundberg L-M, Odén A. Benign and malignant thyroid nodules after neck irradiation. Cancer 1986;58:1219–24.
27. Hanson GA, Komorowski RA, Cerletty JM, Wilson SD. Thyroid gland morphology in young adults: normal subjects versus those with prior low-dose neck irradiation in childhood. Surgery 1983;96:984–8.
28. Hempelmann LH, Hall WJ, Phillips M, Cooper RA, Ames WR. Neoplasms in persons treated with X-rays in infancy. Fourth survey in 20 years. J Natl Cancer Inst 1975;55:519–30.
29. Kaplan MM, Garnick MB, Gelber R, et al. Risk factors for thyroid abnormalities after neck irradiation for childhood cancer. Am J Med 1983;74:272–80.
30. Komorowski RA, Hanson GA. Morphologic changes in the thyroid following low-dose childhood radiation. Arch Pathol Lab Med 1977;101:36–9.
31. Pottern LM, Kaplan MM, Larsen PR, et al. Thyroid nodularity after childhood irradiation for lymphoid hyperplasia: a comparison of questionnaire and clinical findings. J Clin Epidemiol 1990;43:449–60.
32. Satran L, Sklar C, Dehner L, Kim T, Nesbit M. Thyroid neoplasm after high-dose radiotherapy. Am J Pediatr Hematol Oncol 1983;5:307–9.
33. Schneider AB. Radiation-induced thyroid tumors. Endocrinol Metab Clin North Am 1990;19:495–508.
34. _____, Pinsky S, Bekerman C, Ryo UY. Characteristics of 108 thyroid cancers detected by screening in a population with a history of head and neck irradiation. Cancer 1980;46:1218–27.

35. _____, Recant W, Pinsky SM, Ryo UY, Bekerman C, Shore-Freedman E. Radiation-induced thyroid carcinoma. Clinical course and results of therapy in 296 patients. Ann Intern Med 1986;105:405–12.

36. _____, Shore-Freedman E, Ryo UY, Bekerman C, Favus M, Pinsky S. Radiation-induced tumors of the head and neck following childhood irradiation. Prospective studies. Medicine (Baltimore) 1985;64:1–15.

37. _____, Shore-Freedman E, Weinstein RA. Radiation-induced thyroid and other head and neck tumors: occurrence of multiple tumors and analysis of risk factors. J Clin Endocrinol Metab 1986;63:107–12.

38. Spitalnik PF, Straus FH II. Patterns of human thyroid parenchymal reaction following low-dose childhood irradiation. Cancer 1978;41:1098–105.

39. Tang TT, Holcenberg JS, Duck SC, Hodach AE, Oechler HW, Camitta BM. Thyroid carcinoma following treatment for acute lymphoblastic leukemia. Cancer 1980; 46:1572–6.

40. Wilson SD, Komorowski R, Cerletty J, Majewski JT, Hooper M. Radiation-associated thyroid tumors: extent of operation and pathology technique influence the apparent incidence of carcinoma. Surgery 1983;94:663–9.

Fine-Needle Aspiration Biopsy

41. Åkerman M, Tennvall J, Biörklund A, Måartensson H, Möller T. Sensitivity and specificity of fine needle aspiration cytology in the diagnosis of tumors of the thyroid gland. Acta Cytol 1985;29:850–5.

42. Axiotis CA, Merino MJ, Ain K, Norton JA. Papillary endothelial hyperplasia in the thyroid following fine-needle aspiration. Arch Pathol Lab Med 1991;115:240–2.

43. Frable WJ, Frable MA. Fine-needle aspiration biopsy of the thyroid. Histopathologic and clinical correlations. In: Fenoglio CM, Wolff M, eds. Progress in surgical pathology, vol I. New York: Masson, 1980:105–18.

44. Friedman M, Shimaoka K, Rao U, Tsukada Y, Gavigan M, Tamura K. Diagnosis of chronic lymphocytic thyroiditis (nodular presentation) by needle aspiration. Acta Cytol 1981;25:513–22.

45. Kini SR. Thyroid. In: Kline TS, ed. Guides to clinical aspiration biopsy;; Vol 3. New York: Igaku-Shoin, 1987.

46. _____, Miller JM, Abrash MP, Gaba A, Johnson T. Post-fine needle aspiration biopsy infarction in thyroid nodules [Abstract]. Lab Invest 1988;58:48A.

47. _____, Miller JM, Hamburger JI. Cytopathology of Hürthle cell lesions of the thyroid gland by fine needle aspiration. Acta Cytol 1981;25:647–52.

48. Kline TS. Handbook of fine needle aspiration biopsy cytology. St. Louis: CV Mosby, 1981.

49. Lever EG, Refetoff S, Scherberg NH, Carr K. The influence of percutaneous fine needle aspiration on serum thyroglobulin. J Clin Endocrinol Metab 1983; 56:26–9.

50. Löwhagen T, Willems J-S, Lundell G, Sundblad R, Granberg P-O. Aspiration biopsy cytology in diagnosis of thyroid cancer. World J Surg 1981;5:61–73.

51. Miller JM, Kini SR, Hamburger JI. Needle biopsy of the thyroid. New York: Praeger, 1983.

52. _____, Kini SR, Hamburger JI. The diagnosis of malignant follicular neoplasms of the thyroid by needle biopsy. Cancer 1985;55:2812–7.

53. Nathan AR, Raines KB, Lee Y-T, Sakas EL, Ribbing JM. Fine-needle aspiration biopsy of cold thyroid nodules. Cancer 1988;62:1337–42.

54. Nguyen G-K, Ginsberg J, Crockford PM. Fine-needle aspiration biopsy cytology of the thyroid. Its value and limitations in the diagnosis and management of solitary thyroid nodules. Pathol Annu 1991;26:63–91.

55. Nunez C, Mendelsohn G. Fine-needle aspiration and needle biopsy of the thyroid gland. Pathol Annu 1989; 24:161–98.

56. Ramacciotti CE, Pretorius HT, Chu EW, Barsky SH, Brennan MF, Robbins J. Diagnostic accuracy and use of aspiration biopsy in the management of thyroid nodules. Arch Intern Med 1984;144:1169–73.

57. Silverman JF, West RL, Larkin EW, et al. The role of fine-needle aspiration biopsy in the rapid diagnosis and management of thyroid neoplasm. Cancer 1986;57: 1164–70.

58. Suen KC, Quenville NF. Fine needle aspiration biopsy of the thyroid gland: a study of 304 cases. J Clin Pathol 1983;36:1036–45.

Frozen-Section Examination

59. Bugis SP, Young JE, Archibald SD, Chen VS. Diagnostic accuracy of fine-needle aspiration biopsy versus frozen section in solitary thyroid nodules. Am J Surg 1986;152:411–6.

60. Hamburger JI, Hamburger SW. Declining role of frozen section in surgical planning for thyroid nodules. Surgery 1985;98:307–12.

61. _____, Husain M. Contribution of intraoperative pathology evaluation to surgical management of thyroid nodules. Endocrinol Metab Clin North Am 1990;19:509–22.

62. Hapke MR, Dehner LP. The optically clear nucleus. A reliable sign of papillary carcinoma of the thyroid? Am J Surg Pathol 1979;3:31–8.

63. Keller MP, Crabbe MM, Norwood SH. Accuracy and significance of fine-needle aspiration and frozen section in determining the extent of thyroid resection. Surgery 1987;101:632–5.

64. Kopald LH, Layfield LJ, Mohrmann R, Foshag LJ, Giuliano AE. Clarifying the role of fine-needle aspiration, cytologic evaluation and frozen section examination in the operative management of thyroid cancer. Arch Surg 1989;124:1201–5.

65. Kraemer BB. Frozen section diagnosis and the thyroid. Semin Diagn Pathol 1987;4:169–89.

66. Rigaud C. The extemporaneous examination in thyroid pathology. Why and how? Ann Pathol 1989;9:305–7.

67. Rosen Y, Rosenblatt P, Saltzman E. Intraoperative pathologic diagnosis of thyroid neoplasms. Report on experience with 504 specimens. Cancer 1990;66:2001–6.

Staging and Grading of Thyroid Carcinoma

68. Beahrs OH, Henson DE, Hutter RV, Myers MH, eds. Manual for staging of cancer. 3rd ed. American Joint Committee on Cancer. Philadelphia: JP Lippincott Co., 1988:57–62.

69. Hermanek P, Sobin LH, eds. Classification of malignant tumours. 4th ed. International Union Against Cancer. New York: Springer-Verlag, 1987:33–5.

Treatment of Thyroid Tumors

70. Benker G, Olbricht T, Reinwein D, et al. Survival rates in patients with differentiated thyroid carcinoma. Influence of postoperative external radiotherapy. Cancer 1990;65:1517–20.

71. Brooks JR, Starnes HF, Brooks DC, Pelkey JN. Surgical therapy for thyroid carcinoma: a review of 1249 solitary thyroid nodules. Surgery 1988;104:940–6.

72. Cady B, Cohn K, Rossi RL, et al. The effect of thyroid hormone administration upon survival in patients with differentiated thyroid carcinoma. Surgery 1983;94:978–83.

73. Clark OH. TSH suppression in the management of thyroid nodules and thyroid cancer. World J Surg 1981;5:39–47.

74. Demeure MJ, Clark OH. Surgery in the treatment of thyroid cancer. Endocrinol Metab Clin North Am 1990;19:663–84.

75. Griffin JE. Management of thyroid nodules. Am J Med Sci 1988;296:336–47.

76. Lee KY, Loré JM Jr. The treatment of metastatic thyroid disease. Otolaryngol Clin North Am 1990;23:475–93.

77. Maxon HR III, Smith HW. Radioiodine-131 in the diagnosis and treatment of metastatic well differentiated thyroid cancer. Endocrinol Metab Clin North Am 1990;19:685–718.

78. Mazzaferri EL. Treating differentiated thyroid carcinoma: where do we draw the line? [Editorial] Mayo Clin Proc 1991;66:105–11.

Prognosis of Thyroid Tumors

79. Byar DP, Green SB, Dor P, et al. A prognostic index for thyroid carcinoma. A study of the E.O.R.T.C. Thyroid Cancer Cooperative Group. Eur J Cancer 1979;15:1033–41.

80. Cady B, Rossi R. An expanded view of risk-group definition in differentiated thyroid carcinoma. Surgery 1988;104:947–53.

81. _____, Rossi R, Silverman M, Wool M. Further evidence of the validity of risk group definition in differentiated thyroid carcinoma. Surgery 1985;98:1171–8.

82. Carcangiu ML, Zampi G, Pupi A, Castagnoli A, Rosai J. Papillary carcinoma of the thyroid. A clinicopathologic study of 241 cases treated at the University of Florence, Italy. Cancer 1985;55:805–28.

83. Hay ID. Papillary thyroid carcinoma. Endocrinol Metab Clin North Am 1990;19:685–718.

84. Tennvall J, Biörklund A, Möller T, Ranstam J, Åkerman M. Is the EORTC prognostic index of thyroid cancer valid in differentiated thyroid carcinoma? Retrospective multivariate analysis of differentiated thyroid carcinoma with long term follow-up. Cancer 1986;57:1405–14.

Thyroid Tumors in Animals

85. Axelrad AA, Leblond CP. Induction of thyroid tumors in rats by a low iodine diet. Cancer 1955;8:339–67.

86. Doniach I, Williams ED. The development of thyroid and pituitary tumours in the rat two years after partial thyroidectomy. Br J Cancer 1962;16:222–31.

87. Fortner JG, George PA, Sternberg SS. Induced and spontaneous thyroid cancer in the Syrian (golden) hamster. Endocrinology 1960;66:364–76.

88. Furth J, Kim U, Clifton KH. On evolution of the neoplastic state; progression from dependence to autonomy. Natl Cancer Inst Monogr 1960;2:149–77.

89. Goldberg RC, Lindsay S, Nichols CW Jr, Chaikoff IL. Induction of neoplasms in thyroid glands of rats by subtotal thyroidectomy and the injection of one microcurie of I131. Cancer Res 1964;24:35–43.

90. Lindsay S, Sheline GE, Potter GD, Chaikoff IL. Induction of neoplasms in the thyroid gland of the rat by X-irradiation of the gland. Cancer Res 1961;21:9–16.

91. Money WL, Rawson RW. Intrathyroid implantation of chemical carcinogens in the rat. Arch Pathol 1965;79:470–4.

92. _____, Typond P, Rawson RW. The growth and function of thiouracil-induced thyroid tumors transplanted into non-inbred rats thymectomized at birth. Cancer Res 1965;25:423–31.

93. Patnaik AK, Lieberman PH. Gross, histologic, cytochemical, and immunocytochemical study of medullary thyroid carcinoma in sixteen dogs. Vet Pathol 1991;28:223–33.

94. Potter GD, Lindsay S, Chaikoff IL. Induction of neoplasms in rat thyroid glands by low doses of radioiodine. Arch Pathol 1960;69:257–69.

95. Schlumberger HG. Spontaneous hyperplasia and neoplasia in the thyroid of animals. In: The thyroid. Upton, NY: Biology Dept, Brookhaven National Laboratory Symposia in Biology no. 7, 1954.

96. Sinha D, Pascal R, Furth J. Transplantable thyroid carcinoma induced by thyrotropin: its similarity to human Hürthle cell tumors. Arch Pathol 1965;79:192–8.

◇◇◇

INDEX

Aberrant lateral thyroid, 320
Adenoacanthoma, 195, 197
Adenochondroma, 38, **39, 41**
Adenolipoma, 38, **41**
Adenoma, atypical, 38, **42, 43**
Adenoma, follicular
    clinical features, 21
    cytologic features, 31, **32–35**
    definition, 21
    differential diagnosis, 30
    general features, 21
    gross features, 21, **23**
    immunohistochemical features, 26
    microscopic features, 22, **24–28**
    other special techniques, 28
    ultrastructural features, 28, **29, 30**
Adenoma, hyalinizing trabecular, 31, **36–40**
Adenoma, hyperfunctioning, *see* Adenoma, toxic
Adenoma, macrofollicular, 22, **23**
Adenoma, microfollicular, 22, **23**
Adenoma, normofollicular, 22, **23**
Adenoma, oncocytic
    cytologic features, 169, **172**
    definition, 162
    gross features, 162
    microscopic features, 162, **162–169**
    prognosis, 171
    pseudopapillary formations in, **179**
    treatment, 171
    ultrastructural features, 165, **170, 171**
Adenoma, Plummer, *see* Adenoma, toxic
Adenoma, toxic, 40, 44
Adenoma, trabecular, 22, **23**
Adenoma variants, 31
Adenoma, with bizarre nuclei, 31, **35, 36**
Adenoma, with papillary hyperplasia, 38, **41, 43, 44**
Amphicrine carcinoma, *see* Carcinoma, medullary,
    variants
Amyloid goiter**,** *see* Goiter, amyloid
Anaplastic carcinoma, *see* Carcinoma, undifferentiated
    and Carcinoma, medullary, variants
Anatomy, of normal thyroid, 2, **4**
Angiosarcoma
    clinical features, 260
    definition, 259
    differential diagnosis, 264
    general features, 259
    gross features, 260, **262**
    immunohistochemical features, 260, **262, 263**
    microscopic features, 260, **261**
    prognosis, 264
    spread and metastasis; prognosis, 264
    ultrastructural features, 264
Askanazy cells, *see* Oncocytes

Benign, soft tissue-type tumor, *see* Tumors, miscellaneous

Carcinoma, adenosquamous, 197

Carcinoma, anaplastic, *see* Carcinoma, undifferentiated
Carcinoma, angioinvasive, *see* Carcinoma, follicular,
    minimally invasive
Carcinoma, C cell, *see* Carcinoma, medullary
Carcinoma, follicular
    classification, 50
    clinical features, 49
    definition, 49
    general considerations, 49
    general features, 49
    minimally invasive (encapsulated)
        cytologic features, 59
        differential diagnosis, 59, **52, 53**
        gross features, 50, **51**
        immunohistochemical/ultrastructural features,
            56, **60**
        microscopic features, 50, **52–59**
        other special techniques, 59
        prognosis, 61
        spread and metastasis, 59, **61**
        treatment, 61
    widely invasive, 62
Carcinoma, Hürthle cell, *see* Carcinoma, oncocytic type
Carcinoma, insular, *see* Carcinoma, poorly differentiated
Carcinoma, medullary
    clinical features, 208
    cytologic features, 219-224, **225, 226**
    definition, 207
    differential diagnosis, 224
    general features, 207, **210**
    gross features, 209, **210, 211, 215**
    histochemical features, 217, **218**
    immunohistochemical features, 218, **220–222**
    laboratory diagnosis, 208
    microscopic features, 209, **212--218**
    prognosis, 228
    spread and metastasis, 228
    treatment, 228
    ultrastructural features, 219, **223, 224**
    variants, 229
        amphicrine (composite calcitonin and mucin-
            producing), 237, **240**
        anaplastic, 230
        C cell adenoma, 233, **237**
        clear cell, 232, **233**
        encapsulated, 237
        giant cell, 232, **232**
        melanotic (pigmented), 233, **234, 235**
        oncocytic (oxyphilic), 233, **236**
        paraganglioma-like, 237, **237**
        squamous, 232, **232**
        small cell, 231, **231, 232, 234, 235**
        tubular/follicular, 229, **230**
        papillary, 230, **230**
Carcinoma, medullary, familial, **207**
Carcinoma, medullary-follicular, 238, **238–240**
Carcinoma, medullary-papillary, 239
Carcinoma, occult papillary, 96

Carcinoma, occult sclerosing, 96
Carcinoma, oncocytic (Hürthle cell carcinoma)
    clinical features, 173
    definition, 173
    differential diagnosis, 175
    general features, 173
    gross features, 173, **174**
    microscopic features, 173, **175–178**
    other special techniques, 178
    prognosis, 179
    spread and metastasis, 179
    treatment, 179
    ultrastructural, immunohistochemical features, 178
Carcinoma, papillary
    clinical features, 65
    cytologic features, 87, **88, 89**
    definition, 65
    general features, 65, **66**
    gross features, 65, **67**
    immunohistochemical features, 84, **86**
    microscopic features, 68, **69–82**
    microscopic grading, 82, **82, 83**
    other special techniques, 85
    prognosis, 95
    spread and metastasis, 90, **90–94**
    treatment, 94
    ultrastructural features, 84, **84, 85**
    variants, 96
        diffuse sclerosing, 109, **111–114**
        encapsulated, 100, **101, 102**
        encapsulated follicular and related lesions,
            105, **107–110**
        follicular, 100, **103–106**
        macrofollicular, 100, **103**
        papillary microcarcinoma, 96, **97–99**
        solid/trabecular, 109, **75**
        tall and columnar cell, 114, **115**
Carcinoma, pleomorphic, *see* Carcinoma, undifferentiated
Carcinoma, poorly differentiated, 123–128
    insular carcinoma, 123
        cytologic features, 126
        differential diagnosis, 126
        general and clinical features, 123
        gross features, 123, **128**
        immunohistochemical features, 126, **127**
        microscopic features, 123, **124–26**
        nosologic considerations, 126, **129–131**
        spread, metastasis, and prognosis, 126, **127, 128**
    other poorly differentiated, 130, **133**
Carcinoma, pseudopapillary, 230
Carcinoma, sarcomatoid, *see* Carcinoma
Carcinoma, solid amyloidotic, *see* Carcinoma, medullary
Carcinoma, squamous cell, 197
Carcinoma, thyroid, incidence of, 327
Carcinoma, thyroid, staging and grading of, 335
    clinical staging, 332
    pathologic grading, 333
    microscopic grading, 333
Carcinoma, undifferentiated (anaplastic)
    antecedent diseases, 153, **154, 155**
    clinical features, 135
    cytologic features, 150, **150, 151**
    definition, 135
    differential diagnosis, 149

    gross features, 135, **136, 137**
    immunohistochemical features, 143, **145, 147**
    microscopic features, 135, **138–143**
    microscopic types, 146
    other special techniques, 146
    prognosis, 151
    spread and metastasis, 150, **152, 153**
    treatment, 151
    ultrastructural features, 146, **148**
Carcinosarcoma, 135, 142
CASTLE, *see* Tumors, miscellaneous, carcinoma showing
    thymus-like differentiation
C cell, *see* Histology, of normal thyroid
C cell adenoma, *see* Carcinoma, medullary, variants
C cell hyperplasia, *see* Hyperplasia, C cell
Clear cell carcinoma, *see* Carcinoma, medullary, variants
    and Tumors, clear cell features
Cowden syndrome, 21, 65
Cushing syndrome, 208
Cyst, thyroglossal duct, 317, **318, 319**
Cytoplasmic vesicles, in clear cell cytoplasm, 183

Delphian node, 3
Diffuse sclerosing carcinoma, *see* Carcinoma,
    papillary, variants
Dyshormonogenetic goiter, *see* Goiter, dyshormonogenetic

Ectopia, *see* Thyroid tissue ectopia
Ectopic cervical thymoma, 282, **283**
Ectopic harmartomatous thymoma, 282, **283, 284**
Embryology, of normal thyroid, 1, **2, 3**
Encapsulated carcinoma, *see* Carcinoma, medullary
    variants *and* Carcinoma, papillary, variants

Fine-needle aspiration biopsy, 329
Follicle, description, 4
Follicles, of normal thyroid, **8–10**
Follicular carcinoma, *see* Carcinoma, papillary, variants
Follicular neoplasms of undeterminate behavior, 59
Frozen-section examination, 330, **331**

Gardner syndrome, 65
Giant cell carcinoma, *see* Carcinoma, medullary, variants
Giant cell pattern, undifferentiated carcinoma, 135, **141,
142**
Glycogen, in clear cell cytoplasm, 183
Goiter, 19
Goiter, amyloid, 312, **313, 314**
Goiter, benign metastasizing, 61, **61**
Goiter, colloid, 297
Goiter, dyshormonogenetic, 302, **304, 308, 309**
Goiter, parenchymatous, 297
Graves disease, *see* Hyperplasia, diffuse
Ground-glass appearance, 72, **73–75**
    in medullary carcinoma, 224
    in papillary carcinoma, **94, 103**, 104

Hashimoto disease/thyroiditis, *see* Thyroiditis, Hashimoto
Hashitoxicosis, 303
Hemangioma, 282
Histiocytic lymphoma, *see* Lymphoma, malignant
Histiocytosis X, 315
Histology, of normal thyroid
    architectural features, 4, **5–7**

C cell, 7, **9, 11**
follicular cell, 6, **8, 10**
solid cell nests, 12
Hodgkin disease, 275, **275–277**
Hürthle cell adenoma, *see* Adenoma, oncocytic
Hürthle cell carcinoma, *see* Carcinoma, oncocytic
Hürthle cell tumors, *see* Tumors, oncocytic features
Hypernephroid tumor, 186
Hyperparathyroidism, 21, 49, **208**
Hyperplasia, C cell
    definition, 247
    differential diagnosis, 249, **255–257**
    general features, 247
    gross features, 248
    in medullary carcinoma, 209, **216, 217**
    microscopic features, 248, **248–254**
    treatment and prognosis, 257
Hyperplasia, diffuse, 302, **301, 303**
Hyperplasia, nodular, 297, **297–300, 308, 309**
    in thyroglossal duct cyst, 319
    with clear cell change, **191**

Immunofluorescence, procedure, 8
Immunoperoxidase, procedure, 8
Intrathyroidal epithelial thymoma, 286

Leiomyoma, 282
Lipid, in clear cell cytoplasm, 183
Lymphangioma, 282
Lymphatic drainage, of thyroid gland, **4**
Lymphoma, malignant
    clinical features, 267
    cytologic features, 271, **274**
    definition, 267
    gross features, 267, **272**
    immunohistochemical features, 269, **271, 273**
    microscopic features, 267, **268–271**
    other special studies, 271
    prognosis, 274
    spread and metastasis, 271
    treatment, 274
    ultrastructural features, 269
    thyroiditis/other antecedent features, 267
Lymph nodes
    paratracheal, 3
    pericapsular, 3
    prelaryngeal nodes, 3
    pretracheal nodes, 3
    regional, 3
    thyroid inclusions, 323, **323**

Macrofollicular carcinoma, *see* Carcinoma, papillary
    variants
Malakoplakia, 310
Mediastinal nodes, 3
Melanotic (pigmented) carcinoma, *see* Carcinoma,
    medullary, variants
MEN syndrome, 65
Mucin, in clear cell cytoplasm, 183

Neurilemoma, 282
Nodular hyperplasia, *see* Hyperplasia, nodular

Oncocytes, 161

Oncocytic adenoma (Hürthle cell), *see* Adenoma,
    oncocytic type
Oncocytic (oxyphilic) carcinoma, *see* Carcinoma,
    medullary, variants
Oncocytomas, 161
Orphan Annie's Eyes nuclei, 72, **73**, *see also* Ground-glass
    appearance
Oxyphilic cells, *see* Oncocytes

Paget disease, 14
Papillary cystadenocarcinoma, 68
Papillary microcarcinoma, 310, *see also* Carcinoma,
    papillary, variants
Papillary oncocytic neoplasms, 179, **179, 180**
Paraganglioma, 31, **37**, 279, **280, 281**
Paraganglioma-like,
    hyalinizing trabecular adenoma, 31, 279
    medullary carcinoma, 218, 279
Parasitic nodule, 320, **321, 322, 324**
Parastruma, 186
Parathyroid
    disease, 208
    glands, 3
    tumors, 279
Physiology, of normal thyroid, 12
    calcitonin and the calcitonin gene–related peptide, 14
    thyroid hormones, 13, **13**
Plasma cell granuloma, 275, 315
Plasmacytoma, 275
Pleomorphic immunocytoma, 275
Psammoma bodies
    definition, 72,
    in medullary carcinoma, 226
    in mucoepidermoid carcinoma, 195, **196**
    in papillary carcinoma, 68, **75–78**, 87, **89, 113**

Radiation changes, 310, **312, 313**
Rosai-Dorfman disease, 315

Salivary gland type tumor, see Tumors, miscellaneous
Sanderson polster, 4, 31, 298, **299**
Sarcomas
    definition, 259
    general considerations, 259
    true, 149
SETTLE, *see* Tumors, miscellaneous, spindle epithelial
    with thymus-like differentiation
Sinus histiocytosis with massive lymphadenopathy, 315
Sjögren syndrome, 267
Small cell carcinoma, *see* Carcinoma, medullary, variants
Solid/Trabecular carcinoma, *see* Carcinoma, papillary
    variants
Somatostatin, 8
Spindle cell pattern, undifferentiated carcinoma, 135,
    138, 139
Squamoid pattern, undifferentiated carcinoma, 135, **138**
Squamous cell carcinoma, *see* Carcinoma, medullary,
    variants *and* Tumors, squamous features
Squamous metaplasia, 26, 84, *see also* Tumors, squamous
    features
Struma, 19
Struma ovarii, 325
Strumal carcinoid, 325

Tall and columnar cell carcinoma, *see* Carcinoma, papillary, variants
Teratoma, 280, **282**
Thyroglobulin, in clear cell cytoplasm, 183
Thyroglobulin, molecular structure, **13**
Thyroglossal duct, 1, 2, 317
Thyroid gland, anatomy, 2, **4**
Thyroid hormones, 13, **13**
Thyroid, inclusions in lymph nodes, 325, **325**
Thyroiditis, fibrosing (Riedel), 305, **307, 310, 311**
Thyroiditis, (DeQuervain) granulomatous, 305
Thyroiditis, Hashimoto, 303, **305, 306, 308**
    history of, 327
    in C cell hyperplasia, 247, 255
    in hyalinizing trabecular adenoma, 37
    in medullary carcinoma, 207
    in malignant lymphoma, 271
    in nodular hyperplasia, 297
    in papillary carcinoma, 65, 85
    in sclerosing mucoepidermoid carcinoma, 196
    in tumors with clear cell features, 190, **192**
    in tumors with squamous features, 200, **199–201**
    in undifferentiated carcinoma, 150
    with parasitic nodules, 320, **322**
Thyroiditis, multifocal fibrosing, 310
Thyroid tissue ectopia, 317, **317–319**
    component of teratoma, 323,
    lingual thyroid, 317, **318**
    lymph node inclusions, 323, **323**
    mechanical implantation, 320
    parasitic nodule, 320, **321, 322, 324**
    thyroglossal duct cyst, 317, **318, 319**
Tubular/follicular carcinoma, *see* Carcinoma, medullary, variants
Tumor-like conditions, 297
    amyloid goiter, 312
    diffuse hyperplasia, 302
    dyshormonogenetic goiter, 302
    Hashimoto thyroiditis, 303
    histiocytosis X, 315
    malakoplakia, 310
    nodular hyperplasia, 297
    other forms of thyroiditis, 305
    plasma cell granuloma, 315
    sinus histiocytosis with massive lymphadenopathy, 315
Tumors, animals, 335
Tumors, in childhood, 328
Tumors, classification of, 19
Tumors, clear cell features
    definition, 183
    differential diagnosis, 190, **191, 192**
    general considerations, 183
    types, 184
        clear cell medullary carcinoma, 190
        follicular neoplasms, 186, **186, 187**
        lipid-rich adenoma, 189
        oncocytic neoplasms, 184, **184, 185**
        papillary carcinoma 189, **190**
        signet-ring follicular adenoma and carcinoma, 188, **188, 189, 191**
        undifferentiated carcinoma, 189
Tumors, Hürthle cell, *see* Tumors, oncocytic features
Tumors, hypernephroid, 186
Tumors, lymphoid, 275

Tumors, miscellaneous, 279
    benign, soft tissue-type, 282
    paraganglioma, 31, **37**, 279, **280, 281**
    parathyroid, 279
    teratoma, 280, **282**
    salivary gland type, 285
    with thymic or related branchial pouch differentiation, 282
        carcinoma showing thymus-like differentiation (CASTLE), 284, **286**
        ectopic cervical thymoma, 282, **283**
        ectopic hamartomatous thymoma, 282, **283**
        spindle epithelial tumor with thymus-like differentiation (SETTLE), 282, **285**
Tumors, mucinous features, 203
    medullary carcinoma, 205, 207
    mucoepidermoid/sclerosing mucoepidermoid 195, 203
    mucinous carcinoma, 203, **204**
    papillary carcinoma, 203
    secondary carcinoma, 205
    signet-ring adenoma, 203, **204**
    undifferentiated carcinoma, 203
Tumors, nonencapsulated sclerosing, 96
Tumors, oncocytic features (Hürthle cell tumors)
    definition, 161
    general considerations, 161
Tumors, parathyroid, 279
Tumors, procedure for pathologic examination, 331
    description, 331
    example of gross description, 331
    handling, 331
    sections for histology, 332

Tumors, salivary-gland type, 289
Tumors, secondary, 289, **289–295**
    breast carcinoma metastatic to papillary thyroid carcinoma, 289, **294**
    colonic adenocarcinoma metastatic to thyroid, 289, **291**
    lobular carcinoma of breast metastatic to thyroid, 289, **290**
    malignant melanoma metastatic to thyroid, 289 **289**
    mammary lobular carcinoma metastatic to thyroid, 293, **295**
    poorly differentiated adenocarcinoma of lung metastatic to mediastinal thyroid gland, 289, **290**
    pulmonary carcinoid tumor metastatic to thyroid, 291, **293**
    renal cell carcinoma metastatic to thyroid, 293, **294, 295**
    renal cell carcinoma metastatic to thyroid follicular adenoma, 289, 291, **292**
    renal cell carcinoma metastatic to thyroid follicular carcinoma, 289, 291, **292**
Tumors, squamous features, 195
    carcinoma with thymus-like differentiation (CASTLE), 197
    follicular neoplasms, 197, **199**
    medullary carcinoma, 197
    mucoepidermoid carcinoma, 195, **195**
    non-neoplastic conditions, 197, **199, 200**
    papillary carcinoma, 195
    sclerosing mucoepidermoid, 196, **201**

secondary carcinoma, 197
squamous cell and undifferentiated, 195, 197, **198**
Tumors, thyroid, clinical and laboratory evaluation of, 327
computerized tomography (CT) and magnetic
resonance imaging, 328
demographics, 327
family history, 327
Hashimoto thyroiditis, history of, 327
isotopic imaging study, 327, **328**
needle biopsy, 328, 329
palpation, 327
rate of growth, 327,
serum thyroglobulin levels, 328
ultrasonography, 327
Tumors, thyroid, prognosis, 334
Tumors, thyroid, radiation exposure, 329
Tumors, thyroid, treatment of, 334

Ultimobranchial body, development, 1

Ultimobranchial neoplasms, 207

Verner-Morrison syndrome, 208

Weibel-Palade bodies, 264
World Health Organization (WHO)
classification of thyroid tumors, 1, 19
definition of atypical adenoma, 38
definition of insular carcinoma, 126
definiton of oncocytic cells, 161
definition of papillary microcarcinoma, 96
definition of sarcomas, 259
definition of vascular invasion, 50
Wuchernde struma, 123, **123**

Zellballen appearance, 31, **37, 281**